Reproduction Reconceived

REPRODUCTIVE JUSTICE: A NEW VISION FOR
THE TWENTY-FIRST CENTURY

Edited by Rickie Solinger, Khiara M. Bridges, Zakiya Luna, and Ruby Tapia

Reproduction Reconceived

FAMILY MAKING AND THE LIMITS OF
CHOICE AFTER ROE V. WADE

Sara Matthiesen

UNIVERSITY OF CALIFORNIA PRESS

University of California Press
Oakland, California

© 2021 by Sara Matthiesen

Library of Congress Cataloging-in-Publication Data

Names: Matthiesen, Sara, 1985– author.
Title: Reproduction reconceived : family making and the limits of choice
    after Roe v. Wade / Sara Matthiesen.
Other titles: Reproductive justice ; 5.
Description: Oakland, California : University of California Press, [2021] |
    Series: Reproductive justice: a new vision for the twenty-first century;
    5 | Includes bibliographical references and index.
Identifiers: LCCN 2021025580 (print) | LCCN 2021025581 (ebook) |
    ISBN 9780520298200 (hardback) | ISBN 9780520298217 (paperback) |
    ISBN 9780520970441 (ebook)
Subjects: LCSH: Families—United States—History—20th century. |
    Families—United States—History—21st century. | Reproductive
    rights—United States. | BISAC: MEDICAL / Public Health
Classification: LCC HQ535 .M384 2021 (print) | LCC HQ535 (ebook) |
    DDC 306.850973—dc23
LC record available at https://lccn.loc.gov/2021025580
LC ebook record available at https://lccn.loc.gov/2021025581

30 29 28 27 26 25 24 23 22 21
10 9 8 7 6 5 4 3 2 1

The publisher and the University of California Press Foundation gratefully acknowledge the generous support of the Barbara S. Isgur Endowment Fund in Public Affairs.

Contents

Introduction

In August 2018, the *New York Times* published an article about college-educated mothers' stalled re-entry into the United States labor force.[1] The piece featured the research of four economists, who sought to explain why women in the United States continued to outpace men in terms of education when they did not seem to be putting that education to use in the labor market. Women's participation in the workforce hit a wall in 1990—after a rapid increase between 1960 and 1980, it had largely plateaued. The team of scholars—Ilyana Kuziemko, Jessica Pan, Jenny Shen, and Ebonya Washington—offered a multi-part answer to this puzzle.[2] The first part was largely structural: the costs of motherhood began increasing in the 1990s. Child care had become more expensive since the 1980s, breast-feeding was strongly encouraged over formula, creating an exorbitant time cost, and the rise of what sociologist Sharon Hays called "intensive parenting" in the 1990s meant more money and time going towards children's extracurricular activities starting at a very young age.[3] The second part was more psychological: women born in the 1960s through the 1970s, the cohort the economists based their findings on, seriously underestimated "the employment costs of motherhood"—"the time, effort or money" necessary to raise their children while also working. Despite having invested greatly in their professional development and stating that they had every intention of continuing their careers after giving birth, the study found that these same women were more likely to be at home with the kids after motherhood had proved far more costly than they anticipated.[4]

Nearly forty years ago, feminist poet Adrienne Rich cautioned that using middle-class women's white-collar employment as a measure of progress was bound to result in a misdiagnosis of the work that remained. Commenting on the 1980s trope of the white, professional mother whose ability to "have it all" supposedly made feminism obsolete, Rich wrote, "The working mother with briefcase was, herself, a cosmetic touch on a society deeply resistant to fundamental changes. The 'public' and the 'private' spheres were still in disjunction. She had not found herself entering an evolving new society, a society in transformation. *She had only been integrated into the same structures which had made liberation movements necessary.*"[5] Capitalism was willing to accommodate these new workers, so long as they did not let their other job—mothering—get in the way of their paid work. Furthermore, declining wages, the shift towards a service economy, and long-standing racial and gender hierarchies that stratified the labor market ensured that beginning in the 1970s mothers who went to work without briefcases would become a growing share of the nation's poor and working class, concentrated in jobs that comprise the feminized, racialized, and ever expanding "care economy."[6] Rich understood what the economists seemed to have missed: to measure motherhood solely as a drain on one's labor supply and potential earnings took for granted the devaluation of care integral to a society "deeply resistant to fundamental changes." What Rich could not have predicted in 1986 was just how rapaciously "these same structures" would wrest accommodation—in terms of time, earnings, and general way of life—from the vast majority of workers in the United States. What the Occupy movement asserted in 2011 with the slogan "We are the 99%" has only become steadily more visible and applicable: the concentration of income and wealth among the top 1 percent of earners in the United States has reached levels not seen since the Gilded Age. Income inequality has risen in every state since the 1970s, producing a labor market characterized by poverty wages, precarious categories of supposed non-workers such as the "independent contractor," a "culture of overwork," and wage growth experienced almost exclusively by the top earners. Following the recovery from the Great Recession, the top 1 percent captured 91 percent of the income gains between 2009 and 2012, and by 2014 71 percent of American workers earned less than 50,000 dollars a year.[7] As the vast majority of Americans were squeezed, they had to figure out how to take care of their families with less time, less earnings, and less security. While the study featured in the *New York Times* measured the rising costs of motherhood in time spent on childrearing, breastfeeding trends, and child care expenses, recent estimates based on data from the Current Expenditures Survey put the price tag of childrearing at 12,980 dollars annually per child—an unfathomable cost if, like 38 percent of American workers did in 2014, one earns less than 20,000 dollars a year.[8] It was not just that the college-educated mothers in the study had underestimated the demands of parenting, or even that the aspects of motherhood tracked by economists had become more costly. It was that by the twenty-first century, capitalism placed serious limits on most Americans' horizons and required them to resolve on their own whatever aspects of life exceeded those limits.

And all of this is to say almost nothing of the unpaid job women had taken on when they "failed" to make good on their career plans. When economists concluded that "current cohorts of women indeed overestimate their future labor supply," they reproduced the logic of a system that makes reproductive labor invisible, thereby justifying its devaluation even when it is waged.[9] Despite the fact that women repeatedly told researchers how parenting was harder than they had anticipated—evidence of how motherhood *itself* requires a "labor supply"—the study emphasized the cost parenting posed to potential but, ultimately, lost profits. In this way, the study took for granted the disjuncture between the public and private spheres Rich had hoped might be transformed in a society organized around the equal distribution of necessary resources, leisure, and life chances. In contrast to the study's conclusion that family making imperiled women's *real* work, visible as such due to the wage it garnered, socialist feminists have suggested we can think of time caring for others as uncompensated labor that powers the economy through its reproduction of current and future workers. Feminist scholarship has also noted, just as the precarious, low-wage jobs of mothers who work in the fastest growing sector of the labor market providing care make clear, that caring for others is as real a labor market as any other. These interrelated realities—the insistence that family making is not work and the extreme exploitation of care work that is paid—are partially responsible for the inequality that has accumulated over the last forty years.[10] Which raises an important question: if the aforementioned discussion paints a picture of ever worsening working conditions for labor that is paid, what would we find if we looked at the other job working mothers have been doing for the past forty years through a similar lens? What worsening conditions as they relate to family making might we need to account for in order to further explain the untenable inequality that has come to define life in the United States?

Reproduction Reconceived answers these questions by examining the history of family making on the margins. The following pages offer an appraisal made possible by an alternative value system, one that does not devalue the reproduction and care of humans—that sees care work not as a drain on capital but as a boon to it. What I call family making—the practices, costs, and labors of creating and maintaining parent-child relations— is an investment of labor, time, and money that produces and sustains not products, but people who, in turn, create yet more, varied intimacies that make life worth living while also making society itself possible.[11] When it comes to the vaunted realm of the nuclear family, the United States is deeply invested in the idea that the care of one's own children should be, at best, a "labor of love," at worst, a private burden resolved via the market, but should never be accorded the status of invaluable work that contributes to the public good. As I argue in the following chapters, this inaccurate assessment of family has produced immense, varied, and often incalculable costs. But in order to fully reckon with the costs that have accumulated, it is first necessary to understand the conditions that produced them. Neither family making nor our current ideas about it are unchanging. Over the past forty years, the *labors* that comprise family making have been forced to multiply as a result of deepening inequality, while the idea that having a family is an economic privilege has hardened. *Reproduction Reconceived* is a history of these changes and their costs. It is an appraisal of how family making became harder, what costs piled up as a result of such unequal circumstances, and which families have borne the greatest share of them.

ORIGIN STORIES

When it comes to the recent history of reproductive politics in the United States, arguably nothing looms larger than the Supreme Court's decision to legalize abortion in 1973 and the subsequent legacy of *Roe v. Wade*. Over the past seven years, I have described this book to most people with the same one-liner: "It is about reproductive politics in the U.S. since the 1970s." Without fail, my audience assumed reproductive politics meant the right to abortion, and proceeded with a comment or question about the current state of the abortion debate. Despite the growing visibility of the reproductive justice movement, not to mention numerous histories evidencing the expansiveness of reproduction, "reproductive politics" continues to conjure "abortion" in the minds of many.[12]

No doubt one of the reasons for this narrowed focus is the longevity, volatility, and visibility of the abortion debate in the United States. The popular understanding of *Roe*—as a contest between those who believe abortion represents a fundamental right to bodily autonomy and those who see it as the disavowal of the sanctity of human life—is a cleaner version than history would ever allow.[13] Nonetheless, this narrow understanding of *Roe*, and the seemingly intractable nature of the struggle over its future, captures the significance of the decision for those who consider themselves to be involved in this fight and for the many, many more who observe from the sidelines. Specifically, the phrase "reproductive politics" raises the specter of the entrenched terms that define the debate over abortion, where a "woman's right to choose" collides, often violently, with the "unborn's right to live."

But before this view of abortion rigidified into a defense of the quintessential reproductive right on the one hand and the quintessential threat to life on the other, it was sanctioned by a legal decision, *Roe*, that had a specific effect: pregnancy became a choice for motherhood rather than a precondition of motherhood.[14] This statement is not as obvious as it might seem. The dominant framing of the abortion debate, courtesy of the decades-long campaigns waged by the pro-choice and pro-life movements, captures only half of the issue: is the choice to end a pregnancy a fundamental right of bodily autonomy or a fundamental affront to human life? The other possible outcome of that choice, *choosing motherhood*, is left dangling, somehow at a distance from "choice's" legally sanctioned arrival. This gap demands our attention, an investigation of what the post-*Roe* world has meant for those whose so-called choice is not the one the abortion debate pivots around. What happened to ideas about motherhood when *Roe* made it a legal choice? How does this redefinition of motherhood square with what families have faced in the post-*Roe* decades? And why is the ability to have an abortion immediately recognizable, while the ability to have a family—much less family as a right that one is entitled to—so much harder to envision?

To answer these questions, we need to consider the 1973 decision alongside a number of related developments. With the help of other changes that collectively untethered sex from procreation and, more importantly, marriage, *Roe* inaugurated a new understanding of pregnancy. In fact, in many ways, *Roe* is best thought of as the end of the so-called "sexual revolution." Americans' views on abortion were already becoming more liberal before the 1973 decision, a shift made possible in part by the increasing tolerance for contraception and premarital sex that took place over the course of the 1960s. The legalization of contraception in 1965 set in motion an evolving definition of privacy that would also underpin *Roe,* and by 1967 contraception was being sold over the counter regardless of a customer's marital status. These changes initiated a new way of thinking about having children as many Americans came to treat having a family as a question—a choice to be made.[15] A series of Supreme Court cases that declared distinctions between marital and nonmarital children as unconstitutional delivered another blow to marriage's authority. In a very short period of time, norms structuring marriage, gender, and sex were upended. Both legal changes and individual practices helped make previously taboo topics like premarital sex, co-habitation before marriage, and single motherhood more common and openly discussed topics than had been the case just a decade prior. The political stakes of these changes were also made clear by different feminist movements during the 1960s and 1970s. Contraception and abortion to control one's reproductive life, to allow sex for pleasure, and to turn marriage and motherhood into options rather than mandates—these were some of the changes that would need to take place if women were going to gain more autonomy in society.[16]

But only the right to abortion had the power to untether pregnancy from motherhood, to make whether or not to remain pregnant a choice, to decide what one's own body would and would not do—even after it had started down a course of doing. This reality explains why feminists from a variety of movements considered the right to abortion so fundamental to liberation struggles, even if they disagreed about the societal conditions required to ensure abortion was freely chosen.[17] The legalization of abortion made pregnancy an unstable condition in a way that the possibility of miscarriages could not. After *Roe*, the pregnant individual was the major factor upon which a pregnancy hinged. And, as pregnancy became a choice, so too did motherhood.

Choice in 1973, however, was as limited as it was liberating. Importantly, *Roe* delivered legal choice *after* the nation had already made some key decisions about just how much the family should be reorganized to accommodate changing norms around gender roles, sex, and marriage. Two years prior to *Roe*, President Richard Nixon vetoed a bill, despite its bipartisan support, that would have delivered universal child care. Federal government also failed to meet the demands of different feminist movements responsible for popularizing the idea that child-rearing was a job in and of itself, one for which mothers should be compensated, as the National Welfare Rights Organization (NWRO) argued in its efforts to bring dignity and a living wage to poor, Black mothers demonized and neglected by welfare.[18] These and other decisions had material impacts on the feasibility of family making for millions of Americans. But they also signaled the start of a broad-scale shift in political winds that one historian has described as "the moment when liberalism came to seem to many millions of ordinary Americans more like a moral threat than an economic helping hand."[19] Wide swaths of the population were fast losing faith in the tenet that government should play a role, however limited such a role had been throughout the nation's history, in mitigating racial, gender, and economic inequalities. Debates over feminism, sexuality, and the family—alongside those over civil rights, urban rebellions, and law and order—remade the nation in the final decades of the twentieth century. As conservatism moved from the right to the center of American politics, ultimately bringing Democrats along, the liberal welfare state came under ideological and material attack.[20] This is part of the backdrop against which motherhood took on its post-*Roe* features.[21]

When children became a choice women knowingly and actively made, this meant that the circumstances which shaped family making since the 1970s, no matter how dire, also became women's responsibility to overcome. It matters that motherhood became a choice just as more and more families confronted what one historian has called the "Age of Inequality."[22] For many Americans, economic circumstances stressed rather than supported the costs and labors of caring for children. Struggling families in the 1970s confronted stagnant wages, inflation, and job loss especially in manufacturing, an industry whose owners sought relocation to escape union power.[23] These realities pushed ever greater numbers of married women into the labor market to secure a second income to compensate for the family's primary wage earner's deflated or lost wages.[24] The vast majority of such women encountered a dramatically altered labor market defined by precarious, low-wage, service jobs that would come to define the "new postindustrial order."[25] These married women joined single women, many of them also mothers, who had long labored outside the home but had largely done so in the only employment available to them in a market stratified by race and gender: domestic and "pink collar" work that was poorly paid. Despite this dramatic influx of married women into the labor market, working Americans wound up poorer than when the decade began.[26]

The realities of a market increasingly comprised of low-wage, service jobs and the unresolved labor problem of child care fell heaviest on single mothers, as evidenced by their continued participation in Aid to Families with Dependent Children (AFDC) during this period. Throughout the 1960s and into the 1970s, these families increasingly turned to the social welfare program in order to make ends meet despite rampant racial and gender discrimination, inadequate payments, and burdensome work requirements.[27] Whether they looked to the wage economy or the welfare state to make ends meet, single mothers confronted an ideological system that stubbornly refused to recede despite the unfolding economic reality. This ideological system dictated that fathers, not mothers, were the primary breadwinners and that the work women did caring for their families was not work at all. As a result of the worsening economic conditions, the "feminization of poverty" that would mobilize some feminist groups by the early 1980s was already in full swing by the time motherhood became a choice—by 1977 nearly half of all poor families were headed by a single mother, a number that had doubled since 1950.[28] So, what did the immediate post-*Roe* world look like for families?

Writing about the future of the reproductive rights movement in 1981, scholar and activist Angela Davis went so far as to describe the conditions in which poor, women of color found themselves and their families as "so miserable" they could cause women to "relinquish the right to reproduction itself." Here, Davis issued a warning to the majority-white abortion rights movement that reproductive choice could easily slide into reproductive coercion if women felt their impoverished circumstances made it impossible to imagine raising another child that they otherwise wanted. To the movement's argument that abortion "provided a viable alternative to the myriad problems posed by poverty," Davis issued the corrective, "as if having fewer children could create more jobs, higher wages, better schools, etc., etc."[29] Davis understood that capitalism and racism would accommodate *Roe*, producing a terrain where the liberatory elements of reproductive choice were hamstrung by the persistence of exploitative conditions. This was the terrain that confronted families following the legalization of abortion, and one that would become only more treacherous as both inequality and the idea that child-rearing was best left to the private family increased over the ensuing decades. Having children had become a choice at the precise moment more and more families were struggling *and also* were expected to meet the costs of family making on their own.

"Family values," or the politics of sanctifying the heteropatriarchal home, became the ground upon which conservative power was consolidated. But these ostensibly "cultural" politics consistently carried policy riders: fiscal austerity measures that decimated social supports. This devastating and effective political framework helped transform those reliant on government support (rather than on their own economically well-functioning nuclear families) into bad actors who got what they deserved—very little to nothing at all.[30] Gender and sexual politics during the 1970s, 1980s, and 1990s helped remake the welfare state and the breadwinner wage, ultimately turning both into artifacts of a bygone era.[31] It did not matter that the viability of an economy structured around a male provider had never been universally accessible and had largely disappeared before the close of the 1970s—for different reasons, both liberals and conservatives refused to "face facts" with regard to this economic reality.[32] The unforgiving harshness of a politics hellbent on responding to mounting inequality with little more than the mantra of "personal responsibility" is typically illustrated by two prominent plot points when it comes to debates about family making: President Bill Clinton making good on his promise to "end welfare as we know it" and the "unfinished business" of precisely how mothers are supposed to balance work in the home with work in the wage economy.[33] Scholars and journalists have focused on these two sites for good reason. Both illustrate the privatization of dependency that defined the political visions of the vast majority of politicians, regardless of party, by the end of the twentieth century. Both make clear that the costs and labors of family making would not only be borne by individual families but would also be subordinated to "the almost universal adult role" of breadwinner that mothers, whether by choice or coercion, were taking on.[34] One scholar recently described the conditions we have inherited from such policy decisions: "universal free childcare remains a dream, paid family leave is just now moving seriously onto politicians' agendas, and workfare has replaced welfare rights activists' demands for income supports for caregiving."[35] Collectively, these policy decisions and the problems they failed to resolve have helped make work, daycare, and welfare the plot points around which debates regarding the euphemistically phrased "work-life balance" continue to revolve.

There is no doubt that these plot points—which most immediately index the problem of needing both a steady cash flow and a steady labor source in order to ensure children are taken care of—remain key to the story of family making since the 1970s. But as anyone who has participated in the work of family making knows intimately, they are far from the only forces that keep true reproductive freedom out of reach. This book argues that having a family has become *harder and costlier* since the 1970s —especially for those who built families on the economic, racial, and sexual margins of society—due to proliferating and often interconnected factors that are less often associated with "family," "reproduction," or "work-life balance." Specifically, disease, increased criminalization and mass incarceration; medical and legal gatekeeping of the means required for queer people to make and be recognized as "a family"; a racist, for-profit system of healthcare; and the unprecedented reliance on charitable, faith-based organizations to deliver social welfare services have all wreaked havoc on families. As a result, the reproductive labor of family making has increasingly extended far beyond merely how to juggle child care in between work shifts and how to pay for food and rent. As this book shows, these basic but crucial necessities were only the tip of the iceberg for women diagnosed with a life-threatening disease, incarcerated in prisons, who dared to raise fatherless children in lesbian households, or feared their newborn would not live to see their first birthday due to their own lifetimes of medical neglect. The exclusive focus on home, work, and welfare greatly underestimates the barriers to family making erected as a result of broader political and economic shifts that have shaped American life since the late 1970s. In order to capture the full extent of the labors and costs these barriers have placed on families, *Reproduction Reconceived* broadens the scope of what counts as the labor of family making, where it gets performed, and how the state has refused to share in this necessary work.[36] Importantly, state refusal not only ensured that choice would be a fiction for most. It also necessarily produced new forms of reproductive labor through its own negligence. At the broadest register, *Reproduction Reconceived* is a labor history of the work involved in choosing family during a period where meaningful choice for many families was nowhere to be found.

FOREGROUNDING STATE NEGLECT IN REPRODUCTIVE POLITICS

Some caveats are in order. Since the late 1970s, life in the United States has been steadily approaching our current reality, one in which "every family and household has the private responsibility to figure out how to support dependents and enable them to survive and thrive, even as they do so on an uneven playing field constructed by both business and government."[37] Yet it is necessary to acknowledge that this is not a wholesale departure from government's relationship to family making prior to the 1970s. The social movements that captured political life in the 1960s and 1970s were, after all, demanding a radical transformation of both liberal society and the inequality that appeared to them integral to—rather than a grand departure from—the foundational premises of the United States.[38]

American liberalism, even during its most active periods of social welfare, has largely refused to subsidize the labors and costs of family making. It is not hyperbole to say that the moments when the state did expand its safety net, it invested heavily in the white, patriarchal, nuclear family, reinforcing it as both the proper site for social reproduction and the deserving recipient of some forms of social insurance.[39]

This is perhaps best illustrated by programs designed to catch those whose family making fell outside of the nuclear norm, though only on very narrow terms. State-level mothers' pensions meant to aid widows that inspired the federal program Aid to Dependent Children (ADC), made possible by the New Deal, were always conceived as a supplemental rather than a primary wage so as not to undermine dominant gender roles that defined husbands as productive, financial providers and wives as dependent, reproductive caretakers. Even when entitlements such as Social Security were not being funneled directly to the male breadwinner, policymakers had his supremacy in mind. Gender supremacy went hand in hand with racial supremacy, and race-based exclusions, baked directly into federal and state legislation and enforced via administrators of aid, ensured that one's deservingness to receive even the supplementary (read: insufficient) wage of welfare was tied to whiteness and sexual morality.[40] Throughout the twentieth century, this helped keep white, native-born women's motherhood legitimate even when a male provider was absent while denigrating its necessary counterpart—nonwhite, especially Black, women's motherhood—all the while ensuring that family making's value only officially came into view as a wage-less labor of love.

At the same time, it is undeniable that a central feature of the post-*Roe* period was the twentieth-century liberal welfare state's immense diminishment—a change that had significant material and ideological consequences for Americans' access to the "public good." Scholars have demonstrated how a conservative campaign organized around the heteropatriarchal, nuclear family was part and parcel of the economic agenda of neoliberalism: deregulation, slashed domestic budgets, and the superiority of the market to deliver ever dwindling public goods.[41] While these policy changes create systematic insecurity for working people, neoliberalism as a form of governance encourages individuals to see their conditions as individually determined (rather than structurally produced).[42] When it comes to family making under neoliberalism, the very policy decisions that make this already labor- and resource-intensive endeavor more costly morph into bad choices for which struggling families have only themselves to blame. And it is those families who do not conform to the white, nuclear, private household that are encouraged to self-flagellate via public demonization and punitive policies, a shame tax levied most heavily upon poor, single, nonwhite mothers.[43]

Feminist scholarship on the history of reproduction in the United States has shown that the neoliberal regime is only the most recent node in a long history of punishing family making on the margins in order to shore up the idealized norm (itself rife with punitive mechanisms designed to control white, middle-class women's reproduction). From the reproductive and sexual exploitation of enslaved women, to eugenics campaigns targeting indigent and incarcerated women, to the forced sterilization of poor Black, Latina, and Native American women reliant on public health services, to the criminalization of abortion, the history of reproductive rights in the United States is littered with concerted efforts to control different women's reproduction for various ends.[44] Feminist anthropologists, sociologists, and political scientists have demonstrated that the mobilization of reproduction to achieve these varied ends is far from past but remains an ongoing project.[45] Collectively, these works illuminate the many ways different women's reproduction is disciplined through various regulatory frameworks, often in service of broader political aims. Everything from anti-immigrant sentiment to fears about overpopulation to gains for women in the workplace to economic policy intent on state austerity can find expression in punitive campaigns that fall on women's bodies in stratified ways.[46]

Because "neoliberalism" has become so ubiquitous a label that it is now an open question whether or not it still has explicative value, and since harm can be—and, more often than not, is—doled out slowly and subtly, the history that follows is not described in terms of neoliberalism, and it explores the ways family making has been imperiled by neglect just as often as it has been the target of explicit attacks.[47] *Reproduction Reconceived* focuses on the exploitative and "miserable conditions" that Angela Davis drew our attention to forty years ago in her "Racism, Birth Control, and Reproductive Rights," and takes stock of what labors and costs pile up when survival in the face of exploitation and neglect over-whelms one's experience of family making.[48]

When it comes to family making in the United States since the 1970s, what the state has *not* done is as important as what it has done. In order to emphasize the state's failure to act, I gather under the term "state neglect" historically specific conditions that especially shaped the final decades of the twentieth century, such as mass incarceration and the HIV/AIDS epi-demic. Neglect conveys a failure to care just as it implies a responsibility or obligation. Sometimes this failure is deliberate and willful, and sometimes it stems from indifference. Regardless, neglect means someone else has to pick up the slack. The end result is not only the punishment inherent to neglect, but the additional labor the neglected must do to survive. Just as it is "expensive to be poor," it takes more work to survive in the face of neglect. In the instances examined here, this reality meant an expansion of the reproductive labor required for family making, a work burden borne overwhelmingly by women. Neglect can also tell us a lot about what we truly value (if we are able, we usually tend to the things we care about), so we can also think of neglect as one of the primary engines of the devalua-tion of reproductive labor. Indeed, state neglect is a precondition for the fairly common view that having and raising children is a privilege rather than a right. The state's lack of investment ensures family is seen as a pri-vate burden and that those who fail to meet the demands of this endeavor have only themselves to blame.

We tend to overlook neglect because it is often slow and cumulative, comprised of "miserable conditions" that become the everyday ground on which the work of survival must be performed, and which tend to be over-shadowed by more explicit, targeted reproductive rights violations. The shackling of incarcerated women during childbirth, for example, right-fully horrifies many, but the tendency for this dehumanization to pierce far more hearts than the fact that such women are very likely to lose custody of their children by virtue of being incarcerated is what this book wants to trouble. As this book shows, state neglect of family making has often had a broader reach than the regulatory campaigns that explic-itly expose the violence of the state.[49] I hope that this book evidences the immensely punishing strategy of neglect as a deadly force to be mobilized against with the same urgency as overt, targeted acts of violence. Lastly, and without reducing the politics of the family to "flotsam and jetsam floating above the real story of monumental wealth distribution," this history illustrates that sometimes the state simply does not care about the gendered and racialized labor of family making.[50]

The fact that state neglect has served as a driving force in maintaining reproductive inequities since the 1970s demands investigation and attention. In the chapters that follow, I examine how punishment has been doled out through neglect daily, slowly, and in the face of crisis conditions rendered mundane by the state's lack of urgency. In this book, I frame the state's decision to neglect families at the racial, sexual, and economic margins of society as a battle over who should perform the labor of family making and what we value—questions integral to the project of reproductive freedom. Since the 1990s, the reproductive justice movement has made tremendous headway in helping the public see that the conditions in which children are raised are not a matter of private or individual choice but of structurally determined public constraints.[51] The movement for reproductive justice has forcefully declared that this reality should be considered an affront to human rights.[52] While *Reproduction Reconceived* is not a history of the reproductive justice movement, it is in part inspired by the liberatory, Black feminist political framework now commonly referred to as "RJ," conceived of by the Women of African Descent for Reproductive Justice in 1994.[53] It highlights past efforts of individuals who also understood that families were struggling against conditions not of their own making, and who believed combatting state neglect was necessary to ensure women and their children were entitled to healthier, safer, dignified lives.

SEEING STATE NEGLECT

How does one make state inaction visible? This is the methodological question at the center of *Reproduction Reconceived*. The following history is my answer, though it is surely not the only one. It is influenced by certain priorities. I wanted to better understand why explicit, punitive attacks on reproductive rights cause shock and outrage while the slow but potentially deadly devastation of neglect is often tolerated with seeming ease. One way to do that is to examine the experiences and efforts of people unwilling to tolerate such deadly conditions, to excavate their varying diagnoses of and responses to the state's abdication of the rights, intimate ties, and lives of so many families. Neglect engendered conflict, action, and alternative ways of valuing family making. The following narrative is largely driven by different communities' rejection of the idea that families had only themselves to blame for their circumstances and instead believed that local councilmembers, state officials, judges, physicians, federal authorities, and business interests were responsible for families' conditions. They took action to hold these actors accountable and to demand more, and in the process they crafted strategies designed to expose neglect's urgency and prompt change. The mixed outcomes of these strategies documented here are meant to be instructive, particularly in light of the fact that many of the intolerable conditions these individuals fought against have yet to be alleviated, and continue to engender political struggle in our current moment.

I also wanted to intervene in the recurring, mainstream debate over "women's role in the workplace" that frequently operates at a remove from the reproductive issues addressed in this book: Black infant mortality, queer family making, the reproductive rights of incarcerated mothers, the HIV/AIDS epidemic, and pro-life/anti-abortion crisis pregnancy centers. The question of whether or not women can actually have it all has been rightly criticized as most often centering highly educated, professional women, predominantly white—the faces of neoliberal feminism—who have had to choose between tending to their families or the next round of promotions. The very terms of the debate have also been criticized—as the quote from Adrienne Rich suggests, liberation is not a seat on some corporation's board. And socialist feminists have pointed out that the euphemism of "work-life balance" so often attached to this conversation is actually a crisis of care integral to capitalism.[54] To these observations I want to add that even if tomorrow we started actually valuing care work as it is currently defined, whether through a living wage or a more radical restructuring of society, we would miss much of the labor required to maintain a family under varied conditions of neglect. And so, this book follows family making beyond the private household and the workplace, to hospitals and physicians' offices, to prison yards, cells, and children's visiting centers, to experimental drug trials, AIDS service organizations and hearings on women and AIDS, to crisis-pregnancy centers and welfare offices and fundraising efforts, to courtrooms and legal aid organizations, to community meetings, targeted campaigns and spontaneous protests, to living rooms transformed into lesbian feminist self-insemination classrooms, to heroic and taxing mutual aid efforts, to Congressional hearings and city council meetings that serve as a record of lawmakers' priorities, and to support groups where shame and grief were transformed into political action. What may at first glance seem a random assortment of sites is in fact the route one must travel to fully account for just how hard, far-flung, and precarious neglect has made family making since the 1970s.

What did different forms of neglect produce during this period? A proliferation of the *types* of labors required for family making and a ledger of costs created by work that went undone. Family making from inside a prison; after receiving a positive diagnosis of a disease the federal government refused to address; without access to quality, humane prenatal care; whilst hiding from laws incapable of recognizing your parenthood; supported by pro-life pregnancy services deeply compromised by anti-abortion propaganda—the neglect integral to these circumstances created new forms of reproductive labor for families on the margins of society. When this life-sustaining labor went undone, numerous costs were incurred by families and the advocates willing to act when and where the state would not. While families often struggled with barriers readily associated with economic costs (homelessness, food insecurity, the power company turning off the electricity), the following chapters show that the most devastating costs cannot be captured monetarily. The death of an infant in their first month of life, despair over dying of AIDs and orphaning young children, giving birth to a stillborn in a prison van belatedly on its way to the hospital, shame fueled by politicians' blaming the loss of an infant on individual behaviors rather than for-profit medical care—these are just some of the incalculable costs that families were made to suffer as a result of state neglect.

In addition to the clear labor demands engendered by neglect, I also emphasize the work of reproduction to make clear that family making is not "natural" but is instead deeply political. Law and policy shape the bounds of what are considered legitimate familial ties and, therefore, legitimate families. These legal frameworks have indexed legitimacy through race, class, marital status, sexuality, and shared genetics. Casting family making as a "labor of love" tricks us into treating care as an infinite, self-generating emotion rather than as taxing work that can also include love—and this trick is only made possible by naturalizing care as "women's work." The enduring "dual devaluation of care work and care workers," combined with racial ideologies that value white women for producing their own families while valuing nonwhite women for caring for families not their own, has ensured both a persistent "racial division of reproductive labor" and the likelihood that poor, nonwhite mothers are considered to be illegitimate family-makers, especially if they fail to conform to sexual norms.[55] These enduring realities mean that so-called illegitimate families, along with those who advocate on their behalf, have had to work overtime not only to maintain familial ties amidst numerous constraints, but also to even be recognized as "a family." Neglect was not a foregone conclusion, but instead became the prevailing norm through the repetition of decisions that cumulatively limited the state's role in supporting family making. The book captures some of this process by examining five major developments that engendered specific forms of neglect. It begins in the mid-1970s, when lesbians hoping to become mothers through artificial insemination had recently inherited a significant legal development: the late 1960s "revolution" in illegitimacy law that declared distinctions between marital and nonmarital children unconstitutional also preserved the law's interest in establishing paternity in order to attach every child to a male provider. Thanks to guidance on self-insemination distributed by participants in the feminist self-help movement, lesbians of differing race and class backgrounds became pregnant without the aid of private physicians (who had long refused to inseminate single women) and started building families without fathers. Lesbians who endeavored to raise fatherless children, however, soon realized that the revolution in parentage law, having left paternity intact as the singular criterion of a legitimate family, was incomplete. The law's inability to recognize lesbian motherhood—its insistence that lesbian mothers were single mothers whose families were illegitimate so long as they lacked a male provider—left lesbian-headed households vulnerable to *legal neglect*. Chapter 1 charts the additional labor required to overcome this neglect, as well as the costs legal recognition posed to families formed in the shadow of the law.

At the same time lesbians were having children and debating the costs and rewards of legal recognition, "tough on crime" laws that would result in mass incarceration and dramatically increase the number of women sent to prisons and jails were increasingly breaking apart families. Poor women ensnared by harsher sentencing laws were also overwhelmingly the primary caretakers of their young children, and the criminalization of Black women in particular resulted in their overrepresentation in California's state prison. Families were separated by a system of punishment that cared very little about the caretaking responsibilities or reproductive health needs of this new and rapidly expanding population. Chapter 2 charts the *carceral neglect* integral to imprisonment in the United States. It focuses especially on the additional labor required to give birth safely, to mother and retain custody of one's children from behind bars, and the incalculable costs that piled up when such work failed to mitigate the harms of carceral neglect.

The first two chapters capture a neglectful state in transition—those working to make family in spite of incarceration, for example, had some success in enlisting state and federal lawmakers to share in this project, albeit in piecemeal and precarious ways. By the early 1980s, however, arrangements that often relied on a key decisionmaker's good will, quickly gave way to the forceful consolidation of conservative power represented by Ronald Reagan's election in 1980. The next two chapters trace two health crises, both made worse by the various actions municipal, state, and federal lawmakers on both sides of the aisle took and, importantly, did not take. Chapter 3 charts how rates of Black infant mortality had become, by the mid-1980s, a formally recognized public health crisis, with politicians, federal health officials, public health researchers, and advocates debating whether or not expanding Medicaid coverage to pregnant women was a sufficient solution to *medical neglect* and the problem of Black infant death. But before Congress began debating legislative action, activists in cities with high Black infant mortality accused municipal officials of "genocide by neglect" and demanded that quality, culturally competent healthcare be treated as a human right rather than a profit-making venture. This chapter explores how critiques and demands such as those issued by the Third World Women's Alliance in Oakland and the Maternity Care Coalition in Philadelphia hinged on the idea that government had an obligation to take of its citizens, an idea that already by 1980 had lost political purchase. As a result, families and their advocates were backed into narrow, political compromises that purported to solve one problem—medical neglect—while further weakening state support for other sorely needed resources, in this instance, welfare aid. It also charts the additional labor required for day-to-day survival under such neglectful, devastating conditions, and the incalculable toll infant death had on mothers and community members.

Chapter 4 also examines the labor of survival, but it does so in the context of the early years of the HIV/AIDS epidemic. The Reagan administration's refusal to respond in the first, crucial years of the epidemic is well known, and while the chapter certainly accounts for this neglect, it foregrounds the *cumulative neglect* underlying the rapid spread of the disease in poor, Black and Latina women who were also mothers or caretakers of small children. By the time the epidemic hit, these families were already enduring housing insecurity, poverty, depressed wages and welfare aid, substance use, and insufficient medical care on top of the demand of caring for small children. They and their advocates labored not only in order to manage their own risk in the face of the disease when no public health response was forthcoming, but also to secure family-friendly social services, such as housing, and to gain access to potentially life-saving treatment through participation in experimental drug trials. Both of these neglect-fueled crises led to incalculable costs: not only death but also the less discussed toll of shame borne by those who blamed themselves for the death of their infants or for getting sick.

By the early 1990s, where chapter 4 ends, different grassroots efforts had worked to mitigate various forms of neglect through a combination of legal advocacy, pressure campaigns, protest, and mutual aid. Particularly through their commitment to providing some form of immediate support, they knew all too well that the need always exceeded what local networks could provide, and so they continued to demand that government replace its neglect with the provision of resources. For the most part, however, these resources were not forthcoming, and so local networks remained vital if insufficient lifelines.

Chapter 5 turns to a grassroots service initiative that formed not out of a desire to alleviate structural inequality but nevertheless comprised a network of support that played a role in mitigating neglect during the final decades of the twentieth century. Pro-life emergency pregnancy services, now known as crisis pregnancy centers (CPCs), formed to counter the "threat" legal abortion posed to single pregnant women abandoned by their families or would-be male partners. Chapter 5 documents poor, pregnant women's increased reliance on these lifelines of last resort, where necessary pregnancy services and support are doled out alongside anti-abortion propaganda. Contrary to dominant depictions of CPCs successfully tricking pregnant women into thinking they are in an abortion clinic, only to manipulate them into bringing their pregnancy to term, this chapter demonstrates how the strategy of combating legal abortion by providing free but limited pregnancy services necessarily secured CPCs a prominent role in the patchwork of resources that serve as families' last line of defense against poverty, homelessness, and food insecurity. As faith-based, privately funded services, CPCs weathered the slashing of government budgets that fueled widespread conditions of neglect and hampered the organizations documented in prior chapters. Pregnant women who rely on these compromised but necessary services must labor to navigate the strings attached to CPC aid: anti-abortion propaganda, conservative Christian values, and race-based attacks on abortion that stigmatize Black women's reproduction. State neglect ensures CPCs remain relevant and even necessary in the lives of those most in need of support. The chapter concludes by asking whether a more robust investment in family making wouldn't make CPCs obsolete once and for all.

Family making is always work, but those attempting to build family at the margins of society have had to work harder—and labor in different ways—at the close of the twentieth century. The limits of individual and community capacity to make family possible in the face of deadly neglect are evidenced by the varied, incalculable costs tallied in these pages. *Reproduction Reconceived* repeatedly demonstrates an important reality: neglect does not produce an abundance of choice. Instead, it produces more work to navigate and survive one's constraints, which necessarily result in costs when, inevitably, life-sustaining work exceeds one's capacity and resources.

Since the arrival of choice *Roe* is so often made to symbolize, what the state has *not* done for families has been central to ensuring that such choice exists only for an ever shrinking few. If exploitative systems determine "the bounds of the possible" within "miserable conditions," it makes little sense to see family making as an absolute choice.[56] Rather, we need an appraisal of the labors and costs of reproduction that have proliferated under state neglect, a process made possible by our willingness to repeatedly devalue care, no matter the human cost. A decade ago, legal scholar Robin West asked if we were "truly comfortable, morally, with a world that we have created, in which only rich people can parent satisfactorily?"[57] While West marks the creation of this world with *Roe*'s passage, Davis's cautionary tale to the abortion rights movement in the years immediately following legalization teaches us that this moral test is nothing new. In hopes that history can help strengthen convictions that propel current movements for reproductive justice, my book offers a rendering of the last fifty years that debunks the myth of choice inaugurated by *Roe*, centers families that have been struggling at various margins, and concludes that our current value system must be reordered if we want to arrive at more comfortable moral ground. True reproductive freedom demands nothing less.

1 The Labor of Illegibility

LESBIAN AND SINGLE MOTHERHOOD
ACCORDING TO THE LAW

It is important to note one major limitation on our efforts.
Because the heterosexual model of conception, family relations, child bearing and child rearing is so prevalent, much
of our analysis involved the task of transposing lesbian
parenting onto a legal or medical framework for which it is
ill-suited.

Report from the Multidisciplinary Study Group on Lesbians
Choosing Children, 1983

A family portrait staged by lesbian feminist and civil rights activist Cathy
Cade depicts Cade, her lover, Kate, Kate's son, Guthrie, and their room-
mate, Pat. Each woman is clad in overalls or coveralls, and Cade and Kate
stare down the camera with their arms crossed while Pat casually hugs her
knees to her chest. The three women sit apart from one another, each
holding her distinct space in the photo, and while Guthrie sits next to his
mother, they are not touching. The items that represent each individual's
work are displayed in front of them, including Kate's tools, Pat's pottery,
Cade's camera, and Guthrie's trucks. It is 1973 in Berkeley, California, and
the residents of the "Emerson Street Household" have replaced the white,
patriarchal, middle-class nuclear family with white, woman-centered,
queer kinship, romance, and motherhood, mocking the conventions of
family portraiture in the process.[1]

Almost two decades later, a lesbian family portrait of a very different
sort appeared in the *New York Times* to provide evidence of the "lesbian
baby boom" that, by 1989, mainstream media outlets had declared was

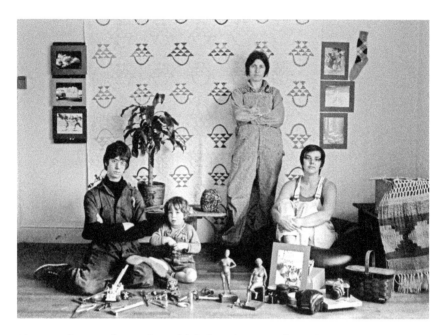

Figure 1. Photographer Cathy Cade's lesbian feminist take on family portraiture, *Emerson Street Household, Berkeley,* 1973. Courtesy of Bancroft Library, University of California, Berkeley.

in full swing. This time, Kim Klausner and Debra Chasnoff are pictured jointly holding their son, Noah. This arrangement consumes the entirety of the frame, though the viewer gets the vague impression that the family is in their home. Both women lean over Noah dotingly as the baby coos. There is no space between either woman or their child, and there is no question about the lines of intimate attachment, both parental and romantic. To be sure, Klausner, Chasnoff, and Noah are redefining the terms of the nuclear family, but this family portrait attests to the success of their self-recognition. There is no trace of ironic distance that might indicate a political critique of the nuclear, domestic bliss that the photo radiates.[2]

The distance between the Emerson Street family portrait and the family depicted in the *New York Times* is only two decades, but these respective photos capture two distinct phases of lesbian motherhood. Still, there is one stubborn, unchanging detail that the camera's shutter fails to

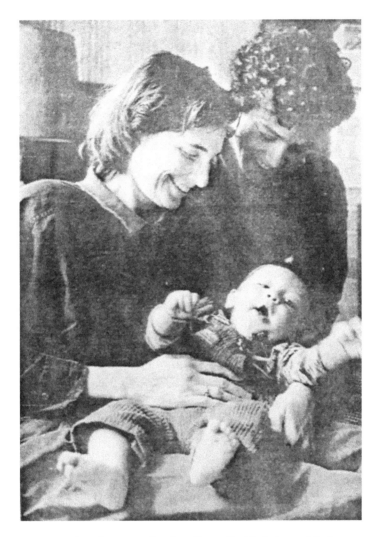

Figure 2. Kim Klausner and Debra Chasnoff with their son, Noah.
Photo taken for the *New York Times* in San Francisco, 1989. Courtesy
of Terrence McCarthy.

expose: both in 1973 and in 1989, these family portraits depict single
mothers. This is not true in the colloquial sense. Kate and Cade were lovers, and Kate's ex-husband was helping to raise Guthrie. Klausner and
Chasnoff clearly understood the decision to have a child and the project of
parenting Noah as a joint endeavor that took place in the context of their

commitment to one another. But lesbians' chosen, familial attachments mattered little to the law. When I say that these two family portraits depict single mothers, I am describing the couples' legal status as such and what that status has meant for their ability to secure sole custody of their children—or not.

What makes these family portraits of concern *legally* is the absence of a father-provider or, to be more precise, paternity. As expectations of traditional gender roles loosened, sped along by feminist and gay liberation movements as well as economic changes, mothers who divorced (or were divorced by) their husbands as well as women who bypassed marriage altogether contributed to the growth of single mothers heading families without fathers.[3] Lesbians were the most intentional in their desire to raise fatherless children, and often the most wary of the repercussions that such an endeavor might bring. They had good reason to worry. Not all lesbians who left heterosexual marriages were as lucky as Kate. Around the time she and her ex-husband divorced, the likelihood that a judge would deny her custody of Guthrie on the basis of her sexuality was the same as flipping a coin, and even the "lucky" ones routinely traded much of their privacy, sexuality, and child support simply to visit their children.[4]

The immense vulnerability of gay men's and lesbians' parental rights that persisted from the late 1960s into the early 1990s profoundly influenced women who pursued motherhood through artificial insemination by donor (AID).[5] Lesbians who made use of the fertility treatment thoroughly rejected courts' findings that having a gay parent was not "in the best interests of the child." But this rejection did not fully alleviate the fear of both the state and individual men that influenced some women's reproductive decision-making. When these women pursued parenthood, they were clear-eyed about the fact that becoming a lesbian mother was threatening precisely because such a status lacked the supposedly essential characteristic of parental fitness: an acknowledged father-provider. As one woman who wanted anonymity from any potential sperm donor explained, "as a lesbian, as a mother, I didn't want some man with his wife and little picket fence to come to some judge and say, 'A lesbian is raising my kid.'"[6] The fact that women were pursuing motherhood outside of marriage *and* heterosexual sex made lesbians pursuing AID guilty of trying to bypass not just individual, would-be fathers, but paternity as well. Paternity was of particular interest to the state as a way of ensuring that the care of children remained a private obligation. Lesbians who turned to AID as a way to make a family feared the repercussions of both trespasses. To insulate their parental rights from both donor and the state, lesbian mothers spent the decade and a half between the Emerson Street staged family portrait and the *New York Times* family photo strategizing how best to thwart the law's desire to attach a male provider to every child.

They had their work cut out for them. First and foremost, women had to find a way to get pregnant without the help of a male sexual partner or a physician. While Klausner and Chasnoff could have used the services of the only sperm bank to openly welcome single women and lesbians, most women had a much harder time accessing the most important part of the process—semen.[7] Fatherless families, much less lesbian mothers, greatly concerned physicians who administered AID through private practice or university medical centers. The treatment was considered appropriate only for married couples—until the fertility industry realized single women were an untapped market in the 1980s. Locked out of institutional routes to pregnancy by physician gatekeeping and hoping to avoid sex with men, lesbians in the women's health self-help movement became experts in what they called "alternative fertilization."[8] Women who built family through this strategy did so by reading medical textbooks, using knowledge of ovulation cycles to increase chances of conception, writing and distributing guides on insemination, and taking on the greatest task of all: procuring semen from willing donors.[9] And they did so at the same time moralizing about the breakdown of the nuclear family led the ascendant conservative movement to elect Ronald Reagan president in 1980.[10] For lesbian feminist activists, self-insemination and its promise of achieving pregnancy on one's own terms was an issue of reproductive liberty just as pressing as the right not to have children. And, at least in the early years, they scorned the "patriarchal laws" designed to control their reproductive and sexual practices.[11] Authors of the 1979 how-to pamphlet *Woman Controlled Conception* were not alone in their assumption that any such recognition would only serve to restrict women's reproductive control, hence the appeal of self-insemination. "The beauty of artificial insemination is that we can do it ourselves, no matter what laws they might pass."[12] Alternative fertilization held the promise of freedom from "patriarchal laws," a chance to create family anew. And yet, lesbians' do-it-yourself (DIY) practices nevertheless had legal ramifications, and navigating the law made the already labor-intensive project of getting pregnant even more laborious. Specifically, because the law had no logic or framework with which to recognize lesbian motherhood—because lesbian motherhood was illegible to the law—lesbian mothers confronted a form of legal neglect that rendered their families vulnerable to state interference. The same year Cade staged her lesbian feminist triumph over patriarchal family portraiture, the Uniform Law Commission approved the Uniform Parentage Act (UPA). Authors of the UPA hoped it would bring state legislatures in line with a series of Supreme Court decisions that declared distinctions between marital and nonmarital children unconstitutional. Specifically, these cases aimed to abolish the legal category of "illegitimacy." But as civil rights and feminist attorneys who fought on behalf of the Black, poor female-headed families targeted by such laws learned, doing away with marital status was not sufficient for eradicating the gender and racial discrimination that rendered these families illegitimate.[13] While the importance of marital status receded, paternity—and its ability to ensure the private care of children by a father-provider rather than the state—remained firmly in place despite the Supreme Court decisions and the UPA's approval. Indeed, the UPA was one of the main laws through which paternity took the place of marital status, and it was this legal quagmire that lesbians raising fatherless children inherited. What relevance should paternity have in families deliberately constructed without a father? How would race and class mitigate or amplify the state's interest in establishing paternity? How did the legal illegibility of lesbian families without a male head of household make these mothers vulnerable to discrimination within a legal regime that affirmed paternity as the singular criterion of a legitimate family?

This legal uncertainty meant lesbian mothers and their advocates labored on three related fronts: to get pregnant in spite of institutional barriers to AID treatment, to do so while fearing the removal of any child thus conceived, and to craft legal solutions that might make their families legible—that is, "recognizable" as a family unit deserving of the same rights afforded those the law deemed "legitimate" families. On the third point, attorneys with the Lesbian Rights Project (LRP) ensured that the

UPA would have to reckon with lesbian motherhood, and the legal aid organization played a large role in overcoming the legal neglect lesbian families faced. The model law contained a clause that nullified a donor's paternity to a child conceived through AID as long as semen was provided to a physician for the purposes of insemination. The family law scholar Harry Krause, who crafted this clause, never presumed that it would be used by anyone other than heterosexual, married couples who wished to conceive a child through AID. But in the hands of LRP attorneys, the clause ultimately enabled lesbian, single mothers to overcome their legal neglect. Working within the terms of the clause, however, meant rerouting lesbians to the very institution that had denied them motherhood in the first place: physician-assisted AID.

Such a solution, now seemingly mundane when one considers the fertility industry's embrace of queers desiring children, was not without costs.[14] Legal structures never intended to legitimate lesbian motherhood did provide protection for some women. But they could not secure the reproductive freedom envisioned by lesbian feminists who hoped that family, built according to the terms desired by each mother-to-be, might become a reality for *all* women. The UPA's ability to negate donor paternity offered the lesbian mother who conceived in accordance with the law an invaluable parental right: privacy.[15] This right was granted in exchange for reproductive decision-making authorized by the physician or the clinic. For this reason, it was more accessible to those who could afford fertility treatment or purchase banked sperm and then self-inseminate. But this was not the only way privacy was more readily available to well-resourced lesbians than their less well-off counterparts. Lesbians' ability to become and remain single mother *providers* was also necessary in order to keep one's family free of state interference. Privacy could easily be replaced with state surveillance and interference, a harm brought more readily upon poor mothers of color. This was made clear by early custody suits involving lesbian mothers whose fatherless families came to the attention of state officials when they applied for welfare. Typically interpreted as evidence of lesbians' vulnerability to paternity suits by donors, I reframe these cases as illustrative of the vulnerability caused by the law's willful failure to recognize lesbian motherhood. Lesbians were perpetually single mothers, and when they became welfare mothers the state was especially insistent that a father be found to make the family whole (and self-reliant).

If what was being worked out in the two decades that lesbians like Cade, Klausner, and Chasnoff insisted on becoming parents was the law's ability to make kinship legible without reference to paternity, then there were consequences for the single mothers who did not adhere to the strategies forged by lesbian attorneys that had the power to transform one's most beloved relations into "family." These costs continue to be borne by queer families who create ties through informal networks, outside of the fertility clinic and in the shadow of the law. The path from the Emerson Street household portrait to the family photo in the *New York Times* is one by which queer family making traded in legal neglect for legal legibility, and some single mothers gained recognition as sole providers as well as the privacy afforded such a status. For families conceived beyond the patriarchal laws some lesbian feminists originally believed could be undermined through self-insemination, however, this limited version of reproductive liberty remains out of reach.

SECRECY AND ILLEGITIMACY UNRAVEL

"Officially, artificial insemination does not exist."[16] Writing in the first edition of *Artificial Insemination*, published in 1964, Dr. Wilfred J. Finegold, Professor of Obstetrics and Gynecology at the University of Pittsburgh School of Medicine, was referring to the absence of legal regulation of AID. Though Georgia would become the exception to Finegold's observation when the state legislated the procedure that same year, the few attempts to regulate AID elsewhere had failed.[17] Instead, legal evidence that the fertility treatment did in fact "exist" could be found in custody cases involving children conceived through AID.[18] Finegold urged regulation of AID, hoping normalization would follow. "The lawyer who claimed that the law's response to artificial insemination will be horror, skepticism, curiosity and then acceptance has diagnosed the situation correctly. We believe that the 'horror' stage has passed and that the public and the legislatures are moving in the area of skepticism and curiosity. Before long, there will be acceptance."[19]

Finegold may have overlooked a recent decision issued by the Supreme Court of Kings County, New York, which suggested that the impending "acceptance" phase had a big hurdle to clear: illegitimacy. In *Gursky v. Gursky*, Stanley Gursky sought to annul his marriage to Annette Gursky. During court proceedings, it was revealed that their child, Minday Gursky, had been conceived through AID, which raised the question of Minday's legal status. The court found that she was illegitimate because her biological father, the sperm donor, was not her mother's husband—Minday was born "out of wedlock." However, because Stanley had consented in writing to the use of AID, the court also found that he was liable for child support, likening his consent to "an implied contract." Further, the court ruled that failing to hold Stanley responsible for supporting the child "would cast a financial burden upon the wife which in equity and conscience should be borne by the husband."[20]

Finegold and other advocates of AID had long rejected the idea that children conceived through AID were illegitimate.[21] Indeed, they were incredibly cognizant of this legal and social risk, prompting Finegold to assure his readers that "no doctor wishes to brand a child a bastard."[22] The social and legal ambiguity surrounding the status of these children was a partial motivator for physicians' insistence that AID remain in their hands. Only they could be trusted to insulate patients from illegitimacy by administering the treatment appropriately and covertly.[23] Legal sanctioning could help society realize that physicians were responsible administrators who would not allow the procedure to be misused. Ushering AID into the "acceptance phase" could be achieved with legislation that adopted the medical establishment's terms: that AID was only appropriate in the case of sterile husbands or husbands with hereditary diseases, that children so conceived were the rightful offspring of the husband, and that only physicians' discriminating expertise could evaluate eligible donors and married couples.

These terms made sure that physicians administering the treatment controlled who would benefit from it. Finegold assured readers that "AI is one phase of medicine in which the physician may honorably refuse to attend to a sick patient."[24] Wives who attempted to seek treatment behind their husbands' backs were relegated to this category, as was the "masculine-aggressive woman" who attempted to force consent from her husband.

Single women who sought AID were considered to be manifesting a different kind of illness, and in at least one case were referred to psychiatric care.[25] The belief that fertility treatment should produce children only for married, heterosexual couples was cultivated and protected by medical practitioners. Neither attorneys nor physicians were eager to see the procedure's potential for exploding the legal category of illegitimacy altogether.

At the same time that physicians were vouching for the legitimacy of children like Minday Gursky, so-called illegitimate families were attacking the discriminatory nature of distinctions that rested on marital status. Beginning with a lawsuit brought on behalf of Louise Levy's children following her wrongful death in 1968, a series of Supreme Court decisions wore down the distinctions between children born within and outside of marriage. Along with individual plaintiffs, civil rights attorneys fought to make such distinctions unconstitutional. Legal advocates hoped to show that laws designed to regulate "morals"—such as nonmarital sex—while race-neutral on their face, were in fact purposefully racially discriminatory. (By the late 1960s, such laws were widely understood as a backlash to civil rights gains.)[26] Attorneys wedded their argument about racial discrimination to the one that proved most compelling and durable to the Court, that children should not be punished for the "sins" of their parents.[27] The first illegitimacy cases to reach the Supreme Court, *Levy* (1968) and *Glona* (1968), along with the Court's ultimate reversal on *Labine* (1971) in *Trimble* (1977), consistently appealed to children's innocence, and the fact that they could not be held responsible for their parents' immoral behavior. For example, in *Trimble v. Gordon* (1977), Justice Powell's majority opinion stated that "parents have the ability to conform their conduct to societal norms, but their illegitimate children can affect neither their parents' conduct nor their own status."[28]

One of the central architects of the Supreme Court's preferred argument was a family law professor named Harry Krause, who helped set the Court's sights on the harm illegitimacy laws brought to innocent children. A prolific and active advocate, Krause published extensively on illegitimacy, making him an influential expert on the topic. In a 1966 article titled "Bringing the Bastard into the Great Society," Krause framed illegitimacy as a necessary front in the war on poverty and racism, pointing out, along with other concerned observers, that "the total number of illegitimate births has increased continuously." Krause considered his attack on illegitimacy to be a battle unfolding "in the private sector," where victory would mean being able "to provide to the illegitimate those private resources that ought to be available to give him an even start in life." For Krause, as for many other liberal advocates, the most valuable private resource were a child's parents, "especially his father," and Krause emphasized that Black children especially had been denied this right.[29] Krause's investment in fathers as private solutions was accompanied by his belief that sex outside of marriage could be regulated by the state, but that existing illegitimacy laws were an ineffective and unjust method of doing so.[30] Krause sought to bring "the illegitimate . . . into the second half of this century" while preserving the role of the male breadwinner as the rightful head of household and keeping the state's interest in regulating sexual behavior unchallenged.[31] The series of decisions handed down from the late 1960s and into the 1970s largely did just that.[32]

Krause considered the Supreme Court decisions invaluable steps towards eradicating illegitimacy-based distinctions. But by 1973, he was increasingly frustrated with state legislatures that had not brought their statutes in line with the rulings. "The old law of illegitimacy is all but a dead letter, but the new law has not yet been implemented."[33] As early as 1967, Krause had himself proposed "a new law," outlining a model statute that would address the numerous state and federal laws imposing distinctions based on marital status. Originally titled "A Proposed Uniform Act on Legitimacy," in 1973 Krause was tapped by the National Conference on Commissioners on Uniform State Laws to draft the "Uniform Parentage Act."[34] The act was approved by the House of Delegates of the American Bar Association in February of 1974.[35] The final language of the act stated: "The parent and child relationship extends equally to every child and every parent, regardless of the marital status of the parent."[36] The Uniform Parentage Act (UPA) ensured every child a legal relationship to *two* parents, but because illegitimacy had by and large nullified a child's relationship to her father, the UPA was really a recognition that paternity mattered regardless of marital status.[37]

Krause's extensive research on the various routes by which the law punished nonmarital children meant that the legal ambiguity surrounding children conceived by AID did not escape his attention. Artificial insemination was included in the earliest draft of his proposed law. At first, Krause allowed for the husband's consent to AID as the path by which any child conceived "becomes the legitimate child of his father."[38] By the time he had written the UPA, Krause's thoughts had evolved to insulate all involved parties. The UPA held that the supervision of a licensed physician combined with a couple's marital status (married only) both secured the legitimacy of a child conceived through AID and severed the donor's rights or obligations to the child.[39]

A searing feminist legal critique issued in the lead-up to the final draft of the UPA pointed out that Krause's proposal "merely substitutes paternity for marriage as the basis for classifying children," effectively maintaining two classes of children through a different marker than marriage—those who could identify their father and those who could not.[40] In their review of Krause's proposed law, Patricia Tenoso and Aleta Wallach charged that the UPA failed to fully abolish illegitimacy. As a result, "the right of women to . . . be free of all forms of male domination" remained out of reach.[41] The UPA institutionalized Krause's belief that a child's access to her father was the key to overcoming illegitimacy as well as the poverty that supposedly stemmed from nonmarital sex. (Tenoso and Wallach offered alternative explanations for poverty, such as racial and gender discrimination in both employment and welfare assistance.) The clause on artificial insemination made clear just how right Krause's feminist critics were about his trading marriage for paternity.[42] In the case of AID, the absence of biological paternity—Krause's solution to illegitimacy—was restored through proof of marriage.[43] When it came to artificial insemination, it was not only that the UPA sought to attach a man to every child (as with children conceived through marital sex). The law also ensured that the very institution it sought to move beyond remained intact to legitimate a husband's legal rights to "his" child, no matter how conceived.

"CHARLATANS," "QUACKS," AND LESBIANS

The UPA clause on AID institutionalized what had long been deemed best practice by fertility treatment specialists: marriage was the baseline requirement for eligibility. For married couples that sought AID as a solution to infertility, this clause promised to protect wives from being found guilty of adultery, protect children from illegitimacy, and protect donors from support obligations. But almost as soon as AID was rendered legitimate by marital status and legal sanctioning, it would be plucked from the physician's office and the nuclear family in the service of ends Krause had not imagined. For lesbians and single women who wished to reclaim artificial insemination from medical and legal gatekeeping, "alternative fertilization" represented the ultimate form of reproductive autonomy. Feminist attorneys may have failed to establish an "independent justification for abolition of illegitimacy" that granted women an absolute "right to self-determination."[44] But outside of the law and the medical establishment, women would begin to enact "the validity of a woman-centered and defined family" that had eluded feminist attorneys attempting to foreground the sex-based harms illegitimacy laws brought to single mothers.[45]

Physicians had long worried about the ease with which AID could be performed, and the possibility that it might fall into the wrong hands only increased their commitment to keeping a tight grip on the procedure. Finegold illustrated just how low-tech AID was with an anecdote in his 1964 publication. In 1952, a woman incarcerated at the Pittsburgh Detention Home for Women became pregnant despite having been incarcerated for several years at the all-female institution. The District Attorney's office was called upon to solve this mystery, and the woman admitted that during one of her fiancé's visits he slipped her a vial of his semen, with which she then inseminated herself using a syringe from the doctor's office. Finegold cautioned that a lack of medical experience was not a barrier to insemination. This reality posed a danger of a different sort. "One of the hazards of the procedure is the ease of its performance. Since very little medical training is necessary and no elaborate instruments are required, A.I. can fall into the hands of charlatans and quacks."[46] Finegold's admission of simplicity evidences that the ability to decide who was and was not fit to parent was a key motivator for physicians' gatekeeping.

Finegold's warnings proved prescient when "seizing the means of reproduction" became one of the signature calls of the feminist health movement that emerged in the 1960s and 1970s, when lesbian activists realized that insemination could deliver "pregnancy without men."[47] The same year the American Bar Association approved the UPA, the lesbian literary magazine

Amazon Quarterly published a piece titled "Radical Reproduction: X without Y." In addition to advocating that lesbians could conceive only daughters through techniques such as parthenogenesis and cloning, Laurel Galana also exposed the medical gatekeeping of artificial insemination. "As usual, the mystique of the medical profession has kept women from taking this tool into their own hands." Demystifying reproductive science was for Galana and other lesbians a path not only to pregnancy without men but female offspring, too. "Why would we want it [selective artificial insemination]? Because the female-producing X sperm are now readily identifiable and we could inseminate ourselves with just these sperm. Two advantages: 1) The chances of a girl would be 100% certain and 2) no fucking required."[48]

Some advocates of lesbian separatism were especially excited about the possibility of controlling for sex, though the dreams of parthenogenesis and cloning faded as lesbian feminist nationalism was expressed in other ways.[49] Of course, not all lesbians, and not even all lesbian separatists, contemplating motherhood were concerned with guaranteeing the sex of their child. And, as evidenced by the diverse kinship arrangements women formed with donors, many lesbians desired some sort of male involvement in their conception and childrearing: it just needed to be on their terms. More often than not, then, feminist publications highlighted how artificial insemination offered a route to family making free of the societal mandate that family be anchored by a patriarchal head of household.[50] Writing in *Lesbian Tide* in 1977, Jeanne Cordova observed that "even now, despite feminism and a liberalization of laws and customs in childraising, the price of having a child, for both gay and straight women, almost always requires having more of a relationship with a man than we want." Artificial insemination seemed to hold the key to overcoming this obstacle. "The *option* of artificial insemination moves womankind one step closer to cutting the patriarchal umbilical cord. . . . Artificial insemination must therefore be an option for every woman."[51]

But the path to this option was also blocked by the same dictates designed to keep women "bonded to men in a nuclear family."[52] At a conference on women and their health held in Boston in 1975, facilitators running a workshop on artificial insemination explained that "one of the reasons for doing artificial insemination at home is that the American Medical Association has tight control over sperm banks and artificial insemination . . . the only way a woman can get around the A.M.A. is to find a sympathetic physician who is willing to say she is married."[53] *Lesbian Tide* also emphasized that "medical protocol now dictates that only married women with sterile husbands may be artificially inseminated."[54] And Francie Hornstein, co-founder of the Feminist Women's Health Center in Los Angeles, recollects that the "one sperm bank in the city" was operated by a physician who "declined to make his services available to women who were not married, not to mention lesbians."[55] Evidencing the long-standing guidance that instructed physicians to treat only married, heterosexual couples, feminist publications contained and circulated stories of women being turned away from private physicians' AID clinics as well as sperm banks.[56]

In the face of this gatekeeping, lesbians needed to address both a procedural issue—how to self-inseminate, and a source issue—how to procure semen. They got to work on both fronts. Publications like *off our backs, Lesbian Tide, Amazon Quarterly, Seattle Gay News,* and *CoEvolution Quarterly* began addressing the procedural issue by printing how-to articles detailing the steps required for self-insemination.[57] They overwhelmingly commented on the ease with which insemination could be performed by the lay-lesbian. A *Conception Comix!* panel illustrating one Bay Area woman's journey to motherhood via self-insemination drove this point home: "Maggie," rushing to make her lesbian teacher support group meeting in San Francisco and having just received the sperm donation from her sperm runner, self-inseminated while crossing the Bay Bridge in her friends' car.[58] By 1979, three lesbian health pamphlets dedicated to reaching "lesbians who want children but do not want to have sex with men" were being distributed by various organizations.[59] One of these pamphlets even opened with an epigraph of Finegold's warning about the hazards of easy insemination, topping off the quote with a smirking "Why, anyone could do it!" The pamphlet explained, "Contrary to what we're told, the mechanics of artificial insemination are as easy as 1-2-3."[60]

The ease of insemination obscures the research, writing, disseminating, and assisting—the work—that went into making "pregnancy without men" available to any woman who wanted it.[61] This was especially true when it came to the source issue: procuring semen. The same publications disseminating advice on artificial insemination make this clear. *Lesbian*

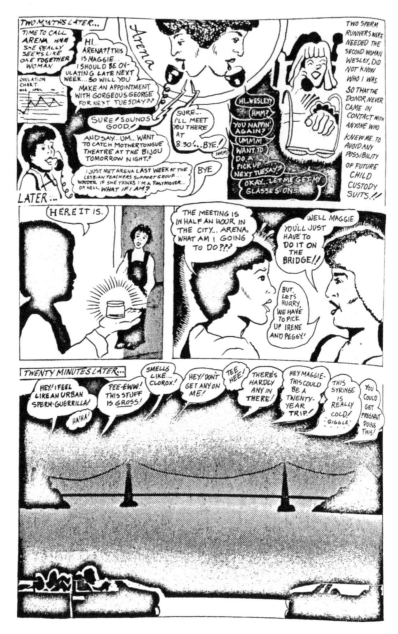

Figure 3. Panel from *Conception Comix!* depicts Maggie self-inseminating as she and her sperm runner cross the Bay Bridge, published in *Lesbian Health Matters!*, 1979. Courtesy of Mary Wings.

Tide reported that "several lesbians report their biggest difficulty in arranging their pregnancy was locating a suitable sperm donor."[62] While many women certainly tried their luck with local physicians and sperm banks, the vast majority turned elsewhere for sperm.[63] By the mid-1970s, two feminist health clinics had begun offering artificial insemination services, securing partnerships with sperm banks willing to act as suppliers.[64] But these projects were still in the early stages and comprised only a small part of clinic operations. As a result, many women turned to informal methods of procuring donors, either through friends or relatives, or through affordable donor networks organized by feminist health activists and supplied by gay male donors.[65]

The informal routes that lesbians devised for procuring semen flew in the face of donor protocols that were considered a major part of physicians' work responsibilities. According to physicians, a key part of their expertise was being able to identify a donor that matched the physical characteristics of the husband so that any child conceived through AID would pass as the married couple's biological offspring. Indeed, this was one of the promises physicians made to their patients, and one of the greatest concerns for couples seeking fertility treatment. This job required immense discretion due to the belief that donors and couples must never be identified to one another—only the physician knew all parties. Locked out of this system of secrecy and forced to create alternatives, lesbians threw open the door to women's having a say in donor characteristics. Long before one could set filters for the traits they hoped to find housed in a sperm bank's online database, Maggie from the *Conception Comix!* panel drew up a "list of desirable traits I would seek in a donor," which included things like "curly hair, no history of family diabetes, and cuddley."[66] Her sperm runner would then try to match as many of these characteristics as possible when looking for donors. One activist who coordinated donors and women required donors to fill out a form that listed "looks and aptitudes, so that women can choose among them."[67] And a woman named JoAnn who eventually used the semen of her gay male friend Paul was confident that "I didn't want to go through a doctor or a clinic as I wasn't willing for someone to control who the donor was going to be."[68]

Donor choice, even in the limited ways it was made available through informal sources, brought with it a set of ethical calculations that lesbians also labored over. Some lesbians, like Maggie, pursued personality traits, but it was the racial and ethnic background of the donor that figured most prominently in early debates about donor traits. Many of the how-to insemination guides that circulated widely during this period were authored by white lesbians, and they urged other white women to use white donors. Maggie followed their lead: she is depicted in the *Conception Comix!* story contemplating how having a "racially mixed kid" would make her responsible for providing "two or more cultural identities for that child" when she only had "one cultural background" to draw on. With some lingering uncertainty, Maggie ultimately decided "not to try to provide a culture I wasn't a part of."[69]

White lesbians who advocated this position invoked an argument popularized by the National Association of Black Social Workers' (NABSW) 1972 position statement that spoke out against transracial adoption and declared that Black children be raised in "black families where they belong physically, psychologically and culturally in order that they receive the total sense of themselves."[70] In addition to robbing children of Black culture, the NABSW maintained that white parents were ill equipped to pass on the skills necessary for navigating a racist society. When white lesbians worried about adding "yet another potential struggle for the child," they were also expressing insecurity about their ability to guide children of color through a racist society, children already made vulnerable to the homophobia that lesbians worried might be itself too great a weight for a child to bear. For some white women who knew their donors, raising a child of color was partially resolved by the donor's presence in their lives. This was the explanation from a white woman who ran a support group for lesbian mothers: her "Jewish-Latin" daughter knew her biological father, a gay man who was her mother's political comrade.[71] Still, how-to guides were more likely than not to express concerns about the inability of white lesbians to provide children of color with their own "culture."[72]

The position was not without critics. One how-to guide described an event at an International Women's Day celebration where a self-identified poor, Puerto Rican woman and her white middle-class lover challenged the wisdom that white women pursue white donors. The couple posited that arguments about culture were hypocritical due to the fact that many white lesbians already resided in "Third World neighborhoods." Furthermore, they predicted that as more and more lesbians pursued motherhood without the security afforded by a white patriarch, they would find themselves in the "same dead-end jobs and on the same welfare and unemployment lines with our Third World Sisters." Such commentary evidences how critiques of capitalism were at the forefront of some lesbian feminist analyses of race, gender, and family during this period. For this couple at least, white lesbians who failed to "face this contradiction" would continue to deny their common struggle with Third World people.[73]

Of course, not all lesbians hoping to become mothers brought such an explicit political analysis to the endeavor, and for women who planned to co-parent, the question of donor background often rested on familial desires that heterosexual would-be parents were rarely made to articulate. Couples who hoped to create "more than just the romantic bond between lovers" used donors who were also relatives so that "genes are kept in the family."[74] The slippage between "genes" and "family" expressed couples' desire to achieve the familial likeness that is imagined as stemming from shared genetics, proof that the child was the offspring of both parents.[75] But such desires expressed even more than this. Shared genetic material—the existence of blood relations—could make a family "real" where a "romantic bond between lovers" who could not procreate supposedly fell short.[76] For example, a *Newsweek* story reported that Bobbi and Lynn "solved the donor problem by recruiting Lynn's brother after deciding that Bobbi would carry the child." Lynn, who supported the family through her job as a postal worker, felt adamantly that she would never be able to have a baby, but was equally strong in her conviction that "I wanted my own blood."[77]

While such desires motivated women of all racial backgrounds, interracial couples like Bobbi and Lynn were more likely to receive commentary that amplified the supposed illegitimacy of their familial formations.[78] A family portrait taken on the cusp of the transition from the Emerson Street family portrait to the *New York Times* photo shows Bobbi, a Black woman, and Lynn, a white woman, jointly holding their baby girl. The accompanying caption reads *"Blood relations"* (emphasis in original), which suggests *Newsweek* either hoped to mock Lynn's claims to "her own blood" or gawk at the specter of interracial, lesbian sex—sex that could not biologically realize the fears of "miscegenation" but nevertheless threatened both the color line and the biological imperative that normalizes heterosexuality.

When the feature on Bobbi and Lynn was published, less than fifteen years had passed since the Supreme Court declared laws prohibiting interracial marriage unconstitutional, and any number of state sodomy laws could have deemed Bobbi and Lynn criminals for their same-sex relationship.[79] Having drawn readers' attention to such tropes, the caption then reestablished the superiority of white, heterosexual procreation within marriage: it read, "Bobbi, *her* baby, Lynn" (my emphasis), and with that singular pronoun the family portrait was made illegible.[80]

As women turned to relatives and friends for semen, they posed the most significant challenge to the medical establishment's strict protocols: using a "known donor." This decision produced the most debate—and anxiety—among women contemplating motherhood. As one woman who had decided to parent explained, "Once you've made the choice to have a child by artificial insemination, the next issue you have to decide is whether the donor is going to be anonymous or known. And that decision indicates all of the rest of the steps you need to take."[81] Indeed, lesbians pursued a variety of "steps" when it came to known donors. In contrast to Bobbi and Lynn, who hoped Lynn's brother would serve as a big brother to their daughter, other women pursued known donors so that they could eventually introduce their children to men some families called "donor friend," others simply "father."[82] A support group comprised of lesbians considering motherhood through known donors in Philadelphia, for example, decided that being able to provide their child with the identity of the donor was important. Charlotte, whose donor was a gay man named Vincent explained, "The child will know that Vincent is the father, and I trust him. . . . The reason I'm going with a known donor is I want to know what I'm getting and because I don't want to deprive the kid of knowing who the father is."[83]

In contrast, women who desired anonymity pursued arrangements that included various degrees of separation between the donor and the woman. The use of a "go-between" was the most common form of protection.[84] *Lesbian Tide* assured readers, "arranging security for your identities is difficult but not impossible. For instance, a friend could ask another friend unknown to the first friend."[85] Oftentimes, this "go-between" acted as both sperm collector and midwife, coordinating their own insemination service. An article detailing lesbian insemination in the Bay Area profiled one such woman, "Lily," who helped women get pregnant throughout the 1970s and

1980s. "Lily" was a midwife named Christmas Leubrie who sometimes inseminated women and attended births in the back of her 1963 VW bus.[86] Leubrie screened her donors for both health history and hobbies. Rather than pay her donors, she asked women to provide monthly gifts related to their donors' interests in order to "bring humanity" to the anonymous arrangement.[87] Other strategies were more expedient. One "East coast gay commune" hosted a party where "men ejaculate into clean jars, the jars are poured together, and women who want children use this mixture."[88] If this approach was not appealing, readers of *Lesbian Tide* might be able to procure anonymous sperm by contacting "Cheri Lesh through the TIDE office," who advertised her services in the magazine.[89] And once again, Maggie from *Conception Comix!* demystified these practices when she detailed the degrees of separation between herself, her midwife, sperm-runner no. 1 (Arena), and sperm-runner no. 2 (Wesley). Maggie explained to readers that "Wesley did not know who I was . . . so that the donor never came in contact with anyone who knew me . . . to avoid any possibility of future child custody suits!"[90]

Maggie's warning about custody suits was a major reason women chose an "unknown" donor. Even those who chose known donors believed that such a choice entailed risk. The woman in Philadelphia who planned for her chosen donor to be involved as a father acknowledged that "there's no protection, there's no legal protection. You just have to find somebody you think you can work out whatever problems arise with."[91] Women's fears stemmed from bearing witness to the onslaught of court rulings beginning in the late 1960s that denied lesbian mothers and gay fathers who had left heterosexual marriages custody of their children. Defense campaigns mobilized by those in the lesbian and gay rights movement on behalf of these parents were a critical piece of the work necessary for reversing judicial bias in some states by the mid-1980s. These political efforts and devastating court rulings circulated through gay and feminist publications, alerting lesbians who were not yet mothers that the state considered their sexuality to be at odds with "the best interests of the child."[92] A profile published in 1980 of a woman Leubrie assisted with insemination made this link explicitly: "In the reality of 1980 America there was a chance that 'they' would want to take Gaea's baby away. All over the country, the courts were trying to take lesbians' children away.

What would they do when they found out lesbians were getting pregnant on purpose? Gaea clenched her teeth. I'm not having this baby so it can be taken away, she said to herself."[93]

Reflecting on the early days of lesbian insemination in 1987, medical sociologist Petra Liljesfraund also highlighted this connection. "The experience of women with children from heterosexual marriages had a significant impact on how these lesbians chose to conceive their children. The fear of custody battles with fathers in a homophobic court system compelled many to choose anonymous donors."[94] Lesbians had taught one another how to seize the means of reproduction, but in order to be assured absolute control over their families, they would be need to wrest some form of recognition from the law.

LEGAL STRATEGIES, FEMINIST SPERM BANKS, AND LEGIBILITY

During these early years of self-insemination, lesbian feminist health activists and women hoping to become mothers developed AID protocols that fit a variety of needs and desires. But fear also loomed large and before too long cast doubt on the reliability of homegrown methods meant to provide protection from state intervention. In addition to ongoing reports of courts denying women access to their children, the practice of self-insemination was exposed by mainstream media at the end of the 1970s, making the question of anonymity even more pressing due to the anticipation of a potential backlash. Sensationalistic media coverage, an increasingly conservative political climate that explicitly targeted gays and lesbians, and the first custody case between a donor and a single woman further stoked concern. Lesbian rights attorneys soon brought their skills to bear on this new reproductive practice and the resulting queer kinship in an effort to identify a legal pathway to motherhood free of interference.

In 1978, an exposé written by undercover journalists posing as lesbians pursuing AID treatment announced the freakish and impossible: "He Makes Babies for Lesbians." The article reported on Dr. David Moss Sopher, a gynecologist in London who assisted lesbians in getting pregnant through artificial insemination.[95] Since 1971, the lesbian rights organization Sappho had been working with Dr. Sopher, sending women who sought their support to him for assistance in procuring semen. The exposure prompted demands from conservative lawmakers and physicians that the British Medical Association limit AID to married couples. In the face of this backlash, Dr. Sopher defended his decision by claiming that he was "not doing anything illegal. A lesbian who wants a baby badly enough could achieve the same result by entering a casual heterosexual relationship." Reinforcing the heterosexual-homosexual binary, Dr. Sopher claimed he was merely "preventing a situation which would be abhorrent to her and cutting down on the risks involved."[96]

Feminist and gay publications in the United States reported on the London controversy.[97] *The Advocate* ran a story about "the fuss" created by the exposé and informed readers that Sappho organizer Jackie Forester had "hoped that thousands of lesbian women would have had babies by AID before it was publicized, for fear that publicity might be followed with attempts to legislate the procedure."[98] *Lesbian Tide* ran an update that the publicity created by the "London baby scandal" had forced Dr. Sopher to stop serving lesbians.[99] These stories coincided with reports from mainstream media outlets in the United States about a court decision in New Jersey that awarded custody to a donor who helped a single woman get pregnant.[100] Physicians were asked for their views on the sudden visibility of single women and lesbians using AID. Dr. Jaroslav Marik reminded readers of the *New York Times* that not all women would be lucky enough to find physicians like Dr. Sopher. While Marik's medical clinic in Los Angeles had "no policy of refusing or accepting them," he emphasized that "we don't like it much."[101]

The British Medical Association ultimately advised doctors that it was ethical to assist lesbians with insemination. Still, *off our backs* was quick to connect the events in London with a New Jersey case that had struck at the heart of the public's disdain for lesbian insemination: "life without father."[102] The New Jersey court granted visitation rights to a sperm donor known to a single woman who had conceived a child through AID. In 1975, the man and woman began a relationship that she said was strictly platonic and casual and he said became romantic and serious. Potentially undermining his claims about romance was the fact that they visited a sperm bank together. When they were turned away, he offered to donate his sperm and she ended the relationship shortly after she became pregnant. She did not allow him to develop a relationship with the child; he subsequently brought suit for visitation rights.[103]

The ruling made clear the legal neglect of a single woman who chose to pursue motherhood outside of marriage *and* sex. The court reasoned: "If a woman conceives a child by intercourse, the 'donor' who is not married to the mother is no less a father than the man who is married to the mother. Likewise, if an unmarried woman conceives a child through artificial insemination from semen from a known man, that man cannot be considered to be less a father because he is not married to the woman."[104] Despite the fact that the woman had covered all costs of the pregnancy and delivery and fully intended to provide for the child on her own, the court reasoned that "there was no one else who was in a position to take upon himself the responsibilities of fatherhood when the child was conceived."[105]

In a section of *off our backs* mockingly titled "legal rights of unwed sperm," Fran Moira drew a through line between Supreme Court decisions in illegitimacy law meant to bolster the rights of nonmarital parents, the custody cases that followed lesbians' dissolution of heterosexual marriages, and the practice of self-insemination. The New Jersey case "carried the paternal rights of the unwed father one step further when it viewed the sperm donor in the same light as the unwed father." Moira made sure to relay the glib observation of an *off our backs*'s staffer that the donor "should be allowed to visit with his sperm any time he felt like it" before somberly warning readers that "it is fairly safe to speculate that if it [the state] could stop lesbians from conceiving and raising children it would." Moira's analysis reprised welfare rights activist and chairperson of the National Welfare Rights Organization Johnnie Tillmon's famous insight that receiving welfare benefits was like a "supersexist marriage" with the state, where women "trade in a man for *the* man," penned in *Ms. Magazine* a decade prior. Moira highlighted the New Jersey donor's battle for custody, reasoning that "it is also fairly safe to speculate that if it [the state] becomes aware of lesbians having and raising children independent of men, it will seek ways to limit such defiance of male control."[106]

Everywhere lesbians looked they could find reasons to believe Moira's predictions were more than "safe." Right-wing conservative leaders had mobilized a dedicated grassroots base by positioning feminism and gay liberation as threats to the nuclear family. Phyllis Schlafly's STOP ERA movement had literally stopped the Equal Rights Amendment in its tracks by 1975; the gay rights movement had lost out to Anita Bryant's Save Our Children coalition, an effort that successfully overturned a county-level anti-discrimination ordinance in Florida by arguing that "homosexuals cannot reproduce—so they must recruit . . . the youth of America"; and progressive movements more generally were on the defensive.[107] In 1979, conservative evangelical preacher Jerry Falwell founded the Moral Majority, helping to consolidate the anti-feminist, anti-gay backlash efforts that positioned feminists (all of whom were assumed to be lesbians) as the greatest threat to the family; he promised to enforce "God's law in the voting booth." In 1980, the religious right helped put Ronald Reagan in the White House.[108] While lesbian mothers' chances of winning custody battles were improving thanks to years of advocacy, such an outcome was far from guaranteed, especially when numerous states had yet to repeal sodomy laws that were used to criminalize gay men and lesbians.[109]

Women began searching for ways to back up anonymous donor arrangements with something more powerful than "go-betweens," and they turned to legal advocates for help. Donna Hitchens, founder of the legal aid organization Lesbian Rights Project (LRP) that cut its teeth representing women whose ex-husbands were trying to erode their ex-wives' custody rights, advised women and male donors to "put their intentions down in writing" prior to conception, even as she admitted that "we don't know for certain whether these contracts will stand up in court since they have not yet been tested."[110] This caveat was reprinted in other articles detailing the practice of self-insemination as a warning to women considering known donors. *The Advocate* alerted readers in 1981, "If you can find a friend who will locate a sperm donor for you, you may be able to preserve your anonymity and thus avoid a future fight over the custody of the child. If he's not anonymous get a written contract detailing custody and visiting rights (if any)."[111] Women who persisted in using known donors confronted what may have been a changing tide. In 1983, Jennifer, new mother to Toby, reported, "our friends told us we were crazy to know the donor. There are all sorts of horror stories about custody battles and fathers who suddenly started demanding more and more time with the baby."[112]

Whether or not "all sorts of horror stories" were actually piling up, the fear they incited was real, and LRP's legal scrutiny of grassroots methods made some kind of formal protection all the more desirable to women considering parenthood. Over the previous five years, the LRP had been contacted by more women seeking legal advice on donor insemination, prompting Hitchens to author a guidance document on AID. The pamphlet was intended to "alert women to potential legal problems that can be avoided through careful planning," and it evaluated existing community practices. A known donor granted women greater control over selection and the possibility of a relationship, but made her vulnerable to the donor developing "paternalistic" feelings that could lead to legal action. Hitchens reported that there were "a number of cases where donors originally claimed they wanted no rights or responsibilities" but later began making demands. Known donors, therefore, posed the greatest risk. The method of mixing sperm from several known donors might prevent such feelings, but Hitchens warned that a new "blood test, called an HLA test," could be used to determine paternity. Using an unknown donor provided a greater degree of anonymity than mixing, as long as the go-between could be trusted, and, perhaps more importantly, was not subpoenaed.[113] Hitchens and the LRP distributed their findings, including at the conference "Lesbians Choosing Motherhood" that was attended by at least 300 women "very anxious to get the information."[114]

Hitchens noted that the women who sought advice from the LRP did so during all phases of the process—prior to insemination, during pregnancy, and after the birth of the child. But they all came with the same worry. "The major concern, of course, is whether a donor will be recognized as the father of the child."[115] Hitchens acknowledged that women were in unchartered legal territory. She told one reporter, "I can read California statutes out of my ears, and none of them will address the questions."[116] But, as LRP staff attorney Roberta Achtenberg told attendees at yet another workshop for lesbians considering motherhood, held in New York City, there did exist a "small sometimes helpful piece of legislation" that comprised "the legal backbone" of the country's existing statutes on artificial insemination.[117] Nearly twenty years after Finegold expressed his hopes that acceptance of AID could be hastened through legislation, only nine states had adopted the UPA, and none of them explicitly addressed the growing practice among lesbians.[118] Still, the LRP took note that when California adopted the UPA in 1975, section b, which nullified a donor's rights to any child conceived through AID as long as a physician oversaw the donation, did not require the woman to be married.[119]

Hitchens and the LRP culled two possible strategies from the UPA. For states where providing semen to a physician nullified the rights of the donor, women wishing to use a known donor might be able to "achieve the benefits of using a known donor without encountering the weaknesses, if a woman can find a doctor who will assist her."[120] The second strategy offered, in Hitchens's estimation, "the best security against any legal problems in the future," but that meant returning donor choice to the physician. "Almost all states have doctors or medical clinics that will arrange AID. The woman is never told who the donor was and the donor is never told who received his semen. There is total anonymity." Hitchens was clear about the weaknesses that accompanied this experimental solution. Even if a woman could find a supportive doctor, the fees would make treatment cost prohibitive for many women.[121] And overcoming these barriers could not guarantee that a court would interpret the statute according to LRP's legal reasoning. Still, the UPA offered a potential route to making lesbian motherhood legible. The medical authority once used to block the route to family making from single women and lesbians now emerged as these women's best hope for making families of their own.

California's family code, and the LRP's strategy, helped make the first sperm bank dedicated to serving lesbian and single women a reality in 1982.[122] The Oakland Feminist Women's Health Center, a family planning clinic, announced that it would begin offering insemination services, complete with semen provision. Barb Raboy, a staff member at the center, was largely responsible for learning the techniques of cryopreservation so that the center could have its own donations on site, as opposed to feminist health clinics that had offered the service earlier but were reliant on outside sperm banks or physicians to supply semen for their clients.[123] The *Los Angeles Times* announced the opening of the sperm bank by declaring, "Feminist Have Own Sperm Banks: They Service Women Who Want Children, Not Husbands."[124] At the opening ceremony the director,

Laura Brown, announced that her infant daughter was a result of the clinic's anonymous donor program, which had been running informally prior to the establishment of the sperm bank.[125] She also told reporters, "It's not up to us to decide who can and can't have children. . . . Lesbians, single women, and women with infertile partners are encouraged to participate."[126] The feminist-run sperm bank consulted with attorney Karen Ryer in order to craft contracts all donors were required to sign. The contract stated: "I understand that I have no legal rights or obligations to the afterborn child pursuant to Civil Code 7005 (b)." What made this contract different from the contracts created between women and known donors, or between anonymous donors and the go-betweens that collected their sperm, was the signature that followed the donor's. All contracts were signed by the physician representing the sperm bank.[127]

Cautiously optimistic experimentation with the UPA solidified into best practice when the LRP's repeated warnings that lesbians "who inseminate themselves at home are legally at risk if the donor, through a paternity action, demands custody or visitation rights to the child" were realized.[128] Two years before the sperm bank opened its doors, the LRP took the first case of a lesbian whose donor sued for paternity, seeking visitation rights. In 1979, friends Mary K. and Victoria T. decided they wanted to co-parent a child together. Jhordan C. agreed to provide sperm for Mary K's insemination. The women wished to protect their privacy rather than involve a physician, and performed the insemination at home, with Jhordan C. acting as a known donor. The women had no intention of involving Jhordan C. in their son's upbringing, but the donor claimed a verbal agreement allowed for his involvement. A California court, citing the state's UPA, ultimately awarded Jhordan C. paternity because the arrangement lacked physician oversight.[129] Achtenberg explained,

> We took a case in Sonoma County for a lesbian couple that didn't know California has a statute governing artificial insemination. They also didn't know that if she didn't use a licensed physician to receive the semen from the donor, she didn't effectively cut off his legal rights to the child. They had only an oral agreement, they didn't use a doctor, they didn't have a contract and when the child was born, the donor sued to be declared the father. Now she has to parent a child with a man who's a virtual stranger to her.[130]

With evidence that at least two courts would defer to the UPA to resolve lesbian mothers' custody rights, the LRP's legal strategy of going through a physician gained steam throughout the rest of the decade.[131]

"THE LESBIAN" IS ALWAYS "A SINGLE" (OR, WHEN THE BULLDAGGER IS THE WELFARE QUEEN)

When commenting on *Jhordan C. v. Mary K.* in print, the LRP emphasized the liberal goal of inclusion that would "get the courts to see that gays and lesbians can be as good a parent as straight people." But the organization was well aware that the case concerned more than Mary K.'s same-sex sexuality. Echoing their feminist forebearers who criticized Harry Krause's fixation on paternity, the LRP argued that the state's physician requirement infringed upon an unmarried woman's right to procreative choice and family autonomy.[132] This argument did not sway a judge reportedly obsessed with securing paternity so as to avoid sticking "that label on him [the child]."[133] The judge was distraught over Mary K.'s membership in another category long associated with "'nonnormative' procreation patterns and family structures": single mothers.[134]

Mary K.'s dual status was not lost on media dedicated to exposing the fact that AID had escaped the bounds of marriage and was supposedly driving up rates of single motherhood.[135] The *Chicago Tribune* broke "unmarried applicants" into three categories: "the career woman, the disturbed women, and the lesbian." According to the article, the lesbian's motivations for insemination set her apart from other single women in her desire to dispense utterly and completely with men. "AID appeals to the homosexual woman because there is no known father to challenge her fitness in a custody battle."[136] But although receiving the nastiest evaluation, she was subsumed under the category of single parent, rather than being placed outside of it. Even friendlier profiles of lesbians pursuing parenthood also emphasized lesbians' inherently single status. The profile on "Toby's mothers" made sure to point out that in spite of the women's plans to co-parent, "Jennifer technically falls into another category—single parent."[137]

The judge presiding over Mary K.'s case was not the only one alarmed by what label would adhere to children born to single women using AID. A major profile on the emerging reproductive technologies published in the *New York Times* asked, "And how will the single women, the 1,500 of them who have babies through artificial insemination every year, explain it to those children?"[138] A medical ethicist quoted in a *Boston Globe* article profiling the rise of insemination among single women put the passive aggressive question more plainly: "It is complicated legally because it has some of the complications of illegitimacy . . . going through a doctor . . . gives the child a certain status. In the case of a single woman, it's lacking, and if the woman does it herself it's especially lacking."[139] Leonard Loeb, chairman of the American Bar Association's family section, concurred. Loeb claimed that a woman who "inseminates herself" might successfully get pregnant, but he cast doubt on what significance such a fact held for her and the child. Likening the act to "a marriage without a clergyman or a judge," Loeb argued, "You must have someone authorized to give it sanctity."[140]

Those "authorized to give it sanctity" also worried as more and more unmarried women pursued insemination. One medical article that conveniently obscured physicians' historical role in dictating the "social values" attached to AID wrote that "when social values are in a process of change, physicians can be presented with management decisions that go beyond their routine practice and training. An example is artificial insemination by donor (AID) for single women . . . whether heterosexual or lesbian." After a review of the literature finding no negative psychological effects of raising children in families without fathers and/or in homes headed by lesbians, the authors ultimately decided that "it is ethically permissible to carry out AID for the single woman in selected cases but not . . . obligatory to do so. A physician has a right to refuse to fulfill a single woman's request for AID."[141] Other physicians also advocated for preserving "the practitioner's judgment" in deciding whether or not to provide treatment, and a year into operation the feminist sperm bank in Oakland was distressed by the scale at which "health professionals absolutely refuse to inseminate unmarried/lesbian women."[142]

Sometimes even "the practitioner's judgment" was not enough, even if supportive, even if women could afford treatment, and especially if a "single" lesbian was in an interracial relationship and hoping to have a child. The case of a couple who sought AID through one of the women's primary care doctor suggests why medical authority was a solution primarily beneficial to single women whose "queer" reproduction most approximated the prescribed norm: heterosexual white mothers bearing white children. While the physician in this case was supportive and assisted the patient in "undergoing AID with the semen of an anonymous donor of the same race as her partner," when the hospital staff and then the local press found out, the couple and the physician were overwhelmed by negative publicity. The physician assessed the implications of both the "ethical aspects of homo-sexuality" and the "ethical aspects of the interracial relationship" in a sub-sequent article, explaining that "the present case ... shocked some who learned of it" because "the couple involved not only were homosexual but also were of different races." Following the negative publicity that deemed their nascent family illegitimate on multiple grounds, the couple ceased requesting AID, at least from this particular physician.[143]

Single women's "nonnormative procreation" was also vulnerable to more official forms of interference when they failed to keep parenting a private cost. In 1983, the *Hastings Center Report* discussed the case of Teresa, who Dr. Franklin inseminated. When single women approached Dr. Franklin to request AID, he interviewed them twice to determine if they were suitable, "medically and psychologically." Once Teresa became pregnant, Dr. Franklin came under fire after the press reported that Teresa was receiving pregnancy benefits and planned to file for AFDC after the child was born. Dr. Franklin never asked for detailed financial informa-tion, but Teresa's situation made him realize that he also did not "want to deliberately tax the system."[144] That same year, *off our backs* reported on a case of a single woman in Milwaukee who, becoming pregnant through insemination, began receiving welfare payments after the baby was born. The state legislature passed a bill that made inseminating a woman who was on welfare or who might become eligible for welfare medical malprac-tice. The governor ultimately vetoed the bill.[145]

While it is not clear whether the women in these cases were *lesbian* single women, the archival record bears out what Cathy Cohen argued in her 1997 groundbreaking essay on intersectional, queer, coalitional poli-tics: whether heterosexual or lesbian, as far as the state is concerned a single mother, particularly one who is poor, Black, and on welfare, is already "queer" due to her "nonnormative procreation patterns."[146] Cohen's article is instructive for understanding that lesbianism was not the sole, maybe not even the primary, "deviance" operating in the aforementioned cases, even if they have typically been framed as such. Most scholars discuss the first custody battles involving lesbians as evidence of homophobic laws unwilling to recognize gay parenthood.[147] Missing from these analyses is what first prompted such a family's contact with the state: when a lesbian mother violated procreative norms of keeping the costs of childrearing a private affair by applying for welfare aid. The first case to grant visitation rights to a former partner and co-parent began when Bobbi and Lynn split up, leaving Bobbi and their daughter with no economic support. When Bobbi applied for AFDC, she was approached by county investigators wanting to know why "the father wasn't paying child support." According to Bobbi's attorney, she explained "there is no daddy—here's the turkey baster," but also identified Lynn to the deputy district attorney. who promptly filed suit for child support. A judge issued Lynn a decree requiring her to pay 100 dollars a month in support on "the same forms usually used for errant fathers." Lynn used the order of support to bolster her suit for visitation rights, a demand Bobbi strongly resisted due to fears Lynn would take the child to her family in Louisiana. Whereas the family portrait printed in 1979 mocked their interracial, queer family, in 1983 the same photo was re-captioned to reflect Lynn's new legally sanctioned status as provider—she is listed as "Father" while Bobbi's motherhood is merely implied. While legal documents did not make explicit reference to either woman's race, it is likely that Lynn's whiteness and class standing further bolstered her role as proper provider in the eyes of the judge— particularly when cast against Bobbi's status as a Black mother receiving welfare aid. Despite Bobbi's fears that Lynn's involvement could result in their child being taken across the country, the judge identified with Lynn's custodial desires, concluding that "simply because there is no specific statue or case that covers the situation, it doesn't follow that there isn't a right that can be asserted by Miss Loftin."[148]

While Bobbi and Lynn's circumstances certainly foreshadowed custody issues that would increase as lesbian couples and co-parents broke up, forcing courts to reckon with same-sex parenting, they also evidenced the legal neglect of lesbian motherhood. The same neglect was at work in the case of Mary K., which was just as much a cautionary tale of state paternalism as it was a tale of the overzealous donor. Mary K. and Jhordan C.'s arrangement was discovered by Sonoma County authorities when Mary K. went on welfare following the child's birth, thereby signaling to authorities her failure to provide for her family through private means. Local officials demanded the name of the child's father, and sued Jhordan C. for child support in order to reimburse the county for Mary K.'s welfare payments. Jhordan C. agreed to pay, was awarded a judgment of paternity, and renewed his ultimately successful motion for visitation rights.[149] While both individual women's pleas and the LRP's legal guidance emphasized the threat of "a man's" potential for paternalism, lesbians' status as single mothers reveal Tillmon's key insight about paternity's integral relationship to "*the* man," specifically the history of a welfare state built on the utter refusal to regard mothering as work or recognize mothers as rightful heads of households—even after the end of illegitimacy. The feminist legal scholars who accused Krause's UPA of trading in marital status for paternity would no doubt have been nonplussed by the legal issues arising from lesbian insemination.[150] "Pregnancy without men" might have been "as easy as 1-2-3," but the legal neglect lesbian mothers confronted in the decades after paternity took the place of marriage would prove more difficult to overcome. In its newsletter to supporters, the LRP declared the historic case a mix of victory and defeat. Mary K. and Victoria T. would have to raise their son with a man they claimed was never meant to have a role beyond donor. But the decision also confirmed legal advocates' bet on the UPA.[151] The LRP assured women that the right to create family anew had been affirmed, with the caveat that they "comply with certain legal requirements. Privacy, procreative choice and family autonomy are alive and well."[152] The legal reach of both "a man" and "the man" could be successfully warded off by yet another "man"—physician authority. Sperm banks and private physicians emerged as the most secure route to delivering single women reproductive choice, where choice held not just the infinite possibilities contained in a donor catalog, but the privacy from state interference afforded the liberal, self-reliant individual.

CONCLUSION

In a 1975 issue of *Quest*, attorneys Nan Hunter and Nancy Polikoff analyzed defense campaigns for lesbian mothers who had been denied custody of children conceived in heterosexual marriages. Their piece promised to assess the "host of tricky political and legal issues" raised in litigating lesbian mother custody cases, but first made sure to cast these women's lot with the "millions of women other than lesbian mothers—welfare mothers, incarcerated mothers, politically radical mothers, heterosexual mothers who are not married to their partners, or simply mothers with jobs outside their homes who also face a daily threat of losing custody of their children." In an analysis that partially anticipated Cohen's coalitional politics based on "one's relation to power," Hunter and Polikoff saw lesbian mothers' "strongest political bond" in "other independent mothers, regardless of sexual preference."[153]

Polikoff and Hunter no doubt understood that the lesbian mother was very often these other mothers, too, a likelihood that only increased as lesbians intentionally built families on their own terms. Almost as quickly as lesbian health activists popularized AID, however, women began searching for ways to neutralize the negative impacts of their "independence" in the face of legal neglect. But some liabilities were more easily mitigated than others. The do-it-yourself strategies developed to make conception a reality in all lesbians' lives who wanted it contrasted sharply with the legal strategies developed in hopes of making that choice legible to the law. Rerouting "woman-controlled conception" through medical and legal structures designed to establish paternity most benefited "independent mothers" whose queer reproduction was the least so: middle-class, responsible providers; white women who birthed white children; and women who ceded their reproductive decision-making to medical authority. For these families, the legal neglect produced by illegibility might successfully be replaced with "privacy and autonomy."

In the 1997 preface to her already classic ethnography, *Families We Choose*, Kath Weston reflected on the full-fledged "gayby boom" and warned that it would be a "mistake" to conclude that such families were "*freely* chosen."[154] This statement is as true for well-resourced, legally savvy, and, with the legalization of gay marriage, married queers who can more readily access formal recognition as for those who cannot, though the costs of choosing from within "the state's long-established practice of wielding the marital family ideal as a coercive tool" are not equally shared.[155] While the fertility industry has capitalized on the vision first conceived by feminists who started the sperm bank in Oakland, legal advocates estimate that informal insemination arrangements still comprise nearly half of all LGBTQ families' journeys to parenthood. Many of these families use known donors without physician oversight, and are more likely to be low-income and nonwhite, factors that compound the likelihood of such families being deemed illegitimate.[156] Some of these families pursue such arrangements precisely because they are "not mediated through doctors, nurses, tests, and sterile instruments."[157] Regardless of the motivating factors, families formed through these unsanctioned circumstances are more vulnerable to state interference than their legally recognized counterparts when relationships end, when state aid becomes necessary, or when interracial families garner skepticism and scrutiny. And while gay marriage has saved the lesbian from perpetual singledom, unmarried women—whether coupled or not—in more than half the country's states must still contend with laws that nullify donors' parental rights only when the woman undergoing AID is married.[158] In short, many families continue to parent in the shadow of "patriarchal laws" that render them illegible and vulnerable to state interference as a result.

Lesbian-headed families that emerged in the space between the Emerson Street household portrait and the *New York Times* announcement of lesbian motherhood's arrival confronted legal neglect that challenged their claim to "independent" motherhood. Their struggles against the medical institutions, welfare offices, and laws determined to preserve the white, patriarchal, self-reliant household even after illegitimacy's end were joined by other families' labor in the face of new impediments to family making. Changes to the administration of punishment through sentencing policy and imprisonment wreaked havoc on the "independent" mothers Polikoff and Hunter instructed free lesbians to align themselves with: incarcerated mothers. Mass incarceration would also remake family and its labors while producing numerous costs as the twentieth century came to a close.

2 The Labor of Captivity

INCARCERATED MOTHERS AND THEIR CHILDREN

> An integral part of serving the families of imprisoned
> mothers was locating and placing children with foster par-
> ents who were supportive of the mother/child relationship.
> This was not a simple task, as local social service agencies
> held the view that incarceration, per se, suggested unfitness
> as a mother.
>
> Prison MATCH/Pleasanton Children's Center Advisory Board
> report, early 1980s

> While in the California Institute for Women, we have seen
> individual cases in which hundreds of collective children
> are taken away from their imprisoned mothers and given to
> the courts, to adoption agencies, or to foster homes.
>
> "Sometimes I Feel Like a Motherless Child," *The Clarion*, 1974

In the early evening of December 16, 1975, during dinner hour at the California Institution for Women (CIW), incarcerated women used rags to ignite a fire in Wilson A Cottage, then gathered the decorations meant to bring Christmas cheer to the otherwise sterile TV room and headed to the administration building. There, they lit the decorations on fire inside of a trash can and hurled the flaming can through Superintendent Brook Carey's office window, scattering broken glass, two Christmas trees, and charred decorations as they moved, according to Carey, "en masse, scream-ing and yelling, from one building to another." While CIW firefighters attempted to keep Wilson A Cottage from burning, dousing women in fire extinguisher fluid in the process, Lieutenant Wolters sent Sergeant Martina to guard the armory and issued "chemical agents" to the other correctional officers defending the rest of the administration building. The officers exhausted their tear gas supply in less than ten minutes, but were quickly supplied with aid from neighboring men's prisons, whose superintendents sent staff, guns, and gas to CIW.[1] Officers of the San Bernardino County Sheriff's department dispatched units to the perimeter of CIW and lent their helicopter so that the entire grounds were illuminated by a circling searchlight. With the prison secured, the mix of state and county officers turned to "the apprehension of the roaming and marauding inmates." The nearly 500 women who participated in the riot did not heed repeated orders that they "lock up," instead brandishing glass and bricks against prison staff. It was not until officers raised their twelve-gauge shotguns to fire warning shots into the air, sending women to their units, that staff declared the situation "clear." By then it was nearly three o'clock in the morning.[2]

In her report to Director of the California Department of Corrections (CDC) J. J. Enomoto, Superintendent Carey seemed to take comfort that the protest was not "a pre-planned course of action on the part of the inmates, but rather a spontaneous release of hostility resulting from the Administration's decision to rescind the privilege of allowing any more outside visitors to come in and bring food for Christmas parties." On the night of the riot, officers had informed the Women's Advisory Council that remaining holiday parties would be closed to visitors due to concerns about security and the possibility of escape risks. The riot, even when filtered through numerous correctional officer reports, make clear that while the "release of hostility" may have been "spontaneous," it stemmed from an accumulation of insults. In addition to keeping women's loved ones away during the holidays, one woman mentioned that they had also been barred from using the telephone, prompting her to threaten, "we'll show you what we can do."[3] The women's rage was driven as much by the punitive removal of so-called privileges as by the neglectful response to their concerns. When Sergeant Searcy tried to quell the protests by telling the women they had made their point and so should return to their cottages, they reportedly responded, "Why should we? You mother fuckers always say, yeah we'll take care of it, but you fuckers never do anything, so we are not locking up."[4] Another woman echoed her peers' sense of desperation and determination. "Kill me, but I won't stop or go to my cottage."[5]

In response to the riot, CIW officials made good on a plan to turn Harrison Cottage into an Alternative Program Unit (APU). Staff felt that they needed to be able to "separate from the general prison population certain women who cause serious problems within the institution," a need made clearer by the riot "which occurred at CIW several months ago."[6] Firsthand accounts from women who had been sent to the APU prompted community concern from outside groups like the State Bar Committee on Corrections and the San Francisco Bay Area-based Women's Prison Coalition, which charged that the incarcerated women assigned to the APU would undergo inhumane behavior modification treatment. CDC director Enomoto deflected these accusations by stating that the APU was still in the proposal phase. As evidence, he included a draft proposal which explained that "there should be no denial of routine opportunities and privileges which can then be earned back by good behavior; rather loss of privileges should be connected to misbehavior."[7] Representatives for the prison assured inquiring state officials that the APU would include "recreation, entertainment, schooling, and other activities," while conceding that there would "be limitation on movement."[8] And Enomoto assured advocates that CIW staff would "achieve a correctional system that is increasingly humane, fair and safe."[9]

The Christmas riot at CIW and the subsequent APU debate provide a window into anti-prison organizing on the threshold of mass incarceration: incarcerated people, supported by progressive social movements, were rebelling against the punishment, neglect, and legacy of rehabilitation that defined captivity in the United States.[10] For incarcerated people everywhere, conditions of confinement entailed a variety of inhumane horrors, sometimes carried out under the cover of "treatment" like the "alternative programming" promised by CIW staff. Such initiatives laid bare critiques of rehabilitation that remain relevant today—treatment regimens administered by the same institution that imprisons human beings as its primary objective could only ever offer truly grotesque contradictions in terms (such as placing trans, queer, and gender-nonconforming incarcerated people in solitary confinement, ostensibly for their own protection). Furthermore, invocations of treatment presumed that incarcerated people themselves—rather than the traumatic and inhumane conditions that characterize incarceration—represented some kind of deviation in need of fixing.[11] By the time the APU was pursued at CIW, an institution that disguised cages as "cottages" in a campus-like environment, prison uprisings had convinced much of the public that the so-called treatment principle was bankrupt. The idea that criminality could be cured through rehabilitation was repeatedly rejected by liberals and progressives alike In a landmark 1971 report, the American Friends Service Committee (AFSC) charged that "the punitive spirit" of incarceration "survived unscathed behind the mask of treatment."[12] The AFSC and others especially took aim at one manifestation of the treatment principle: indeterminate sentencing.[13] Critics charged that when judges and parole boards operated on the mandate to account for the whole individual, not just her crimes, arbiters' prejudices as to who could be rehabilitated resulted in discriminatory sentencing.[14] This critical shift in the perception of prisons forced open the question of what incarceration should become. When Enomoto wrote of an "increasingly humane, fair, and safe" system, then, he was describing one possible *future* rather than the continuation of a successful legacy.[15]

By now, most of the world knows what direction incarceration in the United States took instead, at least in broad strokes. The 1970s law and order campaign struck a death knell to even the "mask" of rehabilitation and in its place a new model took hold: "incapacitation" on a massive scale.[16] This development produced a situation in which the United States imprisons more people per capita than any other nation, housing nearly a quarter of the entire world's prison population.[17] Often described as a "punitive turn" in the administration of prisons, tougher sentencing laws, expanded prosecutorial powers, massive investment in prison construction, and an unprecedented use of solitary confinement characterize mass incarceration in the United States. Between 1973 (two years before the riot at CIW) and 2008, the American imprisonment rate grew fivefold, with the number of women incarcerated in state prisons doubling the pace of growth for incarcerated men.[18]

Growing awareness of mass incarceration in recent years has ensured many Americans are familiar with this narrative. But additional work on incarceration illustrates how one "of the most volatile points of contact between state violence and one's body is the domain of gender," an insight that has yet to achieve the same level of public recognition.[19] Nonetheless, scholars and activists helping to advance this urgent argument have shown how such a statement holds true both before and after the "punitive turn." Sexual violence, sometimes lethal conditions of labor exploitation, psychological torture through forced drugging, discrimination in sentencing and parole, reproductive violence in the form of shackling during childbirth and forced sterilization as well as abysmal healthcare, and the violence of putting incarcerated people in prisons according to their assigned sex at birth (as well as the violence that follows such misplacement) comprise just some of the punishments carried out in the domain of gender as it intersects with white supremacy and capitalism.[20] Scholars have also refuted claims that the criminal justice system is meant to protect from harm the women it so frequently punishes: those who are Black, Latina, Indigenous, poor, immigrant, and do not meet normative expectations of gender and sexuality.[21]

But on the eve of December 16, 1975, the "punitive turn" towards "warehousing" was not yet a foregone conclusion, and women incarcerated at CIW were protesting not just explicit punishment (revoking of privileges, tear gas, shotguns) or the inherent contradictions of treatment (Christmas parties in cage-cottages, "alternative programming"), but also a third, fundamental feature of incarceration: carceral neglect ("you fuckers never do anything").[22] For incarcerated women, neglect—whether through willful failure, indifference, or policy gaps—especially imperiled their caretaking responsibilities and desires. The barring of visitors at Christmas represents how familial ties were necessarily severed by the fact of incarceration, but this punishment went hand in hand with neglect that meant such ties were often permanently extinguished. A social worker might use the cancelled visit as proof of a woman's lack of investment in her child's welfare, for example. The utter failure or refusal to acknowledge the legal significance of such a visit was only the tip of the iceberg. For women taking care of children prior to incarceration, the inability to regularly communicate and visit with their children, much less ensure the legal status of their custody, was due to total neglect of their familial desires and obligations.

Such neglect extended beyond familial ties that had existed before a women's sentence. When Barbara Cardell gave birth to a baby boy eight days after the CIW uprising, the infant was promptly placed in foster care, despite Cardell's objections.[23] Superintendent Carey used the neglectful conditions at CIW to justify the punishment of taking away Cardell's child, explaining that *"CIW does not have the necessary facilities* to provide a proper home."[24] Neglect also brought other forms of devastation to women's lives while confined to prison. When Annette Harris began experiencing vaginal bleeding in the fourth month of her pregnancy, CIW staff ignored her condition for three months until she was rushed to the hospital because her severe abdominal pain had induced vomiting. She gave birth to her son in the ambulance, and he died two hours later.[25]

Women's reproductive labors challenged Superintendent Carey's claim that a prison could not be a "proper home," [26] and together with advocates on the outside, incarcerated women attempted to force corrections to account for the family making that was a fundamental aspect of their lives. The majority of incarcerated women were primary caretakers of small children prior to their criminalization—this reality did not vanish just because families were separated by prison walls. Similarly, women who entered prisons pregnant had distinct medical and legal needs. Women asserted that the loss of their children, whether to the foster care system, to death as a result of medical neglect, or to the distance imposed by the loss of liberty, were egregious violations of their rights and humanity. They argued that their status as prisoners did not preclude the prison from making it possible to continue their role as mothers. Incarcerated women fought to keep their families together in the face of carceral neglect. As women and their children were separated by incarceration in the final decades of twentieth century, the attempts by families and their advocates to restore familial ties forced prison authorities to confront incarcerated women's family making. The ensuing battles and their outcomes evidence how mass incarceration produced new forms of reproductive labor as families fought to remain intact in the face of state punishment and neglect.

Neglect proved a formidable challenge. Incarcerated women and their advocates worked hard to force prison authorities to meet their reproductive needs and desires, thereby dramatically expanding the reproductive labors involved in family making. Those committed to bolstering incarcerated women's ability to have and raise children confronted political hurdles specific to the moment and structural hurdles inherent to neglect. Even though the liberal consensus of the early 1970s held that prisons were not sites of successful rehabilitation, the rhetoric of treatment did not disappear overnight. Women and their advocates got caught between the last vestiges of rehabilitation's political currency—already rife with contradiction—and the unforgiving ascendance of "get tough" logics. Navigating this fraught and shifting terrain meant drawing on political arguments that women only ever had a tenuous hold on, at best.

This precarity also defined the infrastructures, however temporary and imperfect, incarcerated women and advocates built by using such arguments to their advantage. Near-herculean efforts were necessary to make even the barest forms of parenting possible from behind bars. Simply allowing women to see their children once a month in a child-friendly space required an enormous amount of labor by mothers, outside advocates, foster parents, and social workers. Furthermore, such labor hinged precariously upon prison staff participation. Should just one prison official slide back into neglect, the tenuous arrangements built to foster women's intimate ties inside penal institutions would come crashing down. The inherent vulnerability of such arrangements laid bare the destructive force neglect could have on families impacted by incarceration. Prison officials did not need to use violence, the torture of behavior modification, or sexual assault to further erode both their own and incarcerated women's humanity. They could simply not act—refuse the labor critical to family making—and thus bring devastation to women's intimate lives.

FROM MATERNAL "DISTORTIONS" TO MOTHER-RELEASE PROGRAMS

When a group of Bay Area women working in various aspects of the criminal justice system came together to study jail alternatives for women arrested in San Francisco in the mid-1970s, they realized that no one had tracked what happened to women following arrest. Their effort to remedy this gap resulted in "a year-long study . . . one of the first of its kind about women and jail." For the year between 1977 and 1978, they found that the majority of those arrested were young, unemployed, undereducated, and

likely to have been charged with committing victimless crimes like prostitution and public inebriation. Black women were arrested in greater numbers than their white counterparts, just as they were more likely to serve
time in jail. And over a quarter of the women were the primary caretakers
of small children at the time of their arrest. The report emphasized wom-
en's circumstances prior to arrest. The vast majority of women working in
the city were employed, but concentrated in the low end of the "occupa-
tional hierarchy." The report estimated that at least a fifth of the city's families were headed by single women and were most likely "working to stay at
the poverty level." The research team aimed to convince readers that wom-
en's use of "lucrative, though not legal methods, of supporting themselves
and their children" stemmed from necessity rather than innate drivers.
"Traditionally, people seeking to explain the criminal activity of women
have looked for biological and/or psychological reasons . . . little attention
has been paid to the ways in which various other factors, such as local economic conditions, educational and vocational opportunities . . . might
influence women's behavior."[27]

The authors of the San Francisco report were far from alone in their
efforts to elevate and address the problems faced by incarcerated women.
Beginning in the 1970s, newfound attention to the plight of women in
jails and prisons came from radical social movements, women entering the
legal profession and law enforcement in greater numbers, liberal feminists
in the National Organization for Women (NOW), and state-level women's
commissions.[28] While these politically diverse groups parted ways when it
came to solutions, they nevertheless emphasized the structural factors that
drove women to crime. The coalition of activists that organized the defense
campaign for Joan Little, a poor, Black women incarcerated in a North
Carolina jail whose ultimate acquittal saved her from the death penalty,
not only framed Little's case as an act of self-defense against rape by a
white prison guard but also argued that her situation was a product of
"prison conditions for women, including misuse of prison guard authority
to obtain sexual gains; the discriminatory use of the death penalty against
poor people and blacks; and the selection processes which fail to produce
juries of true peers."[29] A far narrower and more economic-focused analysis
was offered by the liberal founders of the National Resource Center on the
Female Offender to explain how women ended up in prison: "The average

woman in prison . . . is typically poor, has little education . . . and few mar-
ketable skills."[30] And in hearings on women and crime organized by the
District of Columbia's Commission on the Status of Women, testimony
highlighted the racism of a criminal justice system that tended "to favor
the white middle class," resulting in a disproportionate number of Black
women in the DC Women's Detention center.[31]

These structural critiques of the criminal justice system depict women
as victims of racism, misogyny, poverty, and violence—both prior to and
during their incarceration. Many—though certainly not all—advocates
hoped that by emphasizing the conditions that drove women to illegal
activity, correctional officials would be convinced that alternatives to prisons (rather than prisons themselves) were the solution to the problem of
so-called female criminality. However, the political aim of amplifying
incarcerated women's plight collided with the dearth of research on wom-
en's experiences in the criminal justice system. When the New York-based
Women's Prison Association (WPA) titled its 1972 report on incarcerated
women "A Study in Neglect," they captured the same sentiment that drove
the women's jail study group in San Francisco to subject the jail to a gendered analysis. In regard to "information on female offenders," the WPA
asked, "Who are they? What crimes do they commit? What happens to
them in court and in prison? And what happens to them when they are
released? It is difficult to find answers for even these relatively simple
questions. Literature on women prisoners is scarce." The WPA laid responsibility for this neglect and lack of information at the feet of "male officials
in the criminal justice system," many of whom deemed the problems of
incarcerated women to be "insignificant."[32]

While many advocates did pursue their own research, they also drew on
what few studies on incarcerated women already existed in order to support their demands for alternatives. Those who were especially concerned
about women's caretaking responsibilities marshalled sociological studies
of mothers incarcerated at the same institution where a decade later
women would demand access to their loved ones: the California Institute
for Women, a prison located in Riverside County, forty-five minutes east
of Los Angeles. Advocates both inherited and built upon the legacy of
rehabilitation that had obscured the punishment and neglect integral to
imprisonment. Contending that prisons and jails were incapable of

administering any meaningful treatment, reformers proposed alternative programs dedicated to fostering women's familial ties, in the hope that such measures would keep women out of prison upon release. Here, advocates walked a fine line between reasoning with what the San Francisco report described as the "too large and arbitrary machine" and getting ensnared in its logics.[33] On the one hand, those hoping to make the gendered vulnerabilities of incarceration more visible succeeded in moving the criminological literature away from pathologizing psychological analyses and towards the consideration of constraints that were not of women's own making. On the other hand, they also placed faith in rehabilitation just as the political mandate to get tough on crime freed prison authorities of this long-compromised obligation. Even as some advocates forged a gendered analysis of rehabilitation in order to secure alternatives for women and their children, its political currency had come to a decisive end. Rehabilitation, however contradictory or ultimately punishing, only held sway when politicians and prison officials felt obligated to depict penal institutions as more than warehouses.

CIW's prominence as the largest state prison for women in the country until 1990 made it a sought-after laboratory for researchers studying rehabilitation in the decades prior to the loss of faith in the idea that incarceration should entail a treatment component. Dorothy Zietz was one such researcher, and in 1960, the CDC contracted her as part of its Corona Project, an assessment effort prompted by concern about how mothers and their children were impacted by incarceration.[34] In her sample of forty cases of women "having child welfare problems," Zietz found that "the inmate mother is dependent upon her family, the institutional staff and community agencies . . . for information about the child's health, behavior, appearance, and growth." This dependence placed her at a great disadvantage, particularly when prison staff regularly worked with representatives from child welfare services without involving the women whose children were under discussion. In describing "a typical approach to legal separation," Zietz explained how women were informed by letter of their children's custodial court hearings, but had no way of attending the hearings to communicate their continued interest in guardianship. When they failed to show up to court, they received another notice saying that the child would be put up for adoption because they had missed the custodial hearing. Further expediting women's loss of custody was the belief on the part of many child welfare officials that adoption was the best option for all children, in part because they were "anxious to move as many children as possible from public support." Zietz also noted that agencies set to work "separating mother and child emotionally, long before legal separation is accomplished," by refusing to answer women's requests for information about their children. In describing one example of this common practice, Zietz emphasized that *"This woman had already surrendered three children for adoption by this same method."* In another case where children were "relinquished by rather questionable means," a private agency placed a child in foster care upon the mother's incarceration and refused to let the woman's husband and child's father see the child. A "petition of abandonment" was initiated on the grounds of the mother's incarceration and the father's lack of visitation.[35]

It is unclear just how many children were stolen from their families as a result of the institutional neglect baked into incarceration and child welfare services.[36] But in an illuminating example that demonstrated why the AFSC indicted rehabilitation as a "mask of treatment" just a decade later, Zietz focused on how family separation was detrimental to women's treatment regimen. In keeping with the dominant views on rehabilitation, Zietz expressed hope that women's demonstrated concern for their child's welfare could be "therapeutically useful"—even if "her concern for her child may be superficial, remote and unrealistically related to her past performance as a mother." The absence of a child-welfare services officer who could assist women in understanding and implementing alternative child care plans was a "deterrent to the inmate's full participation in and use of the institution's programs." Zietz demonstrated this by reporting on a woman who, after a year of repeatedly asking for and receiving no updates from the agency holding her child, "earned 12 disciplinary slips for pilfering, misconduct, offensive language, failure to obey orders and other acting-out behavior." When she received word that her custody had been ended via an "abandonment action," she "handled her feelings again by misbehaving and earning 8 more disciplinary actions." Despite her "history of prostitution, forgery, and drug addiction," Zietz insisted that "she had not legally demonstrated her unfitness as a mother, since she had had no opportunity to care for her child." The woman subsequently refused to participate in group counseling and "wanted nothing to do with a social worker" because, as she told Zietz, "I don't trust them."[37]

Zietz's report vacillated between suggesting that dedicated child welfare counselors could advocate for women whose children had been wrongly taken from them and demonstrating that such supports were necessary to help women adjust to their inevitable loss of rights. In a group counseling session with twelve pregnant women, Zietz fielded questions and comments that demonstrated women's immense anxiety about their parental rights following childbirth. Women expressed fears that "the courts" would take their children away, demanded to know what "their rights were," offered the solution of a prison nursery, and asserted that "it is unfair for the courts to take our babies away from us while we're in here and can't defend ourselves." Zietz was able to answer many of the women's questions and pointed out that doing so alleviated much "unnecessary anxiety and upset."[38] Zietz was adamant that counselors with expertise in child welfare needed to work with women to make alternative child care plans. But because her investment was in women's successful adherence to treatment, rather than shoring up the parental rights women clearly wanted help in defending, she also overstated how much such a plan could alleviate women's incredible constraints. While women considered information about their children critical to their legal standing as parents, Zietz emphasized the therapeutic potential of transparent communication, regardless of what was likely to be communicated: the women's irretrievable loss of their children.

Four years later the CDC teamed up with the Department of Social Welfare to expand on Zietz's findings. Whereas Zietz set out to identify service gaps specific to incarcerated women with children, Serapio Zalba and his research team endeavored to assess more than just "inter-agency cooperation" by asking a central question: "What is the role of the mother while she is in prison?"[39] Researchers spent two years culling demographic data from the 885 Warden's Inmate Cards representing each woman at CIW, researching the situation of all minor children, administering a questionnaire to women in order to "establish a social/psychological profile of inmate-mothers," and conducting interviews with women at CIW as well as relatives, caretakers, and agency employees.[40]

Zalba replicated many of Zietz's findings regarding women's experiences of imprisonment. Despite Zietz's recommendations for better interagency coordination, for example, Zalba's research team found that "sharing of casework information was practically non-existent either between public welfare and/or juvenile probation departments with the California Institution for Women, or between the Institution and public welfare or juvenile probation departments." Furthermore, interviews revealed that women reported being especially concerned about their children's well-being and their own custody rights, leading Zalba to conclude that "the role of the mother is more crucial for the mother herself than is the father's role to him, and that separation from her children . . . more directly strike at her essential personal identity and her self-image as a woman." Yet, to an even greater degree than Zietz, Zalba struggled to believe that women's expressions of concern about their children were genuine. Despite interviewing a total of 124 incarcerated mothers with minor children about the health and welfare of their children, their largely negative experiences with state agencies, and the arrangements they attempted to make for their children upon being sentenced, the report described women's narratives as largely delusional. Women's reports of making arrangements for their children that fell through or were thwarted by third parties, of caretakers and agencies refusing to answer their requests for information about their children, of avoiding public services because "I don't trust state agencies" and of prison staff giving them "a runaround" when it came to family-related problems (or responding to logistical and legal questions about parental rights with the therapeutic directive to "group on it" at the next counseling session) were undermined by interviews conducted with supposedly more reliable caregivers and agency providers.[41] Discrepancies that arose from these respective sources were attributed to "distortions by inmates because of an intense need to depict themselves as having been good mothers who cared, were concerned, and as deeply involved in the lives of their children as circumstances permitted." What researchers really uncovered through interviews with incarcerated women were "conscious or unconscious distortions by inmate-mothers as to the adequacy of the care they gave their children before they were incarcerated, and the inadequacy of the children's care currently provided by others." So great was this distortion that imprisoned mothers who articulated plans to reunite with their children upon parole release were believed to be motivated by "what would gain institutional approval and the earliest parole date," a perversion of the structural barrier indeterminate sentencing posed for women attempting to make plans for reunification.[42] Such a conclusion put women in an impossible situation: the very "maternal concerns" they were expected to demonstrate upon having undergone successful rehabilitation were instead used as evidence of their pathological scheming and manipulation.

By attending to women's maternal concerns, even if for the sake of the treatment regimen, Zietz saw a path to rehabilitation.[43] But Zalba argued that motherhood and rehabilitation were fundamentally irreconcilable, and that incarcerated women should be denied their right to parent their children to the greatest extent possible. The study concluded that what women most needed was support in accepting "separation from her children in the future," especially for those who "could not let go." This latter group was of serious concern to researchers because women who could not accept loss of custody were a potential threat to their children. "Her negative feelings about such plans may result in her sabotaging sound arrangements made for the children." These concerns were amplified by the "deviant behavior other than crimes" that researchers uncovered in their analysis of mother's case files. Seventy-seven percent of incarcerated mothers had histories of alcohol and drug use, prostitution, "overt homosexuality," and/or institutional commitment. Women's marital histories—with many having been married twice or more times—further demonstrated to researchers "a picture of instability and discord."[44] Zalba's study showed that Black women were disproportionately represented at CIW, comprising 27 percent of the imprisoned population but accounting for just 6 percent of the state's general population (while white women comprised the majority of prisoners). While neither Zietz nor Zalba granted explanatory power to women's racial backgrounds in their respective analyses of families impacted by a mother's incarceration, it is likely that dominant theories of criminality influenced their respective conclusions. For example, Zietz's prioritization of rehabilitation may have been aided by the fact that the majority of the forty women she interviewed were white. Zietz likely continued a tradition of penology's disparate application of the treatment principle, whereby white prisoners were seen as better candidates for rehabilitation than their counterparts of color, who were deemed untreatable due to the idea that their criminality was innate.[45] In contrast, due to their overrepresentation among all

prisoners, Black women were also overrepresented in the long-form follow-up interviews with mothers of minor children that influenced Zalba's
conclusions.[46] His analysis emphasized "deviancies" ranging from single
motherhood to poverty to drug use that further linked criminality to
blackness, continuing one of the major through-lines of criminological
thought and penal practice since the nineteenth century.[47] While both
researchers ultimately concluded that mothers' familial ties necessitated
additional support from prison staff and other state agencies, only Zalba
positioned mothers as threats to their children's safety and interpreted
their plans to reunite with their children as schemes.

Immediately following Zalba's work, another study of prison life at
women's facilities was published for the purposes of examining, and
explaining, "rampant homosexuality" at women's institutions. In 1965,
David Ward and Gene Kassebaum, two sociologists at UCLA, once again
turned CIW into a laboratory where they set out to "explicate the character of the pains of imprisonment which women prisoners experience" as
well as "the adaptations made to these deprivations."[48] The sociologists
spent much of the report's 200 pages painstakingly detailing women's
"homosexual adaptation" in response to the pains of imprisonment, mir-
roring the findings of studies conducted in men's prisons.[49]

However, Ward and Kassebaum made a cursory note of one pain
that made imprisonment more of a hardship for women than for men—
separation from their children. So severe was this "uniquely female deprivation" that the report recommended separation of mother and child "only
under extraordinary circumstances."[50] Unlike Zietz and Zalba, Ward and
Kassebaum did not question the veracity of women's maternal suffering,
most likely because it supported their claim that women's same-sex activity was about reestablishing traditional gender roles in the absence of men
rather than evidencing actual lesbian desire.[51]

Collectively, these studies positioned women's concerns about their
children as the most detrimental effect of incarceration. Yet, this assertion
was plagued by a paradox. Researchers found that women's concern for
and separation from their children represented the discovery of a uniquely
gendered "deprivation of imprisonment." At the same time, they agreed
that such concerns were impediments to rehabilitation at best or distortions at worst. Furthermore, for white mothers turned "female offenders,"

such deviancy from racialized gender norms registered as an individual emotional disorder, capable of being remedied by counseling that would help women "interpret" the assault on their rights. Such an analysis sometimes allowed for researchers to question the means by which women lost their children. Black mothers, however, were not even afforded the stigmatizing diagnosis of psychological pathology. Thoroughly defined by an untreatable criminality, their motherhood and attendant concerns about their children were not even legible to researchers, except as a potential threat upon release.

When advocates turned to the plight of women behind bars a decade later, they too zeroed in on women's familial attachments, but unlike earlier researchers they foregrounded the structural barriers that caused women's suffering. Those working in New York City to help women with their legal claims informed correctional officials that women's social and legal relationships to their children was the number one problem unique to female offenders. "Many children of women prisoners are either placed in foster care, unsuccessfully put up for adoption, or are never returned to their natural mothers even in most cases where that would be beneficial to them."[52] The Chicago branch of the American Friends Service Committee informed members that "women's prisons are hotbeds of horror stories of mothers who don't know where their children are," reporting that 80 percent of inmates at Cook County Women's Correctional Facility were also mothers.[53] Publications written by and for women in prison and their supporters such as *No More Cages* and *Clarion* also reported on the "cruel and damaging" process of women's separation from their children.[54]

In order to bolster their claims about the negative impact of incarceration on families, advocates turned to an unlikely source: Zalba's 1964 study. In 1973, Helen E. Gibson published an article in the *Wisconsin Law Review* outlining the lack of resources in women's correctional facilities. Prisons for women lacked most of the programs available to men *and* they failed to account for women's role as mothers: "Zalba, in a 1964 study of women prisoners and their families in California, expressed the view that 'The role of the mother is more crucial for the mother herself than is the father's role to him.' The fact that the majority of women prisoners were also mothers, combined with the lack of infrastructure to support regular visitation, exacerbated the challenges that awaited women upon leaving prison—her task of daily child care and discipline.[55] In Gibson's hands, the recommendation in Zalba's report that children be kept away from their mothers even upon release was repurposed by the legal advocate to make the feminist argument that women in prison be recognized as mothers and reproductive laborers.

Gibson's article was only the beginning. Armed with a structural analysis, advocates wrested what they could from the scant research available on incarcerated women to argue that prisons needed to accommodate women's caretaking responsibilities. A special 1974 issue on Planning for the Female Offender from the American Association of Correctional Psychologists referenced Ward and Kassebaum's study's conclusion that "lack of family ties is a critical deprivation experience for women in prison" to bolster their position that "institutions be near the woman's home community."[56] An article on the parental rights of women referenced the Zalba study to prove that "female offenders who are mothers face a two-pronged sentence. First they must serve the prison term, and second, they must cope with the additional punishment of a temporary or permanent deprivation of parental rights."[57] Another article did the same, to establish the psychological trauma accompanying involuntary separation of mother and child.[58] And in a 1979 article assessing how incarceration impacted women, the same studies helped bolster the claim that "deprivation from family and social structures is more keenly felt by women prisoners than men"; further, the article stated that the "worst problem of prison mothers and their children is enforced separation."[59]

Upon establishing the harm caused by separation and loss of custody, many of these same articles echoed pregnant women's suggestion to Zietz that women be allowed to keep their children with them in penal institutions, particularly during the earliest stages of childhood.[60] Some appealed to the institution's treatment obligation, arguing that such programs would make it "possible to construct a truly rehabilitative atmosphere for incarcerated mothers."[61] Others blended rehabilitation with an acknowledgement of reproductive labor when they envisioned special programs called "mother-release."[62] Modeled after work-release programs aimed at helping prisoners line up jobs prior to parole, a "mother-release" program would allow "the prisoner-mother . . . to use her work-release time for the achievement of her post incarceration duties, performing her parental responsibilities . . . and thus satisfy the child's best interests as well as aid in her own rehabilitation."[63] The Women in Prison chairperson for the California chapter of NOW also endorsed what she called "infant care furloughs" that would release "the new mother and baby to her home community and her other children."[64] Even the director of the women's prison in Washington State suggested she considered mothering to be rehabilitative when she explained, "We believe that mothering is an extremely important role for women with children in our society, and, therefore, should be a vital part of any total rehabilitative program for women."[65]

THE COSTS OF NEGLECT

In articles, studies, and reports, rehabilitation could be used to advocate for incarcerated women's ability to stay connected to their children despite their imprisonment. But advocates hoping to make such programs a reality confronted two political challenges. The first was the well-established, inherent contradiction of rehabilitation—how exactly to extract healing from a site of harm? The second challenge was impossible for advocates to predict. While many criticized the criminal justice system from the left, others began to assert that government's ability to manage inequality was ineffective—from both the center and the right. Rather than paying even lip service to rehabilitation, the new litmus test for prison authorities and elected officials became "getting tough" on social problems that were increasingly attributed to the culture of poor communities of color (rather than a society built on class exploitation and racial hierarchy). Advocates concerned with how incarcerated women could maintain familial ties, how to provide quality pregnancy care from within prison, and how to shore up women's legal rights to their children may have seen political promise in a revamped version of rehabilitation, one largely administered via alternative structures. But they did so in a broader, shifting context in which punitive sentencing became "politically essential" for both Republicans and Democrats aiming to stay in office. While advocates' and prisoners' mobilization of motherhood enabled them to slightly prolong rehabilitation's political currency during this period, ultimately their "soft" approach also lost out to the mandate of toughness that would usher in mass incarceration.[66]

When Superintendent Carey placed Barbara Cardell's newborn son in foster care in 1975, Cardell fought to get him back. With the help of the Women's Litigation Unit of the San Francisco Neighborhood Legal Assistance Foundation and the Women's Prison Coalition, Cardell filed a petition that cited Penal Code 3401, a forty-seven-year-old state law that granted mothers in California prisons the right to keep their children with them until the age of two. Petitioners argued that Section 3401 was evidence of the legislature's willingness to consider CIW suitable for infants and small children. Cardell and her supporters took this logic one step further when they asserted that the statute "created an absolute right in the mother to keep her baby with her while she is incarcerated." Women incarcerated at CIW and their legal advocates built on the petition to bring a lawsuit against the director of the CDC on behalf of Cardell and other similarly situated women at CIW. The suit claimed, "it would be unconscionable to permit the state, by disobeying the provisions of Section 3401 of the Penal Code, to create the very conditions which would subject petitioner to deprivation of the custody and control of her child by the state."[67] The court was not convinced. Because the statute provided the mother only an *option* to keep her child, the court ruled that correctional officials held ultimate discretion over whether or not to adhere to Section 3401.[68]

Despite the loss, the lawsuit prompted the California State Assembly's Select Committee on Corrections to conduct hearings on issues facing incarcerated women. Advocates bolstered their rights-based claims by pointing to the evidence on the gendered harm of separation. A staff attorney for the Women's Litigation Unit explained in her testimony that "the most cruel way in which most women in prison and jail are treated is that they are torn from their children and their families."[69] Attorneys also cited low recidivism rates "for women who keep their children with them," though they did not reference any specific articles. They bolstered their claims about incarcerated women specifically by pointing to the broader, but waning, mandate of rehabilitation: "the cruel irony of the present situation is that the state, ostensibly committed to the eventual social reintegration of inmates, denies prisoners the opportunity of preserving those relationships which have been shown to contribute substantially to her successful reentry into society."[70]

In this way, advocates flipped the script on rehabilitation. It was not that individual women had failed to accept their treatment regimen, per Zietz. Rather, corrections had systematically failed women: "There are at least eight different ways in which a child may be taken from a natural parent. The complexity of these methods baffles the minds of the law review and treatise editors, and does havoc to the individual unschooled in custody proceedings. Often, when a woman is arrested, if she has been unable to make alternative arrangements her children may be brought within the juvenile court's jurisdiction. Until last year, incarcerated parents did not have the absolute right to be present at these crucial hearings, nor a right to an attorney."[71] Such "prison personnel inattention" led directly to incarcerated women's children being "taken away," a clear violation of their rights and humanity.[72]

Advocates in California believed that these issues were best addressed through a more robust version of the outdated statute Cardell and other women put their hopes in. Concerned community members and legislators collaborated on the Mother Infant Care (MIC) program, and in February of 1977, State Assemblyman Terry Goggin introduced Assembly Bill (AB) 512, which mandated the development of a community treatment program for mothers and their children to be administered by agencies contracted by the CDC. To get the bill through the legislature, sponsors reversed the direction of harm caused by separation. AB 512 opened, "The Legislature finds that the separation [of] infants from their mothers, while their mothers are in prison, can cause serious psychological damage to such infants."[73] In the press release announcing the bill, Goggin distanced the innocent children from their criminal mothers. "We should not punish the babies along with their mothers who have committed crimes. My bill will require the Department of Corrections to minimize the tragedies of separating infants from their mothers."[74]

Despite the discursive consequences of this politically expedient framing, advocates considered AB 512 to be an example of the "alternatives to incarceration" they hoped would decrease the power of the criminal justice system along with another central reform—an end to indeterminate sentencing. The same year AB 512 went to the legislature, California joined the nationwide movement to replace indeterminate sentencing laws with fixed sentences. SB 42, the Uniform Determinate Sentencing Act (UDSA), brought the state's sixty-year dependence on indeterminate sentencing to an end.[75] Echoing the sentiment of incarcerated people, prisoners' rights advocates, and expert criminologists calling for the abandonment of rehabilitation, SB 42 stated, "The Legislature finds and declares that the purpose of imprisonment for crime is punishment."[76] On this, diverse interest groups working on criminal justice reform in California could agree. "SB 42's rejection of the rehabilitation model for a punitive one was almost a consensus position, with law enforcement on the one hand, and the ACLU, Prisoners Union, Friends Committee, and criminal defense attorneys on the other, generally concurring that the grand experiment of rehabilitation had not worked," wrote a legislative representative for ACLU of Northern California.[77]

Yet, supporters of SB 42 were deeply divided on what programs should replace treatment. Progressive groups in California were eager to support determinate sentencing legislation, but only on the condition that shorter sentences and more robust alternatives to incarceration were a major component of the "new" wave of criminal justice.[78] Instead, groups like the Prisoners Union watched as the bill became a litmus test for Governor Jerry Brown and other Democrats to prove that they could be tough on crime, a debate that left little room for considering the effects of imprisonment on society at large, much less on those behind bars. Law enforcement spokespersons such as Los Angeles Police Chief Ed Davis stoked public fears about personal safety, saying that SB 42 would trigger the release of thousands of dangerous criminals from prison. The idea that dangerous people should be locked up for as long as possible worked its way into SB 42 through various amendments.[79] A coalition of nine prisoners' rights groups organized a press conference at the state's capitol a year after the bill's introduction to go public with their concerns "about the legislative negotiations." They directed their ire at Brown for giving "carte blanche powers to law enforcement representatives (the district attorneys and police) to draft any provisions they feel are appropriate. Where it was once possible to negotiate with all sides on these important problems, we now find that as long as law enforcement has the governor's proxy there is no room for viable change. We have no choice but to oppose SB 42 and the juvenile bills."[80] The bill passed in spite of the coalition's reversal. Less than two years later the state's prison population had increased by nearly 3,000. By 1981, the CDC was calling for the construction of more than six new prisons over the next ten years in order to keep pace with the projected growth of incarcerated persons.[81]

What advocates hoped would be an alternative-to-incarceration program designed to keep women and children together would instead inaugurate a decades-long struggle against the CDC's willful neglect, some of which was baked in directly to AB 512.[82] The original bill required no legislative appropriation and mandated CDC officials to allocate funds from the existing budget in order to implement the program. The bill even made sure to cap the amount that could be drawn from the General Fund. Unsurprisingly, less than a year after AB 512 had passed, community groups tracking the bill's progress became concerned. The Committee for Women and Children of the East Long Beach Neighborhood Center informed members that "little has been done to implement this legislation. In placing numerous calls to drug, probation and correction institutes, little or no information was available concerning the progress of such facilities." Based on their research, the committee concluded that the CDC "is impeding and disregarding the rights of inmates to have access to an alternative community mother/child rearing program."[83] The recently formed community-based AB 512 task force agreed. The task force showed that the program largely existed in name only. While set to start in January of 1980, by April of that same year there were no contracts with community agencies in place, incarcerated women had not been informed of the program, and no additional funds had been raised.[84] As a result, less than eight women had entered the program since its inception.[85]

Amended legislation designed to address these failings was signed into law in January of 1982, but three years later attorneys with Legal Services for Prisoners with Children (LSPC), a legal advocacy organization founded by Ellen Barry in 1978, learned that the number of total participants in the program was still "extremely small."[86] Widespread negligence on the part of CDC staff kept the program significantly underenrolled. Women were not systematically notified about the program at the time of sentencing, especially women whose first language was not English; those who applied (the majority of whom were told about the program by their public defenders) often waited up to 24 months to learn if they were eligible despite the

30-day timeline outlined in the statute; staff often lost, misplaced, or failed to process applications; most counties lacked a program (by 1985 there were only two MIC "houses"); and limited funds for the programs that did exist meant they were ill equipped to accommodate even the small number of participants. The CDC needn't exhibit "*expressed* opposition to the full implementation of the program."[87] By simply doing nothing, correctional staff ensured incarceration separated women from their children while also violating women prisoners' rights under California state law.

Neglect not only brought the pain of separation. It could also be a lethal force. In addition to not knowing what happened to their applications (assuming they found out about the program at all), pregnant women at CIW also lacked access to regular prenatal care. There was no Ob-Gyn staff on site; the chief medical officer was an orthopedist; there were no directives about routine prenatal care; staff repeatedly ignored women's requests to go to the prison clinic; and women's medical files were routinely lost. And while CIW contracted with Riverside General Hospital to provide prenatal, delivery, and postpartum care, prison medical staff regularly denied requests from hospital staff and women themselves for this outside treatment. Despite going to the medical clinic twice a day every day and speaking with nurses, Annette Harris waited three months before being permitted to see the CIW physician, Dr. Srivastava. Upon his examination the doctor told Harris she was "fine." When Harris's abdominal pain became so severe that she vomited, she was rushed to Riverside General Hospital, and lost her son two hours after giving birth in the ambulance. For two and a half months after Harris's premature delivery, she was not sent back to the hospital for a follow-up exam or the counseling program for mothers who had lost their infants, which was hosted by the Ob-Gyn clinic.[88] Even making it to outside care did not guarantee one's health and safety. When Brenda Jackson finally made it to Riverside General Hospital to be treated for heavy vaginal bleeding, she was diagnosed with placenta previa. CIW staff ignored the obstetricians' directives and at six months she gave birth to a stillborn, joining Harris and other women who had lost their infants that year.[89]

In response to rampant negligence, LSPC and the ACLU brought two lawsuits against the CDC in 1985 on behalf of pregnant women and mothers at CIW. Both eventually ended in settlements, which legal advocates noted allowed for quicker and more comprehensive relief for prisoners than going to trial. The suit against "serious indifference" to pregnant women's medical needs instituted protocols for prenatal care, such as establishing a special Pregnancy-Related Health Care Team, and required prison officials to provide semi-annual reports on all treatment of pregnant women by medical staff, among other oversight mechanisms.[90] Meanwhile, five years lapsed until settlement of the lawsuit regarding the MIC Program, and despite LSPC's best efforts to build oversight mechanisms into the agreement, the program remained underutilized.[91] By 1989, CIW was more than 220 percent over design capacity, which LSPC attorneys noted only exacerbated the institution's "egregious treatment of pregnant and postpartum women."[92]

THE TRIUMPH OF WILLFUL FAILURE

While LSPC and pregnant women and mothers at CIW used the law to wage the battle against neglect in California's largest state prison for women, others labored against neglect's destructive weight at a federal institution nearly four hundred miles from CIW. As AB 512 and SB 42 worked their way through the state legislature, the Federal Correction Institute (FCI) in Pleasanton became the first federal prison to house a children's center. After speaking with women at FCI about what programs were most needed at the prison, two Bay Area women, Yvette Lehman and Carolyn McCall, proposed a daily program in which children and their mothers would spend each day together in a preschool-like setting. This idea was "flatly rejected" by Warden Charles Turnbo, whose counteroffer was to organize special visits for women and children four times a year.[93]

Prison Mothers and Their Children (MATCH) was the compromise. The centerpiece of Prison MATCH was a children's center, staffed by a director and incarcerated women, where women and their children could spend the entire weekend together. MATCH was originally funded as a pilot program by National Council on Crime and Delinquency (NCCD). After the success of the first year, it garnered some funding from the Bureau of Prisons (BOP), which made it possible to add a vocational program in early childhood education for the women at FCI.[94] In this short time, it also managed to win over skeptical prison staff. "I think you've gone from real suspicion—in almost everyone—to folks saying, 'This is a fantastic program. It is helping the mothers. It is helping the kids.'" Prison MATCH's stated aim was to "encourage the correctional system to look at an incarcerated family as a total unit—needing meaningful contact between parents and children during imprisonment and necessitating the coordination of prison and community-based resources for their needs."[95]

Prison MATCH "formed out of a concern for the potential harm to both mother and child when they are separated because of a mother's imprisonment."[96] The program threaded the needle of past advocates' different claims about harm. The damage of incarceration was equally shared by mother and child, but differentially experienced through maternal suffering and the threat of delayed child development, respectively. Thus, the children's center was meant to serve not only as a space where mothers and children could "restore family ties" but also as an opportunity to educate mothers about the stages of child development—they were to become "experts" of their own parental experiences. Credit for this programmatic principle went to the women at FCI. They had "argued for good vocational training in the field of early childhood education" since the "program's inception," demanding "training in an area which bears some perceived relevancy to their lives."[97] Staff on both sides of the bars hoped that the vocational program offering women a Child Development Associate (CDA) certificate would enable them to work in federally funded children's programs such as Head Start upon their release. In a bid for funding from the Women's Educational Equity Act Program within the Department of Health, Education, and Welfare, Prison MATCH staff turned years of stigma cultivated by research on "maternal distortions" on its head. "As any Head Start teacher knows, some of such children are also the offspring of incarcerated parents. Women inmates have stressed that they have as much or more of a right and responsibility to work with these children as anyone in society because of their own unique life situations and sensitivity to the issues involved in teaching public day care children."[98] Incarcerated women's experiences with the criminal justice system signaled valuable expertise rather than stigma or deviancy. The child development framework was not only marshalled as a professionalizing opportunity but also guided interactions taking place between mothers, children, and staff at the center. An evaluation report belies any trivializing notion that the center was merely a child-friendly visitation room. Rather, staff embarked on a radical initiative to adapt "normative" child development models to the challenges of separation caused by imprisonment. "In the traditional children's center, the focus of this age group is on encouraging independence from the mother and the moving to peer contact and relations. Our focus, on the other hand, has evolved as one in which we nurture needs as well as enable the child to build or rebuild trust in their relationship."[99] Center staff also helped small children make sense of the multiple primary caretakers in their life so as to establish a mothers' central role in spite of her absence. For example, a toddler named Michael was born in prison and had never lived with his mother. As a result, he called his foster care parent "mommy." The center director worked with the guardian and Michael's mother to encourage Michael to see his biological mother as a primary caretaker, introducing him to "mommy Carol" (the foster parent) and "mommy Alice" (the biological mother). When Michael was moved to a new foster home, Alice insisted on being referred to solely as "mommy" and having Michael call his foster mother by name. Attentive to the need to help Michael with this transition, the center staff introduced the term "mommy-mommy" for Alice. After a two-month period, Michael spontaneously began calling Alice "mommy" and looking to Alice when he needed help.[100]

Michael and Alice's story illustrates just how much work, care, and collaboration on the part of a diverse cast of actors were required to make Prison MATCH a reality—evaluation reports and program initiatives lay bare the reproductive labor that made family possible despite state neglect. The complex network required to make "mothering from prison" a reality—one that also foregrounded women's parental authority—was astounding. For starters, foster parents had to be willing participants in the program if the children were actually going to make it to the children's center. This was not only a logistical and fiscal challenge given that travel to the prison site often took up the bulk of foster parents' weekend hours, but participation also entailed the emotionally taxing component of learning how to "share" parenting with the incarcerated mothers. Foster parent orientation classes were regularly offered so that guardians and mothers could develop "co-parenting models" for the children participating in the program.[101] Then there was the task of negotiating with child welfare services in order to address aid for the children, unsafe living situations, and custody battles. And a great deal of work was required to ensure Prison MATCH made good on its claim that "programs like this one must be developed from the start with the fullest possible participation by inmates."[102] Incarcerated women served on the organization's advisory board, worked in the children's center, and were involved in decisions ranging from interviewing candidates for the center's director position to developing program initiatives. Because the CDA training did not qualify as a prison work assignment, Prison MATCH also raised funds in order to pay those who participated.[103]

In addition to the more immediate tasks associated with running the children's center, Prison MATCH staff also had to fend off the neglect inherent to incarceration—a battle that consistently tested program capacity. Pregnant women turning to Prison MATCH prompted staff to take on the issue of adequate prenatal care and delivery accommodations for inmates.[104] Desperately needed social services support was also necessary if mothers were going to have any involvement in their child's well-being in between visits and following their release. The program recruited the services of a social work intern on a temporary basis, but the need for a permanent position was clear. Incarcerated staff members echoed participants from Zietz's study when they highlighted this just two years into the program:

> We have recently lost a member of the Center staff who was actively involved giving social service aid to the mothers here. We cannot express emphatically enough the need for a social service component in PCC [Pleasanton Children's Center]. This need has been highlighted at board meetings and at inside staff meetings. We badly need casework assistance in handling such problems as working out custody arrangements for our children, setting up good foster care, making the right decisions for children who are residing in another state while their mother is here, etc. Our immediate concern is that, now that we have identified this need and are planning new program directions, what can we do with the problems that arise in the meantime?[105]

Prison staff also reported feeling "stymied in these cases, not knowing enough about community-based resources for children with problems and, often, not having the particular social service expertise that is needed to even decide what kind of referral to make for a family." Yet, Prison MATCH closely regulated who could be considered experts of maternal incarceration. By highlighting FCI staff's primary, punitive role, Prison MATCH emphasized the specialized knowledge and vested interests required of anyone who might start such a program inside a prison. "Prison staff are not trained to be advocates for families—in fact, their role as guards prohibits it." As they labored to create spaces of family making within prisons, center staff repeatedly confronted the fundamental contradiction of trying to install structures of care within an institutional site of harm.[106]

Despite such challenges, the program garnered attention from those working in corrections. In its second year of operation, Prison MATCH reported that it was "becoming somewhat difficult to balance focusing in on our ongoing concerns at Pleasanton with requests for various kinds of information and assistance from other communities."[107] Requests came from the Michigan Department of Corrections, Maine Department of Corrections, New York Department of Corrections, and various Sheriff's departments in California, among others; whenever possible, Prison MATCH traveled to offer in-person assistance.[108] Between 1978 and 1989, Prison MATCH successfully helped establish programs at federal, state, and county facilities in over seven states.[109]

Whether or not such programs were taken seriously by prison officials, it is clear that incarcerated staff considered outreach work fundamental to raising awareness about their unique circumstances. Writing in just the second quarterly report for the program, they offered their perspective on the differences between sending men and women to prison: "When a man goes to prison, his woman on the outside will usually do everything in her power to keep that broken home together. On the other hand, when a mother goes to prison, quite often there is no husband there on the outside, and we can easily lose contact with our children. Often people in control of our children have little or no interest in bridging the gap between us and our kids. . . . How can we make people understand our needs as women and mothers while we are imprisoned?" For inside staff, participating in workshop discussions and conference presentations was not just about promoting Prison MATCH, but an opportunity to "publicize our needs as imprisoned mothers and the needs of our children."[110]

Lehman and McCall originally approached FCI with their proposal because they had been told federal corrections staff might be more amenable than the staff at CIW. The tip was a good one. After his initial disdain, Warden Turnbo lent his enthusiastic support for the program, allowing Prison MATCH to characterize "the first years, 1978–1982," as "full of growth, change, and excitement."[111] But it is possible such enthusiasm was lubricated by the program's self-reliance. By 1982, NCCD seed money had run out, and Prison MATCH was spending more time and energy on fundraising efforts. Funding issues were compounded by a 12 percent cut to the BOP budget, and Prison MATCH was ranked last on the list of "optional" programs.[112] In an effort to counter this precarity, outside staff decided to lobby Congress for a line item on the BOP budget that would fund children's centers at the four federal facilities housing women.[113] From 1985–1987, Prison MATCH successfully won contracts from the BOP as a result of this line item, though the funds covered only a third of their operating expenses.[114] In another grasp for security, staff began lobbying for an amendment to the Department of Justice Authorization Act that would both mandate funds and do away with the "sealed bid method" of procuring contracts.[115]

Uncertainty for Prison MATCH ramped up for the same reasons that state-level reform efforts faltered—there was little room for rehabilitation in the tough-on-crime mandate. As the Reagan administration declared a "war on drugs" and as Congress responded by passing legislation that brought increased federal penalties, the overcrowding that had prompted CDC director Enomoto to call for immediate prison expansion at the state level in 1981 was repeated for federal institutions.[116] In an attempt to find room for newly sentenced offenders, the BOP began shifting the makeup of its facilities. When double-bunking prisoners and housing them far outside of their jurisdiction proved insufficient, the federal system began contracting with state and county facilities for additional capacity. Federal prisons that had been co-ed transitioned to all-male facilities, and in the process, women were dispersed to all regions of the country.[117]

FCI Pleasanton was not spared from this massive crisis-mode redistribution of prisoners—250 female prisoners were transferred from California to facilities in Washington State and a jail in North Dakota. Being thrust into a new system meant a dramatic disruption in terms of access to penal resources. Neglect rapidly multiplied. In addition to not having the services of Prison MATCH to aid in maintaining some control over their children's lives, women wrote to staff about the absence of law libraries, counseling services, vocational training, and prison jobs. Many of the women had counseling or drug treatment mandated as part of their sentence and were unsure about what their break in treatment would mean for their parole chances. Their ability to alleviate these grievances locally was stymied by local officials' repeated refrain that they were not responsible for federal prisoners.[118] Women, desperate for help, wrote to Prison MATCH staff. One woman explained that her court-ordered visits with her son had no standing in the State of Washington, leaving her with the possibility that she might not see him again before the date set for his adoption.[119] Another expressed her distress at not being able to communicate with her four young children, who she regularly saw at the children's center.[120] Another who was serving a fifteen-year sentence expressed utter desperation caused by separation. "How can I make it not knowing what is happening to my family?"[121]

As their last line of defense, Prison MATCH staff attempted to amplify women's circumstances to those empowered to reverse the changes.[122] They challenged a number of efforts the BOP was undertaking in the face of overcrowding, including the transfer of women to institutions far from their homes and future plans to build new cells for women in highly secure facilities rather than transition them to community-based, alternative units. "Prison MATCH and our many colleagues and related agencies around the country are questioning the wisdom of these BOP practices in light of the longer view needed to improve family ties so as to reduce recidivism." In response to such efforts, the BOP informed Prison MATCH and its sister organization in Fort Worth, Texas that their annual grant would be cut in accordance with the reduced number of women imprisoned at each facility.[123]

In 1989, Prison MATCH was outbid by a different agency that offered to provide services to parents at FCI Pleasanton at a lower cost. Staff surmised that the move was retaliatory in light of the increasingly strained nature of their relationship with the BOP. But in addition to whatever personal vendetta that may have been directed at Prison MATCH, staff most involved in the lobbying also cited a general lack of will on the part of prison officials. "The BOP has said repeatedly to us and to Congress that they view these projects as 'special interests,' and they do not like being told to cater to some groups over others. I guess one way to look at women and children is as 'special interests.'"[124] The strategy of protecting women's familial ties by pointing to their rehabilitative potential, combined with advocates' and prisoners' limited access to power and resources as compared with access by lawmakers and prison authorities, became a valueless currency once the race to punish was underway.

CONCLUSION

A 1977 Law Enforcement Assistance Administration national study of prison programs for women reported that the "newest trend in community-based programs involves residential facilities for mothers and children."[125] Researchers could not have anticipated just how rapacious such a "trend" would need to be to keep pace with the number of women sent to prison over the ensuing decades. The number of women in state and federal prisons increased seven-fold between 1980 and 2000, growing at twice the pace of men's incarceration.[126] Of the two hundred thousand women that were incarcerated in the United States in 2010, over 70 percent were the primary caretakers of minor children prior to imprisonment.[127] Perhaps best illustrated by California's astounding trajectory of twenty-three new state prisons built since 1984, prison construction—not "community-based programs"—defined the nation's response to the astronomical increase in the number of people sentenced to prison during the last two decades of the twentieth century.[128]

The boastful claim about emerging trends was issued just as corrections was turning towards renewing its "punitive spirit." Many prisoners' rights activists were caught off guard by just how swiftly the system's failings became a vehicle for more, rather than less, punishment. In the case of incarcerated pregnant women and mothers, efforts to hold penal institutions accountable for the devastation wrought on families faltered as prison authorities gave up even the pretense of treatment and doubled down on stark retribution. Neglect—both by design and by indifference—

overwhelmed even the most heroic efforts to build infrastructures that supported women's family making.

As incarcerated women, their families, and their supporters know all too well, the costs of the road taken are piled up on both sides of the prison wall. Studies examining women's frequency of contact with their children report that over half of the mothers have not had visits since being incarcerated.[129] As was the case with the women who participated in Prison MATCH, the fact that children of incarcerated mothers are more likely to be placed in foster care or live with extended family makes visitation especially difficult.[130] Prison MATCH can be credited for the child-friendly visitation programs that still exist at some women's facilities, though these pale in comparison to the original children's center at FCI Pleasanton.[131] Mother-child prison visitation has continued to decline since Prison MATCH was formed in 1978.[132]

Such realities illuminate the persistence of permanent family separation as a cost of systems designed to restrict people's movement, whether through prisons, immigrant detention centers, or armed guards policing borders. Just as when Zietz profiled the practices that permanently separated women from their children in 1960, a recent study by the Marshall Project found that one in eight incarcerated parents lost their parental rights between 2006 and 2016. Such outcomes stemmed solely from the fact of the parent's incarceration. Incarcerated women, whose children are five times more likely to end up in foster care as compared to those of their male counterparts, had their parental rights permanently severed most often. One legal advocate captured Zietz's and Zalba's clinical assessments from fifty years ago when she described the process of family separation as a "right" that is stripped "from incarcerated parents so casually."[133] Research on contemporary alternatives is also cause for concern. Not only are community-based programs that allow women to live with their children rare, but research suggests that even these alternatives to incarceration cannot escape "the pull of punitiveness" endemic to penal practices.[134] For children forced to endure family separation, roads often lead back to the prison. Children in the child welfare system, particularly Black children, are more likely to end up in the juvenile justice system due to lack of support from foster parents to "provide private alternatives" that shield white children from state facilities.[135]

While feminist scholars have studied the myriad ways mass incarceration specifically disrupts intimate relations, we have yet to fully recognize
how rampant criminalization and imprisonment has more generally stratified access to family by the start of the twenty-first century.[136] Mass incarceration has ensured that family making became much harder for those
unable to remain beyond the law's reach, a barrier almost exclusively
present in the lives of poor families, and especially so for poor families of
color. Jails now play an outsized role in incarcerated women's lives (where
80 percent of women are mothers) as poverty, racism, and homophobia
intersect to disproportionately criminalize Black queer women. This initial
contact with the criminal justice system triggers a series of events that often
result in permanent separation from their children, further shoring up
racialized and gendered ideas about fit mothers and legitimate families.[137]
As poverty continues to be criminalized, families on the economic, racial,
and sexual margins of society are forced to perform the work of maintaining
legal ties and intimacy in spite of jail cells.[138] This is due to the punishing
nature of mass incarceration as well as the neglect that is integral to conditions of confinement in the United States. Incarcerated women and their
advocates have attempted to make up for the negligent conditions that
pervade every aspect of life on the inside: long-standing policy gaps, interagency disorganization, insufficient medical and legal resources. staff indifference and willful failure. They did so in the face of public contempt for
so-called "criminals" and far too many lawmakers' willingness to destroy
lives for the sake of their political careers. Mitigating such devastation on
family making while laboring in the space of carceral neglect, not to mention the costs that accumulate when such efforts are not enough, largely
remain solely these families' responsibility—and toll.

Legal neglect and carceral neglect produced different vulnerabilities
for families, but together they ensured family making became harder and
costlier during this period. Before the century's end, additional forms of
neglect would take an incalculable toll on families forced to struggle daily
for their very survival. As the next two chapters detail, far too many lost
this fight. The Reagan administration's fiscal policies ensured an already
stressed system of public healthcare was pushed to a breaking point,
which had devastating consequences for two major developments of the
1980s: a growing disparity in rates of Black and white infant death, and

the HIV/AIDS epidemic. By the time the BOP ended Prison MATCH's contract, the nation was embroiled in a debate over who was to blame when Black infants did not live to see their first birthday. Activists who saw infant mortality as an issue of humane, accessible healthcare in the late 1970s struggled to navigate the narrowing political horizon of the 1980s in a fight against medical neglect that exacerbated the health-destroying forces of economic exploitation and racism while extracting yet new forms of reproductive labor necessary for survival.

3 The Labor of Survival

RACISM, POVERTY, AND THE USES OF
INFANT MORTALITY RATES

Sexism + Racism + Profits = High Infant Mortality.

Coalition to Fight Infant Mortality, 1980

To illustrate the issue of East Oakland's high infant mortality rates in the late 1970s, the San Francisco Bay Area-based Coalition to Fight Infant Mortality (CFIM) used the story of a local woman named Carolyn. Eighteen years old and four months pregnant, Carolyn was urged by her older cousin to get prenatal care. After an hour's bus ride from her home to the public hospital, Carolyn spent almost three hours in the waiting room. She was finally seen by a "middle-aged white doctor" who, upon observing her idly playing with the blood pressure cuff when he walked in, scolded her to "leave it alone." Offended and uncomfortable, Carolyn repeatedly asked to see a different physician, preferably a woman. When the male doctor refused her requests, she left without an examination. Not wanting to return to the public hospital, and without insurance, Carolyn was unable to get an appointment with any private physicians for the duration of her pregnancy. It was only when she went into labor at seven and a half months that her anemia and high blood pressure were diagnosed. Her prematurely born daughter had only a "moderate" chance of survival. CFIM asked its supporters to make an impossible calculation: "Were the difficulties and attitudes Carolyn faced due to the fact that she was young . . . or Black . . . or poor . . . or because she is a woman?"[1]

Carrying on the work begun by the Bay Area chapter of the Third World Women's Alliance (TWWA) medical committee, CFIM hoped that Carolyn's story would mobilize community members to combat high rates of Black infant mortality in East Oakland. In their July 1980 newsletter, CFIM explained that despite her story being a combination of several women's experiences, Carolyn's situation was "very real, and too many Carolyns have lost babies, through no fault of their own." Racism, sexism, and a healthcare industry driven by profit were to blame for the fact that East Oakland's infant mortality rate was twice the national average. According to CFIM, these societal factors, rather than their presumed mandate to safeguard "access to health care for all county residents," influenced the Alameda County Board of Supervisors and led to high perinatal mortality rates at its only public hospital, Highland. Just as Carolyn was not to blame for her infant's high-risk birth, CFIM also exempted "the nursing, clerical, and housekeeping staff" from responsibility for the hospital's high rates of perinatal mortality. Instead, CFIM said the county's Board of Supervisors had "neglected Highland." The coalition that formed to combat infant mortality in East Oakland did not mince words in their charge against the board: "infanticide by neglect."[2]

Only sufficient investment, dedication, and care—the opposite of neglect—could reverse the situation at Highland. CFIM pointed to San Francisco General Hospital's turn-around of infant mortality rates just five years previously, explaining that community pressure for additional funding had made possible "the Perinatal Health Project, the midwifery training program, bilingual and bicultural prenatal education programs, and the family addiction center." While CFIM acknowledged that "the quality and sensitivity of care at [San Francisco General Hospital] could be swept away if funds are withdrawn," they insisted that the prenatal programs at San Francisco's public hospital represented "something we must fight to achieve here in Alameda County." At the start of the decade, CFIM asserted that "the fight for the right of people to decent health care is a high priority."[3] If infants were dying in East Oakland's poorest, predominately Black neighborhoods, it was in large part because healthcare remained a business venture rather than a human right. Community activists set out to reverse this equation.

As with any local issue, there was no guarantee that the San Francisco General Hospital's successes could be replicated across the Bay in Alameda

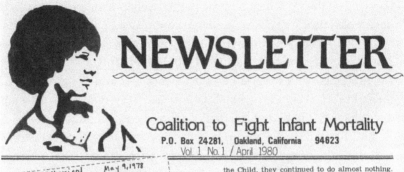

NEWSLETTER

Coalition to Fight Infant Mortality
P.O. Box 24281, Oakland, California 94623
Vol. 1 No. 1 / April 1980

SF Chronicol May 9, 1978

East Oakland's Shocking Rate Of Infant Deaths

By Charles Petit
Science Correspondent

In the Spring of 1978 this headline shocked the community of East Oakland and many other people throughout the State. How is it that 26 out of every 1000 babies born to mothers in our community die before they reach their first birthday? We started to ask some serious questions.

—What causes East Oakland babies to die at a rate twice that of the national average and seven times that of nearby (but wealthy) Piedmont?

—How is it that several third world countries, including Jamaica, Thailand, Jordan, and Hong Kong have lower infant mortality rates than East Oakland?

—In the U.S., medicine is our second largest industry. We spend more on health care than any other nation in the world. Yet, 17 countries have lower infant mortality rates than the U.S.

Something is wrong.
WHO IS TO BLAME?
According to California law, the Alameda County Board of Supervisors has overall responsibility for safeguarding access to health care for all county residents. The County's own infant mortality statistics prove the Board is not fulfilling its responsibility. When these statistics hit the newsstands, the Supervisors had been aware of this problem for approximately two years—and had done almost nothing. And in 1979, the International Year of

the Child, they continued to do almost nothing.

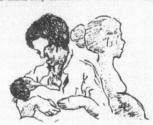

As unemployment and inflation rise, and medical costs soar, the need for public medical services is greater than ever. In Alameda County, Highland Hospital is the only hospital where a woman can go to have her baby regardless of her ability to pay. Highland should have a vital role to play in reducing the rate of infant mortality.

But the Board of Supervisors have neglected Highland. As a result, Highland has an extremely high perinatal mortality rate—that is, the number of children born there who die within one month of birth. In fact, the perinatal mortality rate at Highland is twice that of any other East Bay Hospital.

Highland's high perinatal mortality rate is no fault of the nursing, clerical, and housekeeping staff there, who are generally very dedicated to serving the patients. Highland's problems are a result of poor administration and underfunding by the County.

We charge the Board of Supervisors with infanticide by neglect!

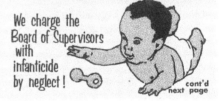

cont'd next page

Figure 4. First issue of the Coalition to Fight Infant Mortality newsletter, charging the Alameda County Board of Supervisors with "genocide by neglect," April 1980. Courtesy of Sophia Smith Collection, Smith College.

County (though providing proof of concept was still a savvy political move). But more so than unique local factors, CFIM confronted a more universal variable: time. When CFIM asserted that healthcare was the government's responsibility, and that the State of California was as much to blame for infant death as county officials, they marshalled arguments that by 1980 were losing ground to conservative arguments that maligned most government provisions. Calls to free both the market and states from federal regulation while also reducing the supposed largesse of federal government that began in earnest in the 1970s declared victory with Ronald Reagan's presidential win in 1980. This political shift did not only take aim at publicly funded healthcare—Reagan famously stated at his inaugural address that "government is not the solution to our problem; government is the problem."[4] Such declarations from the world's most powerful leader made it much harder to demand that healthcare be treated as a right. The administration's 1981 Omnibus Budget and Reconciliation Act (OBRA) codified views about social insurance that economists, some policy makers, and public health specialists had been arguing about for the past decade: principally, that neither government nor private insurance should bear the costs of "life style choices" that led to poor health among some sectors of the populace.[5] CFIM may have blamed the county and the state for Highland's problems, but Alameda County board supervisor Joseph Bort's thinly veiled racist retort that "the problem lies with the East Oakland community and not with the hospital" represented an increasingly dominant view by the time Bay Area residents started debating who was responsible for the local community's high rates of infant mortality.

Those who still believed in government's responsibility to take care of its citizens zeroed in on medical neglect, especially inaccessible prenatal care. Taken up by activists at the local level before congressional representatives and nongovernmental organizations (NGOs) followed suit, this strategy resulted in a puzzling development by the time Reagan entered his second term: the successful expansion of Medicaid coverage for pregnant women. Given popular narratives about the Reagan administration's slashing of the federal budget and penchant for deregulation, any growth of the so-called safety net during an administration infamous for defunding social programs appears to be contradictory.[6] Yet it remains the case that during Reagan's presidency, Medicaid experienced dramatic growth in both program expenditures—which increased by 400 percent—and enrollment. By the early 1990s thirty-five million people were enrolled in the program, up from twenty-five million in 1981.[7]

Funding of prenatal care during a period of American governance infamous for its austerity was achieved through an impossible calculation—a type of illogic that CFIM had warned its supporters against in its early newsletters. The successful expansion rested upon an etiology of infant death that winnowed the many vulnerabilities in Carolyn's life down to her inability to access healthcare during her pregnancy, thereby endangering her future infant This narrow focus on the necessity of healthcare for the sake of Carolyn's unborn child helped paved the way for conservatives' long-desired abandonment of a program that Carolyn also needed for family making, especially after the birth of her infant: Aid to Families with Dependent Children (AFDC). While CFIM dared readers to trace the loss of Carolyn's infant back to a single, isolated constraint, the political compromise that ultimately delivered prenatal care to previously ineligible pregnant women clearly missed the coalition's larger cautionary tale. Medicaid expansion—accomplished in large part by severing the indigent care program from AFDC for the first time in the program's history—further weakened the long-maligned welfare program. Fixing one form of state neglect resulted in the deepening of another.

The consensus among liberal reformers that Medicaid expansion should and could be wrested from the Reagan administration was based on two related arguments: first, infant death, especially Black infant death, had reached crisis proportions due to Reagan's inhumane budget cuts; and second, getting access to prenatal care for poor women of all racial backgrounds was necessary for the health of their future child. How, exactly, was the complex reality of infant death—itself evidence of a society in very poor health—transformed into a single policy demand? In large part, this oversimplified equation found support in the shifting political landscape. The dwindling influence of social medicine that emphasized community participation in healthcare delivery and rising prominence of the demand for personal responsibility in all areas of life ensured that "health" was narrowly bounded in debates over infant mortality.[8] Lack of access to medical care counted as a "clinical risk" to women's health that medicine should be expected to ameliorate. But "social and environmental risks" that also contributed to poor perinatal health outcomes were beyond medicine's purview. Ezra Meharry, chief of obstetrics at Martin Luther King Hospital in Los Angeles, who ran a perinatal regionalization demonstration project in the late 1970s, demonstrated how parsing risk in this way made it possible to divvy up responsibility for poor health outcomes:

> I believe that by the right kind of clinical intervention in high risk situations, we can probably reduce infant mortality by about one-third. That leaves two-thirds of the cases. Their outcome is related to socioeconomic factors, not medical factors. Combine an adolescent pregnancy, plus low or inadequate nutrition, plus a minimum of family and other support services, plus adverse environmental conditions, and poverty and the stresses of unemployment—these clearly add up to increased perinatal mortality and morbidity. It's not a medical question; it's not a clinical question; it's a question for society.[9]

Whereas in the mid-1960s, "society" partially answered this question with initiatives like the Neighborhood Health Center program that combined healthcare with "arrangements for providing employment, education, social, or other assistance needed by families and individuals served," by the time Reagan became president such an answer had been made thoroughly suspect.[10] Politicians and NGOs approached infant mortality as a "clinical question" in the 1980s, debating it within a narrow epidemiological framework focused on standard medical treatment. As a result, Carolyn's story consistently exceeded the bounds within which her life and the lives of women like her were being discussed. Mothers and their advocates working to secure resources from an increasingly neglectful state became experts on just how much was being missed. From their perspective, expanding Medicaid while further weakening welfare benefits was just par for the course. They had already become experts in navigating an insufficient, illogical, neglectful welfare state that routinely required impossible calculations. Their effort to both expose this illogic and secure necessary resources can be seen as another expansion of the reproductive labor required for family making, labor dedicated to surviving the stressors captured in CFIM's calculation, "Sexism + Racism + Profits = High Infant Mortality." As groups like CFIM knew all too well, the cost of piecemeal reforms that offered targeted solutions to broadscale, intersecting problems was very high indeed. It could include the incalculable cost of infant death.

EXPECTING DEATH: DEBATING STATISTICS IN OAKLAND

In some ways, CFIM's assertion that infant mortality was the result of racism, sexism, and capitalism put a Third World, socialist, feminist gloss on the infant mortality rate (IMR) as a standard measurement of public health. Due to the numerous social, environmental, and medical factors associated with infant death, public health specialists for decades treated IMR as a window into the overall health of a given population. Factors that threatened infants' survival were surely a much broader threat, particularly to the women who birthed them. Yet, towards the end of the twentieth century, some within the field began to question the efficacy of treating IMR as a stand-in for population health. While meant to serve as a proxy for assessing (and ostensibly addressing) the whole population's health, too frequently IMR-inspired health policies targeted the outcome of the measure—infants' deaths, while ignoring the rest of the population.[11] This tendency was exemplified by clinical interventions of the sort described by Meharry. Due to both regionalized perinatal programs like the one he oversaw in Los Angeles and advancements in neonatal medicine, infant mortality decreased 41 percent between 1970 and 1979.[12] At the start of the decade, it also looked as if the Black-white disparity that had long characterized infant mortality in the United States might be overcome once and for all.[13]

But as Meharry's comments and other measurements made clear, by the late 1970s the effects of these interventions had run their course. Indeed, the final decades of the twentieth century stood in stark contrast to the preceding two decades, which had seen the most rapid decline in rates of infant mortality.[14] Unfortunately for activists and families, the political currency of the IMR still had a lot of steam. Even with their radical gloss, CFIM was unable to avoid citing the effect (infant death) to illuminate its causes (the conditions structuring women's lives and health) and thereby consistently narrowing systemic critiques into singular healthcare solutions. To make matters more complicated, the IMR was a fairly limited measurement. A population's IMR was widely understood to be an indicator of overall health, but it did not apportion responsibility for said health. The IMR could be used to index society's neglect just as easily as it could be marshalled as evidence of poor, individual decisions.

When a 1978 *San Francisco Chronicle* article announced East Oakland's IMR, activists pursued the route of highlighting society's neglect. In addition to having rates second only to Central Harlem in New York City, the area of East Oakland that stretched from 73rd Avenue to San Leandro along East 14th Street had an IMR twice the average for California, and seven times as high as its wealthier, whiter neighbor immediately to the north, Piedmont. Surrounded by clergy, practitioners, and community advocates, Reverend Michael H. Dunn held a press conference at the East Oakland Family Health Center in May of 1978 to announce that the rate at which Black infants born in East Oakland died before their first birthday was among the highest in the nation.[15] The head of Alameda County's Bureau of Maternal and Child Care, Dr. Allan S. Noonan, also spoke, explaining that East Oakland stood out in the county for its lack of adequate healthcare, low rates of early prenatal care, and nonmarital births.[16] Noonan's merging of structural (lack of healthcare) and moral (nonmarital births) factors foreshadowed the terms of the debate that would emerge over how to decrease the IMR in East Oakland.

CFIM's first newsletter stated unequivocally that the problem was structural in nature.[17] "Racism takes its toll through a system that begins at birth, affects a child's nutrition, extends through an education tracking into a dead-end job and then affects the health of her children in turn. This cycle of overwork, poverty and poor health care produces infant mortality."[18] The coalition concluded its trenchant analysis with a clear assignation of blame. "Our government's refusal to deal with this problem, to actively seek a solution, amounts to an attack on women and minorities." And the organization did not mince words about what such refusal, in the face of systems that produced Black infant death, amounted to: plainly, it was "genocide by neglect."[19]

CFIM's systemic analysis was powerful, but a campaign needs specific demands. The coalition landed on Highland Hospital. Concerns about the quality of care at Highland, particularly its Obstetrics and Gynecology unit, went back at least a decade. In 1973, the hospital lost its accreditation due to a declining number of patients, forcing it to replace the Ob-Gyn team with private physicians who delivered infants on a contract basis. The group of six physicians were majority white, all male, and lived outside of Alameda County. Reports of condescension and hostility, particularly towards patients who did not speak English, began circulating within the community. Accompanying the Ob-Gyn medical team's racism at the interpersonal level were structural barriers to care, especially the fact that Highland was not equipped to address the complications that often accompany high-risk births. A 1975 report on Highland by researchers at UC Berkeley confirmed this deficiency, as well as other concerns, and recommended that unless vast improvements to the Ob-Gyn unit were made, it should be shuttered.[20] An assessment conducted just two years later documented the persistence of complaints about "sensitivity," high turnover among staff, and large numbers of complicated deliveries due in part to "dumping" (private hospitals sending Medicaid patients to public hospitals) of high-risk patients in mid-labor at Highland's doorstep.[21]

In other words, CFIM had set out to improve the life expectancy of infants born in a hospital with a nearly decade-long track record of failing the communities it ostensibly served. In a public statement, Third World Women's Alliance (TWWA) member Leticia Wadsworth charged that the "grim results of the poor, inadequate perinatal care received at Highland Hospital" were the "deaths of helpless infants before the age of one year." She asked, rhetorically, if "the babies and the parents of Third World communities have a lesser right to life and health than the more affluent white community of Piedmont?"[22] CFIM bolstered its indictment of Highland, the chosen proxy for systemic inequality and state-wide neglect, using IMR statistics. The coalition rested its charge on a figure from 1977 showing that Highland had a perinatal mortality rate of 35.3 per 1,000 births, compared to a rate less than two thirds that at Merritt, a private hospital in the Oakland hills.[23]

This IMR was meant to legitimize CFIM's claims that racism and poverty were causes of infant death. But in their campaign against the board of supervisors, quantitative data did little to dull the double-edged sword of social determinants of health. While the coalition invoked Highland's well-documented personnel and economic struggles, county officials pointed to the hospital's patients and their personal health behaviors. Highland's administration, unsympathetic supervisors, and the director of the Alameda County Health Department adamantly rejected the social link asserted by the coalition. The most hostile of the supervisors, Fred Cooper, forcefully blamed women themselves, citing "teenage pregnancy, alcoholism, drug addiction, women who wait seven or eight months to see a doctor," and "women who think hamburgers and french fries are a proper diet to be pregnant on" as the causes for poor outcomes. Supervisor Joseph Bort proffered another theory. "I think it has to do with a basic attitude and approach to life. If you go anywhere in the U.S. and compare black communities to white, black will have a higher infant mortality rate," a difference explained by "a cultural attitude or inherited." Bort's slippage between "culture" and heredity especially signaled how arguments about bad behaviors were often based on an investment in biological racism.[24]

TWWA member Dr. Vicki Alexander made clear that such "irrational, racist bullying" would not stop the Coalition from doing "everything we can to see that this infanticide by neglect is stopped."[25] One of their tactics aimed to strengthen the claim that Highland was responsible for its poor perinatal mortality rate by demanding that the board approve a community-based investigation into the Ob-Gyn department. The demand was partially granted when the board voted to allow a grand jury, rather than community members, to conduct the study.[26] While the coalition resolved to produce their own investigation in response to the vote, the grand jury outsourced the investigation to the California Medical Association, which in turn countered the coalition's use of IMR statistics with a new measurement. The California Medical Association's report claimed that Highland's practice of accepting all patients, no matter their "social state or gravity of illness," meant it was primarily engaged in "crisis management," making "built-in failures" inevitable.[27] To bolster the claim that Highland should not be held responsible for the high-risk population that made up the lion's share of its patients, the report cited supplemental material produced by economist Ronald L. Williams, who had developed a "risk-adjusted perinatal mortality" index that measured effectiveness of care more accurately than crude IMR. Williams examined vital statistics in relation to a number of risk indicators, including race, maternal age, parity, marital status, and pregnancy spacing.[28] Accounting for these varied risks enabled him to produce an "expected perinatal mortality rate" that could be compared to the "observed perinatal rate" for any given area, down to a single facility, such as a hospital.[29]

Williams found that Highland had an expected mortality rate more than double the statewide norm.[30] However, when Williams compared the expected rate to the observed rate of perinatal mortality, Highland actually came in slightly lower than the state average. Alameda County facilities, including Highland, demonstrated a higher quality of care than even some of its wealthier, neighboring counties. Williams concluded,

> much of the high risk status of the Black subpopulation in HSA-5 [East Bay] is likely a result of these risk characteristics as demonstrated best by Highland General Hospital with 15 percent no prenatal care, 13 percent adolescent mothers, 41 percent out-of-wedlock, and with the percent low birth weight . . . among the highest in the State. For this high level of maternal and newborn risk, the observed perinatal mortality rate for Highland is somewhat lower than expected.[31]

By merging structural conditions—such as access to healthcare, with social characteristics—such as teen pregnancy and out of wedlock births, Williams provided an instrument that could highlight either structural barriers or individual behaviors.

The grand jury used William's adjusted IMR to zero in on individual behaviors. "The statistical data show just as certainly that the blame for the high infant mortality rate in certain parts of Alameda County cannot be neatly bundled and dropped at the door of Highland Hospital," which, given the risk, had an IMR "lower than expected." The rate would not decrease "unless women become educated about the conditions that lead to low birth weight babies and [are] impressed with the need of early and continued prenatal care." Highland could not be held wholly responsible for the high IMR, though the report did recommend some changes aimed at supporting its proportion of high-risk patients.[32] In contrast, CFIM's community investigation surveyed 138 community members (78 percent of whom had been pregnant at least once), 5 community healthcare providers, and 22 Highland employees.[33] Responses to the measurement, "Describe any barriers you think prevent women from getting prenatal care," supported CFIM's early calculation of sexism, racism, and profit—

lack of money was the most frequently reported barrier, followed by "discrimination against women and ethnic minorities."[34] Placing responsibility for early enrollment in prenatal care with county officials, CFIM called for a "comprehensive, county-wide, and county coordinated perinatal program" to ensure care to every woman and child, "regardless of . . . ability to pay." And it reiterated its original charge of genocide by neglect by concluding that "the only major barrier to the provision of adequate perinatal care . . . is the lack of a political commitment on the part of county government to poor and minority communities in order to provide that care."[35]

When the grand jury and CFIM went before the county board of supervisors to discuss their respective reports on September 16, 1980, some supervisors highlighted their own, similar recommendations (both acknowledged the need for greater coordination of county services, for example). But CFIM rejected such comparisons. At issue were Williams's instrument, which accepted at least some infant death, and the grand jury's recommendation of "piecemeal programs." In contrast, the community demanded a higher standard, that "not even one baby . . . die needlessly," and called for comprehensive programs "which are culturally relevant and accessible."[36] For the coalition, infant death evidenced state neglect, not individual failings, and could therefore be cured by political will and financial investment.

While the board of supervisors ultimately accepted many recommendations issued by both reports, its subsequent action—to abstain from a financial commitment—would define CFIM's protracted fight to make healthcare a right. CFIM reported on the accumulation of state neglect that unfolded over the next couple of years: the suspension of delivery services at a private hospital in Oakland formerly offered to indigent pregnant women on a sliding scale; a new credit policy at the Children's Hospital in Oakland that would bar children from outpatient services if they lacked cash, private insurance, or Medi-Cal; the county board of supervisors pursuing a three million dollar cut to county healthcare funding; and the kneecapping of legislation meant to fund community-based perinatal services when Governor George Deukmejian cut 1.6 billion dollars from the 1983 state budget.[37] As 1983 came to a close, the coalition informed supporters that "the Board . . . continues to place a low priority on meeting the health needs of poor and third world women and children."[38]

The early battle in Alameda County demonstrates the political difficulty of using IMR data. Whereas the coalition used high rates of Black infant death to indict systemic neglect, county officials used Williams's adjusted measurement to normalize the costs of said neglect. High-risk conditions blurred into high-risk behaviors to make some infant death expected rather than shocking. As the debate over infant mortality garnered greater attention, the IMR's pliability would aid stakeholders willing to push for "piecemeal programs" that had been the object of CFIM's derision. Like CFIM, those who understood there were no quick fixes to the accumulation of neglect struggled to keep multiple, intersecting causes in view.

CAUGHT BETWEEN SERVICE, ADVOCACY, AND OVERWHELMING NEED IN PHILADELPHIA AND BEYOND

If the fight in East Oakland was defined in part by what measurements could be used accurately to assign blame, a concurrent battle in Philadelphia was defined by the myriad consequences of that stalemate. The Maternity Care Coalition (MCC) formed in 1980 in response to high rates of infant mortality in some of Philadelphia's poorest, predominately Black, neighborhoods.[39] Its first task was addressing the blame that insidiously burrowed its way into women's assessments of themselves. MCC's executive director Louise Brookins, an experienced organizer with the Philadelphia Welfare Rights Office (PWRO), was firm in her belief that the coalition's major aim should be "making the community itself become involved in the very thing that was destroying them which they didn't know what to do about. The babies were dying and they didn't know why the babies were dying." Brookins described the reality—obscured both by political slogans and sanitized statistics—of what happened when "not knowing" collided with neglect. "If they were pregnant, well, that's it. They didn't know the nutritional value they need. They didn't know what type of maternity care was out there. They didn't know they could be concerned with what doctors were giving them as medicines. . . . They had no one to talk to that knew anything."

The unfamiliar and overwhelming experience of pregnancy combined with difficulties navigating medical care were compounded by grief, silence, and shame when a woman lost her infant. Brookins was firm in her belief that freeing women of this shame through consciousness raising was of vital importance—community mobilization would never emanate from a place of self-blame:

> The other thing was getting people to talk. People weren't talking. It's almost like if I lost a baby there was something wrong with me and I was stigmatized. Or if my baby was born and lived two or three months and it died, it was because I didn't treat it right. The system looked at it like you might have abused the baby instead of looking for the real cause of why the baby died. They wanted to hide like some people want to hide being on welfare. So when we started to meet on a four or five person basis or on a one to one basis, people began to come out and say: "I lost my baby. I don't know why my baby died but my baby died." After you get the small meeting going, they begin to feel it wasn't my fault that my baby died but it was because of lack of education/not knowing what to do or where to turn.[40]

As various individuals debated causes in order to assign responsibility, those most impacted absorbed the messaging of stakeholders eager to blame women themselves. At Brookins's urging, the MCC set out to redirect women's self-blame towards the structural conditions that made pregnancy such a costly endeavor.

Brookins's investment in a process of politicization reflected MCC's belief that active participation by poor communities of all racial backgrounds in their own medical services had transformative potential.[41] But as Brookins pointed out, many women did not know what kinds of pregnancy programs were available to them: "they didn't know to ask," and some "wouldn't even go to the hospital for care" after hearing that they would be turned away if they lacked the ability to pay.[42] Her insights about the necessity of *personal* transformation prompted the coalition to incorporate service advocacy into its organizing model. Due in large part to Brookins's insistence, MCC's board concluded early on that "we cannot organize people without giving them some kind of service when they need it."[43]

And so, MCC embarked on an effort always intended to be equal parts advocacy and service provision in the tradition of mutual aid. While members helped women and their children enroll in Women, Infant, and Children (WIC) benefits, they also initiated shaming campaigns against hospitals that refused to treat women who lacked access to payment.[44]

When women came to them with issues for which no aid existed, MCC staff triaged, hunting down food supplies and getting women's household gas turned back on.[45] This emergency case management was performed alongside the group's outreach to more than 6,000 North Central and Mantau neighborhood residents, interviews with more than 400 women about their birth experiences, membership drives, training sessions for maternity patients about knowing their rights, and evaluation tours of both city hospitals and birthing centers—all of which happened within MCC's first six months.[46]

Like the coalition in East Oakland, MCC's overarching aim was better delivery of quality healthcare. MCC believed that what was needed to address low participation in prenatal care and high infant mortality rates in Philadelphia's poor, majority-Black neighborhoods was a "Model Maternity Plan." MCC member Sister Teresita Hinnegan, a midwife and social worker, conducted extensive research on neighborhoods with the worst perinatal health outcomes and noted that accessibility to maternity services was hampered by the lack of outreach programs, support mechanisms, and inter-agency coordination. MCC's plan focused on maternity centers designed to meet the needs that community members prioritized, but Hinnegan was clear-eyed about the limits of healthcare solutions, however community-minded, in the face of "poverty and social deprivation." Still, she seemed to hold out hope that Philadelphia's high IMR rate could be improved in spite of broader inequalities. In one assessment, she noted intractable "global problems" versus those problems "amendable to change." Whereas MCC could not hope to reverse the larger problems of poverty and unemployment, Hinnegan listed the high incidence of infant mortality in the local community as a problem the organization might be able to change.[47]

But in real life, inequalities that contribute to poor health do not abide by neat lists. MCC's commitment to organizing through the provision of services ensured that it became increasingly well acquainted with this reality throughout the 1980s. In 1981, Pennsylvania took advantage of the Maternal and Child Health block grant contained within Reagan's Omnibus Budget and Reconciliation Act (OBRA) that gave states broad discretion in program implementation. The state decided that Maternal and Infant Care program funds should no longer go to women who were ineligible for Medicaid, but instead should be used exclusively for preventive care, leaving in-hospital costs like delivery up to women or hospitals to cover.[48] As hospitals absorbed the costs of more and more uninsured women's inpatient stays, they tightened the purse strings. Some began asking for payment up front. Others cut off Maternal and Infant Care patients informally or made it official hospital policy.[49]

MCC consistently attempted to stem the tide of state retrenchment through both service and advocacy, but overwhelming need ensured that service provision became the lion's share of the organization's work.[50] During a five-month period, MCC's client advocacy project served 131 clients who had run into roadblocks, assisting them with welfare aid issues, WIC, medical access, food stamps, food insecurity, housing, and mental health support. One woman who was eight months pregnant came to MCC with no medical coverage and no source of income because her welfare case had been closed when she failed to submit a continued eligibility form that she had never been sent. Her repeated efforts to reach her caseworker had gotten her nowhere, an experience repeated for MCC advocate Judy Thorton when she attempted to reach someone at the welfare office. Only after her third attempt was Thorton able to make her client an appointment that got her back on public assistance. Upon delivering her baby prematurely at eight months, the hunt for funds for a breast pump started, taking Thorton through the social worker at the hospital (who told her the client must pay), to other support organizations (both of which said no) before landing at a pro-life pregnancy services center that provided her with the money. Thorton noted the herculean efforts required to secure services supposedly designed to aid pregnant women. Brought in as reinforcement after women tried and failed to persuade caseworkers to respond to their issues, Thorton would first spend an hour counseling clients before beginning a multi-day effort, with repeated calls and letters to negligent service providers. She also accompanied clients to their various appointments. Thorton invested in counseling so that her clients might "solve their problem without our intervention" in the future, but MCC's vigilant watchdogging was no doubt a major reason most women secured aid at all.[51]

Thorton's experience was not unique. Infant mortality initiatives that had a service component were quickly overwhelmed by the challenges confronting women and their families. When Vanderbilt University initiated a

Maternal and Infant Health Outreach Worker (MIHOW) Project in partnership with rural community health leaders in 1982, its 1983 interim
report commented that helpers were introduced into the field a year earlier than planned due to "the magnitude of need uncovered during home
visiting in the first year." At all four of the field sites, the workers repeated
Thorton's steps. They assisted with applications for Medicaid, WIC, and
AFDC, confronting the poverty that daily produced unstable housing, utilities issues, lack of transportation, and inadequate food and clothing. Less
than a year in the field had left outreach workers demoralized. A report
explained that even though outreach was performed by longtime residents
of the communities, home visits had "stimulated a new awareness of previously unnoticed poverty. The scarcity of services and people charged with
dealing with problems of the poor has pushed the workers to the brink of
despair at times." Their new awareness, combined with their inability to
meet the need, drained workers' resolve.[52]

In their willingness to try and mitigate the immense insecurity that
drove poor pregnancy outcomes, advocacy groups were perpetually pick-
ing up the slack created by negligent state agencies and officials. When
Philadelphia's first Black mayor, Wilson Goode, released the city's "Health
in the Eighties" report, the nearly two to one racial disparity in Black and
white rates of infant mortality received the greatest attention. Goode even
established a special committee charged with overseeing the implementation of relevant recommendations. But the MCC was not even cautiously
optimistic about such developments because "most of the recommendations lack enough specificity to make clear what the City Health
Department and others are expected to do."[53] In their formal response to
the report, the MCC asked "where does the concerned Philadelphian turn
to for designing, advocating, and implementing the various actions and
programs which collectively hold great promise for improving pregnancy
outcomes? As should be obvious, there is no 'somebody' to turn to."[54] Five
years later, MCC member Walter Lear reflected on what happened when
"somebody" like the coalition entered the scene of state neglect: "Ironically,
the more successful direct services of this type, the more likely do they
distract attention from the causes of the need." Such was the bind of combining political advocacy with service provision in the face of neglect—
even when such efforts foregrounded user empowerment.[55]

SERVING WOMEN THROUGH "UNBORN CHILDREN": THE
POLITICS OF MEDICAID EXPANSION UNDER REAGAN

However pessimistic the MCC was about Mayor Goode's intentions, his report nonetheless joined a growing chorus from other locales alarmed about rising IMRs in Lexington, New York City, Los Angeles, Chicago, and Detroit, but such findings were hardly groundbreaking.[56] Already in 1978, the Department of Health and Human Services had identified 564 areas in the country with excessively high infant mortality and had noted with alarm the disparity between rates for white and nonwhite infants.[57] That same year, Congress passed legislation that convened a select panel to assess children's health, but, as with community efforts, timing was not on the panel's side. The idea that federal government should play a greater role in providing healthcare to the poor, even if the majority of those living in poverty were children, invited handwringing about cost rather than about children's futures. Medicaid played the supporting role to such performances. By the mid-1970s, Medicaid costs had far exceeded projections (and enrollments).[58] In addition to the price tag, rising unemployment, which increased the number of uninsured Americans who did not meet state eligibility requirements, made it seem as if the program were failing to provide widespread coverage. By 1976, Medicaid was providing medical care to nearly twenty-three million people.[59]

The select panel acknowledged the narrowed political horizon when it delivered its report to lawmakers in December of 1980, stating that "even though we discovered much agreement on what needs to be done . . . it soon became evident that our very mandate was bucking widespread feelings of alienation from Government, and a rising tide of cynicism and hostility toward all social programs."[60] It met this mandate by issuing recommendations in keeping with a not-so-distant past where a nationalized health program seemed within reach—universal family planning, universal prenatal care, and comprehensive care for all children up to the age of five would comprise a "national child health strategy" at the cost of 4.6 billion dollars.[61] A 1980 Government Accountability Office (GAO) report tasked with investigating how to curb rising rates of infant mortality also foregrounded prenatal care as a possible solution.[62]

How to make prenatal care more accessible, however, still needed to be fleshed out. In contrast to the select panel's suggestion for universal programs, the 1980 GAO report floated Medicaid expansion as a possible route. The suggestion was supported by findings that state eligibility restrictions, such as North Carolina's rule to not cover first pregnancies, kept many women from receiving care before they went into labor.[63] From this perspective, increasing access through Medicaid required addressing one of the system's central features: that delivery of healthcare benefits hinged on the delivery of welfare aid.[64]

Since its start in 1966, the majority of families gained Medicaid coverage through their participation in Aid to Families with Dependent Children. The resulting moniker "welfare medicine" quickly fueled efforts to distance the healthcare program from its much-maligned counterpart.[65] The GAO report's findings were far from revelatory. Medicaid coverage for pregnant women was imperiled by many of the same mechanisms states had used to restrict families' eligibility for AFDC since the program's inception.[66] Restrictive eligibility, such as limiting participation to very low income levels, had been made worse by inflation, and welfare payments were on the decline even before Reagan's first budget took further aim at the program.[67] Through cuts implemented in 1981, more than 400,000 families lost Medicaid coverage when they were removed from the welfare rolls.[68] If prenatal care was going to be expanded through Medicaid, the healthcare program needed to be severed from the long-denigrated welfare program.

If Medicaid expansion was less likely to invite the "hostility . . . towards all social programs" highlighted by the select panel than would universal prenatal care, the Black IMR offered the perfect vehicle with which to make it a reality. A coalition of stakeholders, brought together by Congressman Henry Waxman, began to see the Black IMR as a viable path to Medicaid expansion.[69] Congressional hearings dedicated to the topics of infant mortality, children, and maternal and child health that took place throughout the early 1980s evidence advocates' formula of attributing poor health outcomes to the Reagan administration's budgetary decisions while simultaneously decrying the hypocrisy of and mimicking its pro-life rhetoric. Advocates honed a strategy whereby women's inability to access prenatal care was presented as evidence of the administration's neglect of "unborn children"—a phrase liberal stakeholders routinely invoked in their discussions of inaccessible healthcare. For example, at a 1982 hearing on the impact proposed budget cuts would have on children, Congresswoman Barbara Mikulski testified that prenatal care was necessary to "protect her life and the life of this unborn baby that we cherish so dearly." Other testimonies detailed women in labor being turned away from hospitals because they had no ability to pay, physicians refusing to accept Medicaid patients, medical centers slashing prenatal care budgets in response to the stoppage of federal monies, and babies being born in hospital hallways.[70]

It was at the 1982 congressional hearing that stakeholders levied the political power of the IMR. In his opening remarks, Senator Lloyd Bentsen explained that newly released data demonstrated an uptick in 1982 of infant mortality rates for nine states. Bentsen declared that "there is no doubt in my mind that the 1982 reduction in federal child and maternal health funding played a major role in the rising tide since then of needless infant deaths." The Children's Defense Fund (CDF) also presented its not-yet published findings on the growing number of women giving birth without ever receiving prenatal care.[71] Shortly thereafter, an administrative petition presented to Secretary of Health and Human Services Margaret Heckler by Public Advocates, a public interest law firm in San Francisco, officially laid Black infant death at the feet of the Reagan administration.[72] It took Heckler five months to respond, and her decision to appoint a commission to study the health disparities between Black and white Americans did not appease stakeholders. While the Congressional Black Caucus urged Congressmen John Dingel and Henry Waxman to convene hearings dedicated to highlighting the racial disparity Public Advocates tapped local advocacy groups in Oakland, Philadelphia, New York, Los Angeles, and San Francisco to hold simultaneous press conferences.[73] News coverage of the Black-white disparity in infant death was swift, with the *Washington Post* reiterating the pro-life hypocrisy talking point in an editorial that asked readers "Do Only the Unborn Matter?"[74] At a press conference in Philadelphia, Maternity Care Coalition put the point even more strongly: "Walter J. Lear, M.D. and Viola Sanders . . . today charged the U.S. Department of Health and Human Services with killing black infants in Philadelphia and throughout the nation by inaction on proposed improvements in Federal programs which finance and regulate services for low-income pregnant women and infants."[75] Local municipalities were not solely to blame for "genocide by neglect." Despite the fact that hearings on infant mortality rates just four years earlier had shown Medicaid, Maternal and Child Health programs, and WIC to be rife with administrative and funding problems, stakeholders were laser-focused on Reagan.[76] Congressman Waxman opened hearings on infant mortality rates, subtitled "Failure to Close the Black-White Gap," with a full castigation of the administration. "As you can see from the chart of existing health programs the administration has tried to cut or eliminate every single one of the programs we know that works: Medicaid, food programs, health clinics, and even immunizations."[77] Congressional Black Caucus chair Julian Dixon then made the link to Black infant death in order to indict the administration's anti-poor, anti-Black policies: "Although the problem, in reality, is a result of poverty—not race—the statistics show that black infants in America are twice as likely to die before their first birthday than are white infants." Whereas the Coalition to Fight Infant Mortality and the select panel suggested universal healthcare was necessary to address the alarming statistics, Dixon introduced stakeholders' solution of Medicaid expansion as a "targeted" policy that could close the gap between birth outcomes for Black and white infants. Stakeholders did not aspire to fully reverse OBRA 1981, much less amplify demands that healthcare be treated as a human right. Medicaid expansion that would benefit unborn children by way of delivering prenatal care to ineligible pregnant women comprised the congressional-level strategy.[78]

In a repeat of the debate in Alameda County, national stakeholders' narrative of the IMR as evidence of the neglect disproportionately falling on poor, Black people was contested by administration officials' interpretation of the data. In his testimony, Assistant Secretary for Health Edward Brandt urged caution when attempting to understand both the phenomenon of infant mortality generally and the Black-white gap specifically. Brandt emphasized research provided by the National Center for Health Statistics that suggested race and poverty might have been confounded in advocacy groups' studies. Research looking at low-birth-weight infants born to Black and white women for 1981 showed that even when both groups were college-educated, married, ages 25–29, and had begun pre-natal care in the first trimester, Black women had greater than twice the rate of low birth weight babies than their white counterparts. Brandt highlighted the finding and expressed hope that the evidence made clear "the black/white disparity represents much more than a simple phenom-enon." In response to Dixon's call for "targeted policies," Brandt cautioned against "single focused approaches" that would likely fail to address the complex and multiple causes of the disparity in birth outcomes.[79]

Advocates had little patience for the suggestion that race be treated as a sole indicator. Angela Blackwell, an attorney with Public Advocates, dis-missed the findings presented by Brandt as a distraction from the issue of providing healthcare to America's poor:

> Mr. Brandt alluded several times to the fact that even when you look at col-lege educated, middle-income black women, their low birth weight rate remains twice that of white women. In his testimony, he actually cited that 5.6 percent of the babies born to this group of well-educated black women still produce low birth weight infants. . . . I am sure most low-income black women would say, yes, we will certainly take that 5.6, while there may be need for studies that examine low birth weight to find ways to reduce that 5.6 to the 2-point-something that was cited for white women, we already know that prenatal care could bring down the current 12.5 for black women to 5.6, we need to get on with that business of making that prenated [*sic*] care available.[80]

Representing the Children's Defense Fund, legal advocate Sara Rosenbaum also reiterated the link between poverty and infant mortality, pointing out that "minority mothers and infants were overrepresented among the nation's poor and uninsured."[81]

Stakeholders were understandably skeptical of Reagan officials. But there were likely other reasons advocates were weary of race-based claims. Ronald L. Williams, the economist who contributed to the Alameda County's grand jury report, mentioned an outlier statistic on the final page of his study. At two hospitals, for a large percentage of Black births both high low-birth-weights and high mortality rates were recorded—independent of other maternal risk factors. Williams conjectured that "Black ethnicity is associ-ated with low birth weight independently of such factors as prenatal care, marital status, and maternal age," a speculation about racial differences being rooted in biology that undoubtedly advocates were eager to disavow. Furthermore, any research that challenged the link between early initiation of prenatal healthcare and healthier pregnancy outcomes necessarily complicated stakeholders' indictment of the Reagan administration as well as their goal of Medicaid expansion. Rosenbaum's testimony threaded requisite needles while avoiding others. "We know that poverty places a pregnant woman at higher risk for herself and her baby. Yet, as a result of this administration's policies, AFDC may no longer be provided to indigent women pregnant with their first child until their final trimester of pregnancy, and their *unborn children* cannot qualify for assistance at all."[82] Stakeholders' strategy amplified what was politically useful—pro-life rhetoric, the administration's racism and disdain for the poor, AFDC's restrictive eligibility levels—and avoided what could complicate their ultimate goal of Medicaid expansion—universal healthcare, race-based claims, and women's precarity before and after pregnancy.

Stakeholders secured their first win in 1984, and Congressman Waxman and CDF especially had cause to celebrate. The Tax Reform Act of 1984 ushered in their long sought Child Health Assurance Program (CHAP), which countered categorical restrictions to Medicaid coverage on the basis of familial status. States were now required to cover single women pregnant for the first time, pregnant women in two-parent families where the primary wage earner was unemployed, and children in two-parent families through their first year of life. CDF estimated that these mandates would extend coverage to 500,000 children and nearly 200,000 pregnant women.[83] However, state AFDC income eligibility levels remained the greatest barrier to Medicaid coverage. Additionally, as unemployment rose, so did the numbers of uninsured families who previously had been able to access healthcare through the private market. CHAP was a start, but Medicaid as the delivery mechanism for prenatal care remained hampered by AFDC income eligibility restrictions.

By 1984, local and national mobilizations around infant mortality unplugged a dam, and the issue reached "crisis" status. Despite disagreements on display at the congressional hearings, Brandt, at the urging of the Public Health Service's (PHS) low birth weight working group, informed all state health departments that provisional data for 1984 indicated a "general slowdown in the rate of decline in IMR." A task force of experts was made available to assist states in reversing the trend.[84] That same year, the Southern Governors' Association formed the Southern Regional Task Force on Infant Mortality and published findings that ten of eleven southern states had the highest rates of infant death in the nation.[85] Their landmark "Final Report: For the Children of Tomorrow" urged the federal government to amend Medicaid so that states could provide coverage to families without having to also make AFDC payments.[86]

At the same time, the Black-white disparity, along with data showing a five-year gap in life expectancy between Black and white Americans, finally forced Secretary Heckler to convene a panel on minority health. What came to be known as the Heckler Report, published in 1985, identified infant mortality as one of six causes of death that accounted for the racial disparity in life expectancy.[87] A year later, the Institute of Medicine (IOM) published a report that established low birth weight as the leading factor associated with infant mortality and endorsed early initiation of prenatal care as the most important step towards curbing the problem.[88] In his 1985 award-winning *Scientific American* article, C. Arden Miller, an IOM committee member and leading expert on maternal and child health, popularized both the IOM's findings and stakeholders' claim that Reagan-era cutbacks were responsible for the slowdown in infant mortality decline.[89] And also in 1985 as part of his work with the Southern Regional Task Force, Congressman Lawton Chiles of Florida introduced a bill that would establish a National Commission on Infant Mortality with the aim of developing a national policy.[90]

As infant mortality became a bipartisan issue, arguments about the cost savings of providing prenatal care to high-risk women replaced indictments of the Reagan administration. The IOM report legitimated what advocates and physicians had been saying for over a decade: that most of the decline in infant mortality during the second half of the twentieth century was due to keeping low birth weight babies alive through neonatal technologies—an exorbitantly expensive approach to curbing infant death. It also offered a cost-benefit analysis that lawmakers on both sides of the aisle would make use of. The report estimated that reducing the incidence of low birth weight infants through additional investment in prenatal care would save money overall.[91] The Southern Governors' Association also emphasized cost. The congressional hearings dedicated to establishing a national commission emphasized that "the annual cost of neonatal intensive care in the United States exceeds $1.5 billion" and highlighted research recently completed at Harvard that found treating the consequences of low birth weight to be three times more expensive than funding WIC.[92]

If liberal stakeholders used the IMR to focus on the so-called unborn children a hypocritical pro-life administration had abandoned, the bipartisan uptake and growing national attention brought certain mothers into view, particularly Black teenagers. Despite the IOM's findings that "teenage mothers have many other risk factors that could be responsible for an adverse pregnancy outcome," maternal age became one of the most discussed risk factors for low birth weight and infant mortality.[93] For example, the *Washington Post* interviewed pediatrician Dr. Robert L. Johnson, who informed readers that "a large proportion of infant deaths among blacks . . . is a result of the high pregnancy rate among teen-agers who do not know how to care for themselves or their infants."[94] The Southern Governors' Association also did much to solidify the link between teen pregnancy and infant mortality. Representative Chiles attributed southern states' outsized rates of infant mortality directly to teenage pregnancies, while other governors repeatedly emphasized that it was this factor that alerted them to the problem of infant death in the first place.[95] In turn, mayors and foundations began to look at teen pregnancy, which incentivized advocacy groups concerned with infant mortality and dependent on grant-based funding to do the same.[96] Local task force reports began routinely recommending a reduction in rates of teen pregnancy as part of the solution to addressing infant mortality.[97] And the Children's Defense Fund began campaigning to make teen pregnancy a national concern.[98]

The widely accepted assumption that teen pregnancy caused poverty also meant that conversations about poor children were centered on Black welfare recipients. In 1985, the *New York Times* reported that 22 percent of Americans under the age of eighteen were living in poverty, a nearly 10 percent increase from 1970, with over half of these children living in households headed by single mothers. Arguments about the failure of African Americans to achieve the patriarchal, nuclear family structure fashioned during debates over welfare in the 1960s persisted through the 1980s. A chief architect of such arguments, Democratic Senator Daniel P.

Moynihan, told the *New York Times* in 1985 that "a family is formed when a child is born. When an unwed teenager gives birth, a broken family is formed."[99] He was far from alone in his thinking.[100] The fact that family making so out of step with the traditional nuclear family would result in poverty and infant death seemed almost axiomatic to those disturbed by the decline in males as heads of households—outpaced by unmarried, young Black mothers.

With the financial cost of neonatal intensive care and the moral cost of teen pregnancy both securely attached to infant mortality, the bipartisan stakeholders were at last able to free Medicaid from the constraints of AFDC income eligibility levels. Reagan's Omnibus Budget and Reconciliation Act (OBRA 1986) gave states the option to raise income eligibility thresholds for Medicaid coverage above AFDC levels for pregnant women to as high as the federal poverty level. Within one year of the initial effective date of the law, half of the states had expanded eligibility to 100 percent of the federal poverty level. OBRA 1986 initiated a series of legislative victories that slowly but surely increased pregnant women's and children's access to Medicaid through mandates. And with the implementation of OBRA 1989, states were required to cover pregnant women and children up to six years of age at 133 percent of the poverty level.[101] Reflecting on Medicaid expansion in 1989, Congressman Waxman explained that the legislation reflected "a strongly held conviction on the part of many in the Congress that the nation must invest in the health of its children, and that the Medicaid program is an effective investment vehicle." By framing prenatal care as the panacea for infant mortality, one that was effective because it was prudent, a diverse coalition of stakeholders succeeded in disentangling Medicaid and welfare. Significantly, this newfound "investment vehicle" was a precise instrument that carved out some of the population as deserving of medical care while leaving the deservingness of anyone who was not a pregnant woman, a child over six years of age, or who continued to receive Medicaid via AFDC vulnerable to scorn and neglect.[102]

While Medicaid expansion represented a significant feat given the Reagan administration's strategy of scapegoating poor, Black mothers to justify slashing social programs, a return to the local level demonstrates the limits of targeted programs that leave the parsing of populations intact. In 1989, a health advocacy group in Pennsylvania released their findings from an investigation into the state's Medicaid expansion initiative Healthy Beginnings. The report found that information about the program was poorly disseminated, that workers in county assistance offices were reluctant to provide details about the program and often did not mention (or provided inaccurate information about) the program, that only twenty-seven of Pennsylvania's sixty-seven counties had presumptive eligibility providers, and that enrolling in the program required two trips to the assistance office. The report also assessed Medicaid provider capacity and found that for the state as a whole only 18 percent of physicians qualified as "active" participants in the program. Eligibility may have expanded, but service delivery mechanisms remained corrupted by the profitability of private health insurance and overall negligence.[103]

Such administrative hurdles to Medicaid expansion simply added to the task advocacy groups faced in stemming the tide of insecurity that had dramatically expanded women's reproductive labor during this period. By the late 1980s, one of MCC's longtime outreach coordinator was assisting hundreds of women per year to obtain not only medical care but also welfare, WIC, support with utilities, and, increasingly, access to emergency housing.[104] The MCC understood this work to be "risk reduction" and deemed it necessary to achieving its goal of reducing "the number of high-risk pregnant women who suffer from acute stress and deprivation as the result of sudden, unanticipated loss of food, housing, clothing, medicine, basic living money."[105] Of course, the irony of severing Medicaid from AFDC for the purpose of delivering prenatal care was that medical care—and a very specific, limited form of medical care at that—was the sole intervention for conditions worsened by AFDC's continued inaccessibility.

Activists in Oakland had also confronted the problems raised by the severing of AFDC and Medicaid. Not only had a focus on the effect (infant death) ensured that the solution (prenatal care) was narrowly focused there as well, but the pliability of the IMR made it possible to justify a number of different narratives. Advocates invoked social conditions to press for greater support from health officials, while conservatives and liberals alike linked the IMR to unmarried teen pregnancy. And public officials had often dumped the task of remedying societal conditions back into advocates' laps. Philadelphia city health commissioner Dr. Maurice C. Clifford, for example, defended his administration's limited action on infant mortality by casting it as a larger "societal problem" rather than "the city's problem. I view infant mortality as an index of poverty. My feeling is that until there are stronger programs of social welfare in the broadest sense there is likely to be a continuation of the high level of infant mortality."[106] In Clifford's assessment social welfare programs were not within his purview. As a result, the city was justified in sitting on its proverbial hands while advocates and the families they worked with picked up the slack resulting from government inaction.

UNTANGLING VARIABLES AND CONFRONTING RACISM

Beginning in the early 1980s, some health researchers set out to see if they could develop more precise measures of risk in hopes of clarifying the relationship between social and biological health. Some did so by wading into one of the more politically charged maternal indicators linked to infant mortality—teen pregnancy. Teen pregnancy was considered a risk factor for two reasons, one biological (teenagers are biologically immature, which ostensibly complicates birth outcomes) and one social (teenagers may fail to start prenatal care early in their pregnancies out of ignorance or irresponsibility). In 1986, Arline T. Geronimus, a white public health researcher, published an article in the December issue of *American Journal of Public Health* that took aim at both assumptions. Echoing the IOM report, she established that biological immaturity was at best a partial explanation for the relationship between teenage pregnancy and poor birth outcomes. What she described as the "confounding of the age/mortality association" revealed that pregnant teenagers under seventeen were more likely to be Black, to live in rural areas, and to receive inadequate prenatal care—things she classified as environmental indicators. She also noted that had teenage pregnancies been removed from the data set, the racial disparity in mortality rates would have barely changed. This necessarily undermined the idea that teen pregnancy was a causal factor in the racial disparity. Lastly, Geronimus found that Black women in their twenties and thirties had *higher* rates of low birth weight and neonatal mortality than white teenagers older than fourteen and Black teenagers older than sixteen.[107]

Cutting through the tendency to imprecisely narrate risk factors, Geronimus posed a clarifying question: "What do maternal-age variables measure? Do they measure true age effects or are they proxies for social or environmental factors that are related both to age at first birth and to neonatal mortality?" Geronimus's query struck at the cordoning off of risk. Such distinctions did not only apply to policy debates, but shaped entire fields of health knowledge and had resulted in "a meaning of teenage childbearing that restricted comprehension of the physiologically mediated social processes that may lead to excessive neonatal mortality in the United States."[108] In other words, researchers did not truly understand how the "acute stress and deprivation" highlighted by the MCC operated *through the body* to shape one's odds of birthing an infant that would not live to see their first birthday.

Geronimus took inspiration from two researchers who aimed to rectify this knowledge gap with what they called a "proximal determinants framework," which suggested infant mortality be understood as "the ultimate consequence of a cumulative series of biological insults."[109] Specifically, Geronimus saw a way to explore how researchers had confounded maternal age (teen pregnancy) with environmental disadvantage (racism, poverty, region, healthcare access). Despite the fact that teenage pregnancy was explicitly and implicitly associated with both blackness and poverty in popular discussions and policy debates, maternal age was so widely accepted as an independent risk variable that Geronimus had to make the following claim: "In the United States the populations with high rates of teenage childbearing are the same populations most subject to predisposing risk factors for neonatal mortality and that are least able to obtain adequate medical service." Ignoring this reality meant researchers might have missed far more significant risk factors for infant mortality.[110]

An article published by Geronimus in 1986 (on teenage childbearing and neonatal mortality) refuted the commonly held idea "that excessive neonatal mortality among Blacks is due to the greater frequency of teenage childbearing among Blacks."[111] This study showed that Black women in their prime childbearing years (twenties through early thirties) exhibited *higher* rates of low birth weight and neonatal mortality than their younger counterparts, both Black and white.[112] The body of work by Geronimus and some of her colleagues led to a conclusion that further

challenged the status quo: teen pregnancy was not a cause of infant mortality, and indeed, being a teenager might actually *increase* Black women's
chances for a healthy birth outcome. Health disparities between Black
and white women as well as differential access to medical care likely
accounted for some racial disparity in birth outcomes. For example, the
fact that twice as many Black women as white women entered their pregnancies with preexistent chronic hypertension surely was more relevant
than maternal age at first birth.[113] Moreover, researchers suggested that
such health disparities would worsen over time. "We expect all women,
black or white, to experience decreases in health status as they grow older,
but we see indications here that the health of U.S. black women (who are
more disadvantaged than white women as a group) . . . deteriorates more
rapidly than that of white women."[114] Whereas the Bay Area economist
who created a measurement of "expected IMR" had suggested that "Black
ethnicity" might be the key to low birth weights, these researchers honed
in on racism and poverty as factors that negatively impacted health.

Geronimus was not the only researcher to challenge common assumptions about teen pregnancy during this period, but she did assert her
position "forcefully" and publicly.[115] She was met with equally forceful
criticism. Her detractors balked at the suggestion that there might be a
health advantage to teen pregnancy. Karen Pittman, a Black advocate with
the Children's Defense Fund, accused Geronimus of getting her facts
wrong and worried about the "perverse" implications such an argument
might have for policy development.[116] For Pittman, who believed young
Black women were "drawn to parenthood like a magnet," education and
employment initiatives were necessary to "buy the girl time."[117] The CEO
of Planned Parenthood of Washington, DC, accused Geronimus of depict-
ing teen pregnancy as "a positive" choice.[118] And Colbert I. King, a Black
editorialist for the *Washington Post*, accused Geronimus of racism by likening her argument to that of a "slave owner" who believed Black women's
only role was to have babies.[119]

That Geronimus's critics believed her research was saying something
about a lack of will on the part of young, poor, African American women,
rather than highlighting the circumstances that structured their lives, illuminated in part the extent of her critics' investment in the ideal of a nuclear,
middle-class family, purportedly achievable (and supposedly desirable) for

both Black and white Americans with the right mix of government programs and personal responsibility. In response, Geronimus defended her
research in a variety of venues, and called out her critics for their own misleading distortions and omissions.[120] She also refined her statements. In
her 1991 article for *Family Relations*, Geronimus dropped the language of
rationality and sensibility that had been twisted into willful choice and
instead foregrounded the conditions of marginalization that demanded a
different metric for evaluating costs: "Consideration of these health issues,
along with others, suggests that there may be heretofore unrecognized
advantages, along with lower costs, of early fertility among members of
extremely disadvantaged groups." These advantages were primarily about
besting the biological effects of inequality—younger women were in better
reproductive health than their plus-twenty-year-old peer group because
they had spent fewer years accumulating insults to their health.[121]

Ultimately, Geronimus laid out the theory that would become the defining contribution of her career: "weathering." The idea that "length of exposure to life conditions" either undermined or promoted one's health to
a cumulative effect was invoked to suggest that the entirety of an individual's advantages and disadvantages determined their health—and by
extension, their birth outcomes. When Geronimus suggested that "the
'whole' of the impact of racial discrimination or other socioeconomic disadvantages on infant income may be importantly larger than the sum of its
identifiable maternal health-related parts," she echoed activists in Oakland
who cautioned supporters against parsing Carolyn's intersecting vulnerabilities. She also sided with outreach workers who knew all too well the
limitation of targeted tinkering when she suggested that "significant lasting reductions in black infant mortality rates would not be achieved
through an exclusive focus in the content or distribution of prenatal care."
Pittman was right that Geronimus's results had significant policy implications, but they exposed the perverse impact of societal neglect while lending quantitative support for the broadscale changes activists believed
could bring an end to such costly vulnerability once and for all.[122]

Such views proved prescient. While a 1991 GAO report showed that
Medicaid expansion had significantly increased the number of women
receiving prenatal care, research evaluating the effect of increased enrollments on low birth weight and preterm births showed that prenatal care

had done little to improve these indicators.[123] By the end of the 1990s, more women were accessing prenatal care, but low birth weight and pre-term births were on the rise, with the Black-white disparity still firmly in place. As one researcher put it, albeit with the benefit of hindsight, "it could be argued that in the US the decrease in infant mortality rates that has occurred in spite of rises in the rates of low birthweight and preterm births reflects the failure of public health approaches and, conversely, the success of high-tech medical advances."[124] Medicaid expansion was marshaled to target the IMR, but the dismal conditions the measurement gave expression to were still being triaged with expensive, invasive medical care rather than targeting their roots.

CONCLUSION

In 1989, Bill Clinton, then chairman of the Southern Corporate Coalition to Improve Maternal and Child Health, espoused the logic that had made Medicaid expansion possible under the Reagan administration. "Infants die daily because they and their mothers are not afforded the luxury of medical attention. . . . Many of these deaths can be prevented simply by providing comprehensive health care for nine short months during the mother's pregnancy."[125] What the Coalition to Fight Infant Mortality insisted was a human right in 1980 and what the Maternity Care Coalition believed could only be justly administered with patient-consumer participation, healthcare instead had become a "luxury" item poor women deserved only when pregnant with "unborn children."

Confronted with unequivocal data on the limits of prenatal care, by the mid-1990s health researchers and organizations began championing "pre-conception care"—getting women healthy *before* their pregnancies—as the solution to stubbornly persistent low birth weight and premature birth.[126] At the same time, legislators continued to place barriers between families and good health. When President Bill Clinton signed the Personal Responsibility and Work Opportunity Reconciliation Act in 1996, he and other lawmakers understood that as long as AFDC and Medicaid were intertwined, the aid program benefited from "welfare medicine's" cover. This pairing was severed with welfare reform, a separation that the legislative decisions of the prior decade laid the groundwork for by weakening ties between Medicaid and the cash welfare system.[127] The oft quoted "end of welfare as we know it" meant that AFDC recipients who continued to access Medicaid by way of welfare rolls would join "expansion-eligible" women who qualified for coverage only upon proof of pregnancy. Researchers assessing the impacts of welfare reform on Medicaid access would ultimately conclude that low-income pregnant women had a harder time accessing medical coverage prior to pregnancy—the period of "preconception care" researchers believed was vital for healthy birth outcomes.[128]

The IMR proved to be a formidable organizing tool. Risk factors could be isolated in misleading ways and narrated to wildly different ends, and solutions tended towards treating the effect (infant death). Families and their advocates attempted to make such solutions as expansive as possible, proposing care that addressed things patients themselves considered essential for their health. Such care was not forthcoming. Instead, stakeholders that achieved Medicaid expansion bracketed women's health into "nine short months" of prenatal care that was meant to prevent infant death. This outcome was aided by more than the pliability of the IMR. Broader political and economic trends also set limits on political will: shifting views about government's role in addressing racial and economic inequality, the dominance of pro-life ideology, rising healthcare costs; strapped local and state budgets, anxiety about the dissolution of the nuclear family, and racism that vilified Black, teen mothers. Together, these forces made providing women prenatal care palatable precisely because it did not pose too great a challenge to any of the aforementioned viewpoints and trends.

Reflecting on a decade of work, MCC member Lear wrote, "no sooner is one systemic problem solved then several new ones emerge."[129] Lear's observation conjures an image of plugging a hole in a dike just to have another plume of water burst through somewhere else. In the case of Medicaid expansion, a repair—prenatal care—came at the cost of an ever-widening crack —welfare. Advocates working with pregnant women at the ground level experienced firsthand the futility of separating medical care from social programs from cash support. And even without Geronimus's measurements, the advocacy coalitions CFIM and MCC understood racism, poverty, sexism, and neglect intersected to exact a biological toll on the health of mothers and their infants. Indeed, CFIM's example of

Carolyn's encounter with a dismissive, prejudiced physician anticipated research on the deadly effects of medical racism and sexism for Black women regardless of socioeconomic status.[130] But such systemic, intersectional analyses were continuously elided by debates over the IMR and the pressure to make impossible calculations about what most imperiled poor, Black women's health. As families and their advocates expanded the reproductive labor of family making to include day-to-day survival under state neglect, they suffered the incalculable costs of that neglect—the loss of an infant, which often lead to self-blame.

The fight over how to curb infant death was one of two developments that underscored just how deadly neglect could be. Families at the margins were pushed further still by the arrival of the HIV/AIDS epidemic and the criminally negligent response of the Reagan administration to its devastating effects. In the face of this public health crisis, and with no federal response forthcoming, mothers, caretakers, and their advocates quickly learned that they would be responsible for managing their own and their families' risk and illness. As the 1980s came to a close, the HIV/AIDS epidemic remade reproductive labor yet again as families confronted cumulative neglect, pushed past the breaking point by disease.

4 The Labor of Risk

OR, HOW TO HAVE A FAMILY IN THE
HIV/AIDS EPIDEMIC

If you put a catastrophic illness on women who are
on welfare, you get a crisis.

Testimony from a woman with AIDS, San Francisco, 1990

In 1985, the Public Health Service (PHS) Task Force on Women's Health issued a report titled, simply, "Women's Health." Assembled two years earlier, the task force was charged by Assistant Secretary of Health Edward Brandt with assessing women's health in the context of rapid changes to women's expectations and roles in American society. "In recent decades, women in the United States have undergone a revolution in their self-perception and their traditional relationships to work, money, marriage, and family." With this "panoply of opportunity," Brandt believed, came the necessity of identifying the new and different "health risks . . . most striking in today's environment."[1]

Brandt was not wrong about women's new roles, though many women would likely have disagreed with his characterization of the mid-1980s as offering a "panoply of opportunity." It was true that by the early 1980s a greater percentage of the nation's lawyers, judges, and physicians were women, though those increases barely made a dent in the male-dominated professions.[2] Poor and working-class families, however, could speak of no such a "panoply," as "the results of Reagan-era policies were very quickly grim." Between 1980 and 1984, the bottom one-fifth of American families saw their incomes decrease by 9 percent, and African American families made up close to a half of this quintile.[3] This trend was especially pronounced for families headed by women. By 1983 families headed by single mothers comprised three-quarters of all poor, Black families. For the women who could actually find consistent work, racism and sexism in the labor market greatly curtailed their earning power, and neither the available work nor wages ensured that getting a job was worth the stress (and expense) of figuring out child care.[4] When wages had not been sufficient to make ends meet a decade prior, women had relied on welfare checks. But by 1985, the real value of aid provided through AFDC had declined 33 percent over the past fifteen years. Federal allocations for day-care programs were also cut during Reagan's first year in office, making it harder for poor and low-income mothers to "balance" care work with wage work, however limited.[5] These constraints were piled on top of massive reductions in federal contributions to Medicaid via Reagan's first budget discussed in the previous chapter, ensuring that an already over-strained public healthcare system was made weaker still.[6]

Brandt's report did acknowledge poverty as a significant barrier to women's health—he allowed that "the relationship between poverty and ill health cannot be overemphasized." But it was women's undeniable membership in the category of "worker" that the report believed necessitated an updated assessment of women's health. In light of this new role, Brandt made sure that the task force did not focus "strictly on the diseases and problems unique to women in the traditional sense—that is reproductive problems." Instead, the report claimed to be a clear-eyed assessment of women's health "in the context of the lives women in America lead today." Osteoporosis, diabetes, hypertension, cancer, arthritis, cosmetic surgery, and the importance of exercise were given their due alongside pregnancy, childbearing, sexually transmitted diseases, and women's disproportionate child care responsibilities. The diverse list of "striking" health issues attempted to convey Brandt's acknowledgement that, by 1985, women could and should be more than just mothers. But the persistence of women's caretaking responsibilities made this a sticking point. The task force, implicitly acknowledging the "feminization of poverty," a term coined by sociologist Diana Pearce in a 1978 article, explained that "women now living in poverty are unable to break a cycle in which financial demands are complicated by unanticipated events and the available resources in the family budget are stretched beyond their capacity." This situation was even more pronounced for single mothers responsible for the "sole support of her family."[7]

Whether the report imagined these "unanticipated events" as health-related, the insight perfectly described how one health issue—disease—collided with poverty to threaten families' survival. This was what happened with a health concern that, despite being omitted from the report, was certainly "most striking" in some women's lives by 1985: the arrival of HIV/AIDS. Shortly after Brandt's report, for example, the percentage of women who had gotten AIDS through heterosexual contact more than doubled in a four-year period. Whereas this group comprised 12 percent of cases in 1982, it had reached 26 percent by 1986. The vast majority were Black or Latina women of childbearing age.[8] Reagan's infamous refusal to utter the word *AIDS* publicly until 1986 offers a partial explanation for the task force's omission.[9] The stories physicians, epidemiologists, and public health officials told the nation about the disease during these critical first years shed additional light. In spite of the fact that theirs were among the earliest cases reported, in 1985 women still had not been designated an official risk group by the Centers for Disease Control (CDC), due to the overwhelming consensus that HIV primarily infected gay men.[10] When the CDC finally did investigate seroprevalence in women, authorities limited their studies to sex workers because of the prevalent, if unfounded, belief among medical professionals that drug-using sex workers were the inevitable and exclusive source of transmission via heterosexual sex.[11] The official CDC definition of AIDS created in 1982 was based on manifestations of the disease found more commonly in men than in women, which left out many women living with HIV as well as those who had died from AIDS undiagnosed (and uncounted) for at least the first fifteen years of the epidemic.[12] Such was the dominant epidemiological construction of AIDS and its perceived risk groups during the first decade of the epidemic.

In other words, Brandt's task force was hardly alone in its omission. Then again, maybe the decision to omit AIDS from the list of "health risks most striking in today's environment" was strategic. Just as the issue of working women's concomitant child care responsibilities threatened to do, a discussion of the epidemic among women would have foiled Brandt's overarching aim to move the nation beyond a conception of women's health rooted in reproduction. The life-threatening reality of the epidemic was an "unanticipated event" that stressed families already on the margins like few other constraints had. The women to whom such a weighty task fell would return again and again to "reproductive problems"—supposedly outmoded by the mid-1980s—due to the mountain of reproductive labor required for their own and their families' survival. As evidenced by the brief epidemiological tour above, survival necessarily included a task stemming directly from officials' neglect of the epidemic generally, and its impacts on women specifically: women's work now included managing their own and their families' risk in the face of a deadly disease, a risk few others were willing to assess accurately.

Accurate designation and construction of risk were the missing links. Feminist scholars have shown how epidemiological reports, media accounts, and treatment interventions positioned women not as a risk group in and of themselves, but as a group that *posed* risk to other populations. Those struggling to spark a response to women's experiences of illness in the early years of the epidemic often used the language of invisibility to describe research, treatment interventions, and media coverage that was intent on cordoning off middle-class, white, heterosexual women from risk of infection. But such invisibility was paired with the positioning of women as vectors of risk and infection, a representation that resulted in women's hypervisibility.[13] Writing in 1994, AIDS activist and theorist Cindy Patton described this latter tendency bluntly: "When women are not vaginas waiting to infect men, they are uteruses waiting to infect fetuses."[14]

There is truth to this frame, to be sure. Both in the egregiously irresponsible media coverage and the very architecture of epidemiological categories, the only women who received attention as the exceptions to the "gay" epidemic were framed as sex workers, drug addicts, or monstrous mothers. Women were identified as transmogrified vectors of disease rather than potential victims of infection. But this frame also prioritizes sexism and racism in their most explicit manifestations, making it harder to see the ways women were harmed by rampant neglect. If the media-fueled specters of contagious hookers and selfish mothers were made to do the cultural work of (inaccurately) representing risk for a fearful and ignorant public, women with HIV and AIDS were made to do the work of managing a variety of risks wrought by the epidemic and exacerbated by unabated state neglect. Much of this work centered around issues of reproduction: the day-to-day caretaking of sick children and partners, possible teratogenic effects of experimental treatments, and raising children while themselves terminally ill. These challenges certainly were made harder by sexist and racist tropes that inevitably shaped public responses to and women's experiences of the epidemic. But they were also hard for the simple fact that women were left to manage these often-unacknowledged risks on their own.

Reproduction repeatedly reared its head in the epidemic because the disease pressed upon aspects of women's lives that had been consistently undervalued and deliberately neglected before the arrival of HIV/AIDS. The negligent response to the epidemic only exacerbated vulnerabilities produced by cumulative neglect. That those who fell ill were largely abandoned by government officials collided with a belief, fostered by the Reagan administration, that a single mother's destitution was a result of irresponsible decision-making, and thus hers to weather alone.[15] Neglect, as always, both narrowed the available options and created more work for reproductive laborers, and the new task of risk management amidst a public health crisis often entailed impossible calculations about survival. The AIDS epidemic and the nation's response further stratified family making. State neglect in the face of the terminal illness that ravaged different marginalized communities ensured that accessing and maintaining family became more difficult as the twentieth century approached its end.

EXPANDING THE TERMS (AND LABORS) OF RISK

"The growing number of women with HIV disease parallels a rise in cancer, drug use, homelessness, incarceration, and poverty among women."[16] By 1990, when the *Women, AIDS, and Activism* anthology written by women and AIDS activists in New York was published, ACT UP member Risa Denenberg's assertion was hardly controversial. What many described as the "changing demographics" of the epidemic had garnered greater attention by the early 1990s. By this time, women, particularly poor and low-income Black and Latina women of childbearing age, made up the fastest growing population of newly infected individuals.[17] Furthermore, advocates, by now armed with more research on infection indicators and disease progression in women, were suggesting that HIV/AIDS had always been high in poor communities of color but had gone undiagnosed as a result of inaccessible and unaffordable healthcare.[18] Articles with titles like "The New Face of AIDS" and "Black Women and AIDS: The Second Epidemic" illustrated how identity indexed risk and infection and announced a distinct shift from gay, white men to poor, women of color. In the eyes of some AIDS activists, this shift opened up a different context for understanding the disease. Poverty, racism, inaccessible healthcare, homelessness, drug use, and sexism—constraints largely absent from the lives of the so-called original "face of AIDS"—were helping spread the disease and quicken its effects in this already vulnerable population. Some physicians examining HIV in women agreed. A 1989 article in the *Journal of the American Medical Association* asserted, "control of HIV infection in this population can only be accomplished if the social ills that feed the epidemic are addressed concurrently with the medical problem."[19] AIDS activist Judy Gerber, writing in 1991 about Black women with AIDS, put it more succinctly. "Its [AIDS] impact on a community is defined not by T-cell counts, but by social and economic conditions."[20]

Before widespread acknowledgement of the "second epidemic," gay and lesbian communities responded to the disease when it was clear that official recognition, much less significant federal aid, was nowhere on the horizon. As ACT UP member Vito Russo put it at a 1988 demonstration, the silence from both lawmakers and the public at large made "living with AIDS . . . like living in the twilight zone. Living with AIDS is like living through a war which is happening only for those people who happen to be in the trenches . . . you look around and you discover that you've lost more of your friends, but nobody else notices. . . . And only you can hear the screams of the people who are dying and their cries for help."[21] The extraordinary efforts of early, volunteer-run AIDS service organizations (ASOs), and their varied limits, are well documented.[22] The conditions that drove the percentage of women officially diagnosed with HIV steadily upward throughout the 1980s—from 3 percent in 1981 to 9 percent in 1989— have received less attention.[23] The so-called new face of the epidemic did not occur overnight, but was hidden and then fueled by the disease's collision with other preexisting insecurities as well as early decisions about how to respond to HIV/AIDs in that first decade.[24] For poor and low-income women of color who made up the disproportionate number of women who contracted HIV in the early years, these insecurities comprised the stuff of survival: housing, food, income, healthcare, welfare, child care—basic necessities that had not been forthcoming from strapped municipalities even before the arrival of AIDS.[25] Both illness and state neglect exacerbated these realities, adding a new task to women's caring labor: managing risk for themselves and their loved ones. The first years of the epidemic, then, were comprised of grassroots interventions attempting to combat not only governmental neglect of the epidemic, but also longer-standing inequalities that had set women up for greater vulnerability to infection and death. The task at hand was at least twofold. Women needed to become epidemiologically legible, capable of risk in their own right; and women's "risk" needed to be broadened dramatically. It was not sufficient for risk only to index infection. It should also encompass one's proximity to various forms of insecurity produced and exacerbated by the cumulative neglect of women's caretaking roles, in particular. Long before poor, Black and Latina women were officially recognized as the "new face" of the epidemic, the conditions in which they first confronted the disease ensured this would be their fate.

When Laurie Hauer attended the second national forum on AIDS in Denver in 1983, there were no workshops on women and AIDS. She posted a note inviting women doing AIDS work to meet in a hotel room, and by the time the forum ended a founding statement drafted by the thirty-five women who responded to Hauer's call made the Women's AIDS Network (WAN) official.[26] The group of mostly white healthcare and legal professionals was conceived as part resource development, part member-based education. Those working primarily with gay men diagnosed with HIV hoped to counter the lack of information about women just as much as they sought to educate themselves on what issues they had yet to consider. As the network approached the end of its first year, members agreed that their main goals remained "monitoring and encouraging the development of resources for women" as well as the "education of ourselves and others about women and AIDS."[27]

In contrast, women incarcerated at Bedford Hills Correctional Facility in New York experienced the issue of the epidemic in women firsthand when a woman died of AIDS in 1985. She spent her last night alive in the infirmary unit, effectively quarantined because no medical or correctional staff were willing to assist her for fear of infection. Six women responded to the "the accelerating incidence of acquired immune deficiency syndrome and related conditions" documented in a correctional report by forming the AIDS Counseling and Education (ACE) program, which, after a period of stonewalling on the part of the prison, became active in 1988.[28] ACE asserted definitively that "there are women who are incarcerated who are dying of AIDS" while also contextualizing the epidemic within prior constraints. ACE made clear that "the crisis faced by our community is broader than the number of women who are formally diagnosed as having AIDS at any given moment."[29]

Service providers working in New York and New Jersey also saw the impact of the epidemic on women firsthand—even though women who fell ill and died rarely received an official AIDS diagnosis. This growing trend prompted women in New York to form the Women and AIDS Project (WAP) in 1986 in order to share more and better information about the epidemic in women. That same year, the Women and AIDS Resource Network (WARN) also formed in New York to serve as a support group for women of color diagnosed with HIV or living with AIDS.[30] Such early responses were not limited to coastal cities. The Feminist Women's Health Center in Atlanta added testing for HIV/AIDS to its services during this same period, and in 1987 center staff member Dázon Dixon Diallo created the Women with AIDS Partnership Project (WAPP) to provide education to the poor, Black women who were disproportionately being infected with HIV in the Southeast.[31] Two years later, Diallo would found SisterLove, the first HIV/AIDS organization dedicated to serving women of color in the region.

Early projects focusing on women with AIDS were motivated by the realization that although the lives of women and children were being "so disastrously affected by AIDS and ARC [AIDS-related complex]," few others seemed willing even to acknowledge this fact. It was hoped that advocacy would bring an end to "operating in nearly total isolation."[32] Projects focused on women with AIDS stepped into the public debate about the epidemic that was being shaped in equal parts by silence about women's risk and wildly misleading information about transmission. Setting to work correcting this situation in various parts of the country and through different tactics, advocates were largely united by a belief that the epidemic should be approached from the perspective of those most impacted.

More AIDS cases in women were emerging in both the Bay Area and the Southeast; New York, New Jersey, and Florida were seeing their already high numbers continuing to grow; and it was becoming clear that the majority of women who contracted the virus also struggled with poverty, unstable housing, drug use, intimate violence, and child care. This compelled early AIDS projects focused on women to grapple with overwhelming material realities, which had been shaped by intersecting and multiple layers of neglect. At the federal level, the epidemic's first decade was defined by the Reagan administration's refusal to request the necessary funds required to meet the scale of the epidemic, its willingness to allow even those funds allocated by Congress to go unspent, and internal debates among administration officials over how to address AIDS that delayed public health guidance.[33] As a result, one of the first roles these varied grassroots efforts filled was producing and disseminating accurate information about the disease, transmission, and risk. The Women with AIDS Partnership Project (WAPP) hosted "Do It Safe" parties in public housing projects, drug treatment programs, and homeless shelters, while the Women's Aids Network (WAN) distributed a pamphlet to fill the information vacuum on the disease.[34] So vast was the vacuum that six years after WAN's 1983 formation, it was still receiving requests for materials on the epidemic in women from public health officials in other states.[35]

Getting out accurate AIDS education in the crisis was vital but addressed only one component of the existing need. In addition to insufficient budget allocations at all levels of government, the fact that AIDS had first been constructed as a "gay disease" greatly impacted women's eligibility for disability payments. The battle to expand the CDC's definition, and thus to open up public coffers, would not make aid available to women until the early 1990s. In the intervening years, the neglect specific to the epidemic collided with widening inequalities. Not mentioned in Brandt's discussion of the "feminization of poverty" was how the administration of which he was a part fueled the trend. For example, Reagan's cuts to the Department of Housing and Urban Development (HUD) ensured women and children comprised a significant portion of the homeless for the first time in the nation's history.[36] The administration also levied drastic cuts to the budgets and staff of federal civil rights programs, such as the Equal Employment Opportunity Commission (EEOC), which resulted in far less litigation and governmental disciplinary action to remedy instances of discrimination in housing and employment.[37] As women attempted to mitigate increasing precarity by engaging in illicit economies, they faced greater criminalization, which then moved them from one space of neglect (economic insecurity) to another (prisons and jails, the subject of chapter 2). The administration's heavy reliance on block grants—which gave states less money and more discretion in spending—dramatically curtailed healthcare services for the poor. Medicaid took a hit, but so did preventive health programs, health resources, health services, and alcohol, drug abuse and mental health programs.[38] These multiple constraints meant that women waited until they were in "a crisis state . . . out of money, without housing or hope," to seek medical help. Further complicating matters was the association between AIDS and same-sex sexuality, and the fact that ASOs were largely ensconced in gay communities. Women were unlikely to access emergency services through an "AIDS door" that in both public perception and services rendered was open widest to gay men.[39] Lastly, women's caretaking responsibilities were carried out with greatly diminished public support. The Women's and AIDS Resource Network (WARN) put it best when they explained that women's "day-to-day problems—with housing, jobs, medical and social services, child care, and bills—are intensified beyond description by AIDS and HIV infection."[40] State neglect for the bare necessities was greatly magnified by the epidemic, leaving poor and low-income women of color with children especially vulnerable to the additional precarity of illness.

In sum, advocacy groups quickly learned that examining the epidemic from the vantage point of women meant unraveling a thread of neglect spun long before the arrival of AIDS. The fact that the disease "disproportionately affects women with the fewest resources and those least able to bear its burdens" meant both women and the early projects focused on their needs confronted a reality in which constraints multiplied to ensure risk, infection, and death were unequally distributed.[41] WARN's profile of the women it served in New York City made this clear: "Primarily African-American and Hispanic women, with a high school diploma, unemployed or underemployed, head of household, 4.5 children, with a history of substance and/or physical abuse."[42] A positive diagnosis did not even warrant mention. At hearings on AIDS/ARC–related discrimination, WAN member Nancy Stoller Shaw told the San Francisco Human Rights Commission that the problem of AIDS in women was compounded by the city's existing health and social service system, an infrastructure "already inadequate to meet their needs."[43] Upon learning that three more women in San Francisco had been diagnosed with AIDS in 1986, WAN members noted, "There is no place for a woman with a drug problem, with kids, with or without AIDS or positive anti-body status to go in this city."[44] The epidemic exposed and exacerbated but did not create the already insufficient support structures available to women struggling on the margins.

Amidst these various issues, women's familial obligations repeatedly emerged as the most pressing concern. The list was long. First and foremost was the reality articulated by WARN. "These women—predominately women of color/Third World women—must cope with their own illness and the illnesses of their spouse, sibling, child or grandchild."[45] Women living with HIV and AIDS often put the care of loved ones before their own health. The lack of family-friendly services was also a major issue. No residential treatment programs in San Francisco, for example, would accept a woman in the late stages of pregnancy because such facilities were not equipped for infants. When WAN attempted to make residential services at larger ASOs available to women and children, they were told by one that "children would have too much energy and be too difficult to live with."[46] WAN also fielded complaints from mothers whose children were removed from daycare once providers found out they were HIV-positive, in accordance with the San Francisco Department of Public Health (SFDPH) guidelines that directed public daycare providers to keep children with HIV and AIDS out of group settings.[47] The organization also worried about how different county foster care agencies were handling positive diagnoses of children already in foster care, as well as the long waiting list of ill children in need of placement.[48] Women caring for children living with ARC or AIDS had to shoulder more of this labor—and if they were also housing insecure, figure out where to do it—after the Reagan administration's new system of Medicare and Medicaid reimbursement placed limits on how long a patient could be hospitalized.[49] Depending on a child's severity of

illness and symptoms, such care was emotionally, physically, and finan-
cially taxing, a task that could not be met by one person alone, much less
added onto whatever wage work a woman might be doing.[50] And while
WAN was invited by the SFDPH to submit a proposal outlining "needed
AIDS-related services for women," the 1986 AIDS Report/Plan issued by
the department included none of the organization's recommendations on
the necessity of residential services for women and children affected by
AIDS.[51] The fact that in order to enter housing programs for people with
AIDS women often had to give up their children made this an especially
important issue for WAN and demonstrated the impossible situation facing women with AIDS. "This appears to be a recapitulation of the theme in
many women's lives: to get something that is needed, you must give up
something that is needed."[52]

Of course, *all* ASOs were struggling with underfunding—neglect was
not specific just to AIDS projects focused on women. Sometimes the scarcity engendered collaboration. For example, as the number of AIDS cases
in San Francisco grew while the SFDPH budget stayed the same, WAN
joined other ASOs in alerting officials that "the waiting lines are getting
longer and longer."[53] But the funding issue also threatened such collaboration because it increased the pressure on already strapped operations.
Governor George Deukmejian's 1987/1988 budget undercut the legislature's recommended allocation for AIDS by nearly 25 million dollars.
Included in these cuts were funds dedicated to the development of additional housing for people with AIDS.[54] Such developments increased the
pressure on Shanti Project, an ASO running a residency program for people with AIDS, to dedicate some of its units to women with children. When
the board of the Shanti Project expressed concern about what the organization would do with children if their mother died, WAN member Priscilla
Alexander had little patience. "Shanti should not just serve nice, middle
class white gay men. If a mother with AIDS needs help deciding what to do
about her children, Shanti should assume responsibility for helping her
with that decision, as it helps single people with AIDS make analogous
decisions."[55] Thanks to WAN's pressure and internal advocacy on the part
of Shanti Project's residence program director, the board directed staff to
amplify WAN's concerns to the SFDPH but stopped short of making units
available.[56] Nearly two years later, WAN was still reporting that "in San

Francisco, women with AIDS who want to live with their children only have available hotels through the welfare system, instead of the home-like setting available for women without children."[57] In New York City, WARN was also "increasingly involved in identifying appropriate apartments, negotiating rent, and lease agreements with landlords as a result of the increasing incidence of homelessness and displacement among our clients."[58]

Meeting the responsibilities of caregiving under extreme conditions of neglect and misinformation about the disease in women could and would, in WAN's assessment, cost women their lives. When WAN member Ruth Schwartz presented testimony at the Democratic Party Platform Hearings in 1987, she attempted to counter the dual forces that made the epidemic such a costly toll. Reports that men typically lived longer after an official diagnosis had produced yet another misleading theory about being "a different disease in women than in men." Schwartz aimed to set the record straight by sharing the story of "Betty, a typical woman with AIDS. Betty is 25 years old, Black, mother of 3 children. Her boyfriend shoots drugs. Betty has used drugs off and on herself. When she starts feeling sick, she doesn't pay much attention—she's busy taking care of everyone else." Schwartz explained how Betty's boyfriend started losing weight while her one-year-old stopped growing and fell ill often. He was eventually removed from daycare. By the time Betty was diagnosed with ARC after developing painful abscesses on her legs, she had been feeling sick for two years, and her boyfriend was dying of AIDS in one hospital while her child was dying in another. She spent her time between the two hospitals and home, where her other children lived. Betty died just four months after her own official diagnosis, right before her scheduled eviction from her apartment. Schwartz hoped that Betty's story would make clear that "AIDS is the same disease for women as for men—there are simply some additional social consequences." Those social consequences had not only cost Betty her loved ones. They also ensured that her own death was hastened by her efforts to take care of her family through terminal illness, poverty, drug addiction, and "long histories of poor health and little access to health care."[59]

If advocates involved in early projects focusing on women with AIDS felt like they spent the first six years of the epidemic screaming into a void about these costs, by 1988 the reality they had been describing was becoming harder to ignore. This was due in part to a shift at the federal level. By 1987, Reagan's advisors were brainstorming how the president could display leadership with regard to the epidemic. The result was Reagan's AIDS Commission, and in June 1988 members issued their final report, calling "on the federal government to increase dramatically the resources it devoted to AIDS." Even though the recommendations were not implemented, the commission and its report acknowledged the public health crisis.[60] Additionally, the "new face" of AIDS was undeniable. In New York and New Jersey, AIDS had become the leading cause of death for Black women aged 15–44.[61] Risks and patterns of transmission for poor, Black and Latina women were published in academic journals and more popular publications.[62] Project Inform, an early AIDS organization that distributed information about experimental drugs, reported that 30 to 40 percent of the 4,000 calls they received to their hotline in May of 1988 were from women; they hoped to recruit more female volunteers to work the phones.[63] Board members of Shanti House, the organization WAN had been negotiating with over housing for women for years, finally made units available.[64] And the International Working Group on Women and AIDS addressed the 4th International AIDS Conference with a statement, "Women, Children, and AIDS," that reiterated much of what early groups had found once they started examining the epidemic in women:

> Worldwide, the burden of unpaid health care falls on the wives, mothers, grandmothers, sisters, aunts, daughters and women friends. In industrialized nations, volunteerism is increasingly sought as an answer to the underfunding of care for those infected by HIV. . . . Furthermore, AIDS offers a paradigm for all the critical issues impacting on women . . . [including] deeply engrained societal racism, sexism, and discrimination by economic status . . . absence of appropriate affordable housing, particularly for female headed households, the impoverished, and the working poor and insufficient child care facilities and support services for childbearing of well and HIV affected infants and children.[65]

This growing recognition did not, however, mean a reversal of state neglect, something AIDS activists understood all too well as they neared the end of Reagan's second term. Writing for *Socialist Review*, WAN member Nancy Stoller Shaw captured the ethos of those who mounted a response to the epidemic when elected officials refused to. "It is this widespread, federally sanctioned complacency that has helped lead me to the conclusion that local community organizing efforts, based in the communities with the most serious risks of infection, are the most immediate route to saving lives and creating networks of compassion."[66] The problem, of course, was that community-grown "networks of compassion" were a far cry from the scale of response the epidemic and years of state neglect demanded, especially in light of a growing consensus that poverty, homelessness, drug addiction, racism, sexism, and inaccessible healthcare should be treated as co-factors. "Networks of compassion" could also come dangerously close to Reagan's signature vision by which "voluntarism" would "give the government back to the people" so that federal government could provide as little security as possible to those unable to provide it themselves. While Stoller Shaw and other AIDS activists understood that such efforts at the local level helped to protect the administration's deadly vision, most felt there was little choice but to act in the face of enormous need—and enormous national neglect.[67]

And so, early projects focused on women with AIDS helped the women most at risk for HIV navigate a patchwork of services, often funded with limited, private monies as state budgets tightened, while also trying to make sure closing one gap did not create another. In the Bay Area, Golden Gate Ministries announced a child care program that could offer sixteen hours a month, provided by volunteers, for women with AIDS and/or children with AIDS, while San Mateo County secured a single year of funding to run a polydrug abuse recovery program for women, aimed at stopping the spread of AIDS in this population.[68] These limited, temporary, and often private initiatives happened alongside state budget cuts to family planning clinics that were likely to be low-income women's "only contact with AIDS education and prevention information," as well as access to HIV testing.[69] Both women's health and AIDS organizations asked Governor Deukmejian to restore funds in light of the fact that "the second wave of the AIDS epidemic in California is emerging among intravenous drug users, their partners, and their children."[70]

As recognition that the epidemic had entered a "second wave" grew, early advocacy groups for women with AIDS attempted to help the existing infrastructures take on the perspective they had committed to years prior.

Whereas WAN had repeatedly lobbied Shanti Project to extend its services to women and families, by the end of the decade Shanti staff was asking for WAN's help in figuring out why women underutilized the organization.[71] And when the San Francisco General Hospital struggled to recruit women into its community clinical trials, WAN explained that it was because they were looking in the wrong place. Most women with AIDS did not come through the AIDS ward, Ward 86, but through the methadone maintenance ward, Ward 96.[72] But helping the infrastructure of AIDS care to overcome these limitations was not sufficient for meeting women's needs. When WAN hosted information sessions to hear directly from women about what resources were most important, they were repeatedly told about the burden of caretaking while poor, the stress of living hand to mouth. One woman reported, "I'm a long-term AIDS survivor since 1982 and I've seen few changes since then. We need basic thing like childcare. I have a 10-month grandson to take care of and some days I'm too sick to take care of him." Another said, "We're talking about acute survival needs that no one's funding." And yet another put it bluntly, "The reality is we already have support groups. We need money. I don't have money for my daughter's needs. Our standard of living drops to poorer and poorer. If you put a catastrophic illness on women who are on welfare, you get a crisis."[73] In response to women's repeated demands for "survival subsidies," WAN started an emergency fund to be distributed to women with AIDS, granting individuals in need 50 dollar checks.[74]

In response to such realities, two early projects for women with AIDS eventually built an "AIDS door" that a woman would actually walk through in hopes that her "poorer and poorer" standard of living might be reversed once she was inside. But contrary to the participant who highlighted the need for money, not more support groups, these robust service projects claimed that it was in those spaces where poor, women of color first shared their experiences that eventually made such services a reality. WARN, founded by Marie St. Cyr, a Haitian immigrant activist with a background in social services, was likely New York City's first organization dedicated to women of color impacted by AIDS. Through support groups, self-help efforts, and leadership development, WARN worked on helping women with HIV and AIDS move through a process that overcame stigma and embraced empowerment. For St. Cyr, this was a deliberate, intentional process that made change possible. "Having women represent themselves was key, that women were finally able to stand up and say I am a woman and I am HIV-positive and I am deserving of service . . . when women started speaking up across the city in their own voice that's when we began to really see changes."[75] Like other ASOs, WARN struggled constantly for funding but managed to maneuver around financial challenges by working in coalition with the predominately white, professionals that comprised the Women and AIDS Project (WAP), who often tapped their networks to make sure money flowed to WARN's coffers.[76] WARN eventually established Iris House in East Harlem, a comprehensive ASO— complete with residential services—dedicated to providing family-focused support to women of color affected by HIV/AIDS.[77] In its first year of operation, the organization was equipped to serve fifty women but ended up stretching resources to serve the more than three hundred women who showed up at its door. In addition to the case management and support groups that WARN had worked to make available on a small scale, Iris House provided units of housing where women could live with their families, child care for when women were attending appointments, a kitchen for workshops on nutrition, as well as meal provision, psychological services, legal services, and a community education program that targeted East Harlem residents.[78]

Dázon Dixon Diallo also saw self-help as integral to overcoming the "thick" stigma surrounding HIV/AIDS for women, and she was particularly attentive to the needs of African American women who were also often poor.[79] Diallo's "Do It Safe Parties," which she ran through the Feminist Women's Health Center in Atlanta, put this principle at the core of the outreach project and took the tools directly to the program's target population of women at higher risk of infection. Staff often visited participants at hospitals, transitional halfway houses, battered women's shelters, homeless shelters, and housing projects and discussed risks associated with intravenous drug use, how to safely share needles, and safer sex practices. Workshops were "non-judgmental" spaces where women could discuss sex, risk, their bodies, and pleasure while learning from one another and staff in a "nonhierarchical context."[80] Inevitably, discussions also concerned women's living conditions, such as self-help sessions where "it seemed like everybody in the room was having a problem with being treated badly in the homes where they were living, or near homeless."[81] In 1989, after the clinic phased out the Women with AIDS Partnership Project, Diallo decided to start her own organization. SisterLove continued the education and outreach work begun at the feminist health clinic, and, in keeping with what Diallo knew to be true about the needs of women with HIV/AIDS, also established LoveHouse, the first HIV/AIDS housing program in the Southeast, where women could live with their children. Like Iris House, LoveHouse attempted to provide the wraparound services that women in support groups had made clear were vital to their survival. In addition to self-help retreats, LoveHouse also provided transportation, child care, and advocacy services.[82]

In a variety of ways, early projects focused on women with AIDS attempted to share in the labor of managing women's multiple risks: to infection, to poverty, to homelessness, to being overburdened by caretaking, to violence, and to succumbing to the tremendous weight of state neglect. In the second decade of the epidemic, a different set of actors would shoulder more risk management work, but of a different sort. As women with HIV demanded access to treatment strategies more often accessible to HIV positive men with health insurance, the task of managing one's reproductive risk further expanded women's labor under the AIDS epidemic.

DISTRIBUTING THE COSTS OF RISK

In 1989, researchers published a clinical account of what Ruth Schwartz had attempted to make clear in her story about Betty and the costs of the epidemic. The researchers' account explained that "The survival interval of women with AIDS has been studied. In general, women have a shorter mean length of survival between the diagnosis of AIDS and death than men (298 days for women vs. 347 days for men). Specifically, black women who were IV drug abusers who died of Pneumocystis carinii pneumonia in New York City had the 'least favorable' survival of any group of AIDS patients."[83] As early AIDS projects had argued, the fact that poor and low-income women of color already in poor health succumbed to AIDS faster than their male counterparts was proof that "survival" required more than a successful AIDS treatment. Still, it would be inaccurate to suggest that those committed to women and AIDS work did not take up political struggles over treatment. Both HIV-positive women and their advocates understood that experimental drug treatment was just as vital as access to it was unequal. As the epidemic entered its second decade, federal and state negligence was confronted by a formidable opponent the direct-action AIDS movement. Treatment, particularly the development, funding, testing and distribution of experimental drugs, became one of the most visible battlefields in which AIDS activists and governmental officials sparred over how to address the epidemic.[84] For those committed to exposing how the disease exacerbated existing inequalities that disproportionately structured women's lives, this battlefield entailed an additional hurdle well known to earlier AIDS projects, and the women who had fallen ill: reproductive labor, this time in the form of managing reproductive risk.

Before AIDS activists learned that women's reproductive capacity would become a sticking point in their battle to make experimental drug treatment more accessible to women, a powerful women's health lobby and the Congressional Caucus for Women's Issues joined forces to push women's health to the front of domestic politics by 1990. They were not motivated by the AIDS epidemic. Not until the mid to late 1990s would consensus form around the idea that AIDS was a women's health issue. Rather, this group was concerned with "women's health" writ large. Due to the history of institutionalized sexism in medicine, this group argued that women's health was underfunded, underresearched, and poorly understood. What interest in women's health *did* exist had for too long been focused on reproduction. All of this resulted in women suffering worse health outcomes compared to their male counterparts. The lobbying initiative especially focused on one of the key findings published in the 1985 report by PHS's Task Force on Women's Health: the severe lack of medical knowledge regarding disease manifestation in women. Biomedical research rarely accounted for gender differences, which meant that most diagnoses and treatments were predicated on research findings specific to men.[85]

In response to recommendations put forth in the PHS report, the National Institutes of Health (NIH) instituted a policy to ensure the inclusion of women and minorities in research study populations. In this gesture, congressional representatives Olympia Snowe and Patricia Schroeder saw an opportunity for leverage. The congresswomen initiated a Government Accountability Office (GAO) report which found that in the five years since the change, the NIH had not made much progress with regards to the policy.[86] The report noted that "although the policy first was announced in October 1986, guidance for implementation was not published until July 1989, and the policy was not applied consistently before the 1990 grant review cycles."[87] Attempting to curb the political fallout caused by negative findings, NIH director William Raub announced the creation of an Office of Research on Women's Health and tasked the agency with ensuring women's adequate representation in clinical research.[88]

The focus on increasing women's participation in clinical research dredged up a fraught history of medical experimentation, particularly the thalidomide tragedy of the late 1950s. The drug had been marketed to pregnant women to help alleviate morning sickness but caused birth defects that impacted thousands of children. While Germany suffered far more impact than the United States due to its much wider distribution of the drug, the episode nevertheless "transformed the field of teratology and expanded scientific interest in testing for teratogenic effects"—damage to the developing embryo or fetus.[89] The thalidomide tragedy prompted passage of the Kefauver Harris Amendment to the 1962 Food, Drug, and Cosmetic Act. For the first time in FDA history, drugs would have to be proven safe and effective before receiving approval. Subjects of experimental testing were suddenly vulnerable to harm, and pharmaceutical companies faced the relatively new possibility of litigation.[90] While few other cautionary tales of teratogenic effects were felt as strongly as thalidomide's, the lack of protections for vulnerable research populations was raised again and again in the revelations to the public about the harmful effects of diethylstilbestrol (DES), the intrauterine device Dalkon Shield, and the racist, long-running Tuskegee study. The response was more regulatory action, specifically the creation of the National Commission for the Protection of Human Subjects of Biomedical and Behavioral Research, contained in the 1974 National Research Act. This commission singled out the fetus and pregnant woman as especially vulnerable subjects in need of protection.[91] In 1977, the FDA demonstrated how protection was achieved through exclusion when it advised researchers against the inclusion of "women of childbearing age" in clinical trials until animal reproduction studies had determined the effective drug was not also a teratogen.[92]

Women's capacity for pregnancy had, since 1977, been used as the reason to exclude them from clinical trials testing experimental treatments, though their informal exclusion was routinely implemented well before that. Having exposed the NIH, Representatives Snowe and Schroeder set their sights on the FDA's policies with a second GAO report. Its findings were no more encouraging. Women generally were underrepresented in trials, and even studies with sufficient numbers of women had not been analyzed for gender-based differences.[93] The 1977 guideline was a perfect example of how women were reduced to their reproductive functions at the expense of a wholistic approach to their health and illness. As long as the 1977 guideline was in place, any recommendations to examine disease manifestation and treatment in women were empty. Getting rid of it became one of the women's health lobby's central goals.

By the late 1980s, the direct-action AIDS movement was also laser-focused on federal health agency policies and practices that they deemed too cautious or discriminatory in light of a terminal disease that had no cure. These efforts were motivated by a belief that getting "drugs into bodies" as quickly as possible was the best hope for extending and saving people's lives. By 1990, the FDA had approved only one AIDS drug, AZT. Participation in clinical trials was the best route to other treatments that were in development. The accessibility of this treatment strategy, however, varied widely depending on one's race, class, gender, and insurance status. The majority of trial participants were white men with access to private healthcare.[94] ACT UP made overhauling treatment protocols one of its major priorities during this period, and the activist organization zeroed in on those exclusionary practices that had kept this treatment strategy out of women's reach. For example, the New York City chapter of ACT UP provided detailed records of how federally funded AIDS Clinical Trial Group (ACTG) sites excluded women.[95]

ACT UP's Women's Caucus was aware that the FDA guideline contributed to women's exclusion from trials, but it was an HIV-positive woman named Mary Lucey who ensured that direct-action AIDS activists would join the women's health lobby's reversal efforts. Around the same time Congress announced the results of the GAO report detailing the FDA's exclusionary practices, the HIV Law Project (HLP), a legal advocacy organization providing legal aid to low-income HIV-positive people in Manhattan, took on Lucey's case. Lucey had experienced extreme side effects when prescribed AZT. Her doctor instructed her to enter a clinical trial testing Tat inhibitors, drugs designed to inhibit certain proteins and freeze replication of the virus. Those running the trial, however, informed her that she could begin participation only after undergoing sterilization. Upon refusal, Lucey was barred from entry. The company cited the 1977 FDA guideline in defense of its decision to exclude her from the trial.[96]

HLP helped Lucey gain access to phase 2 of the trial and used the suit as a platform to take on the 1977 FDA guideline. Along with a number of other organizations working on civil liberties, women's rights, and AIDS, HLP filed a citizen's petition on December 15, 1992 that characterized the guidelines as gender discrimination.[97] The petition emphasized how HIV and AIDS were "a matter of life and death for women whose only hope of treatment was enrollment in a clinical trial."[98] The coalition claimed that women were entitled to the same treatment strategy popularized by well-resourced, white, gay men. The direct-action AIDS movement framed women's access to experimental drugs as a right as well as a matter of survival, just as it was for anyone with a positive diagnosis.

With both the petition and the GAO report now a matter of public record, the efforts of the women's health lobby and AIDS activists amplified attention to the FDA guideline. Women's participation in clinical trials became a major topic of debate, though women quickly discovered that they were not the only research subjects under consideration. Rather, two decades of pro-life activism had done much to establish the fetus as an entity in need of protection from women themselves. The debate over access to clinical trials, then, hinged on the question of fetal protection. Feminist lawyers writing at the time went to great pains to allay researchers' and pharmaceutical companies' fears of legal liability, arguing that informed consent would protect against the chances of being sued by either a female participant or her future offspring.[99] Spokespersons for pharmaceutical companies promptly rejected this legal reasoning. The executive director of Bristol Myers Squibb argued that "a change in federal law would be required to decrease any sponsor liability" due to the fact that most states allowed suits on behalf of the fetus.[100] Invested physicians one-upped pharmaceutical executives' liability concerns by invoking the problem of lack of medical knowledge about women's health. One reminded executives that the persistent exclusion of women from trials not only lacked "sound logical foundation" but also "had grave consequences for the advancement of knowledge of disease in the female."[101] The FDA was ultimately forced to weigh in on the debate, and Ruth Merkatz was given the job. Merkatz steered the FDA through the minefield of abortion politics that persisted just below the surface of liability concerns by reminding onlookers of the cautionary tales that prompted greater protections. Thalidomide and other studies gone terribly wrong not only demonstrated "the checkered history of clinical research in this country" but also made one "wonder why women might wish to be included in clinical trials" at all.[102]

External pressure proved strong enough to make the FDA choose sides, and in July of 1993, the agency ceded to arguments about women's autonomy. Announcing the guideline reversal, the FDA conceded that "the 1977 guideline, seen from the viewpoint of the 1990s, has appeared rigid and paternalistic."[103] It was not the only win claimed by the women's health lobby. The passage of the NIH Revitalization Act and the creation of the Office of Women's Health, to be housed in the office of the FDA commissioner, followed on the heels of the FDA's initial announcement. The year 1993 proved to be momentous for the lobby dedicated to women's health. With the authority of her new position as director of the Office of Women's Health, Merkatz proceeded to announce the guideline reversal widely. Ever cautious of appearing too nonchalant about potential fetal harms, Mekatz reiterated the FDA's "paternalism" but firmly stated that "nothing has changed at the FDA with respect to the important and justifiable concern for fetal protection."[104] With initial publications in *Academic Medicine* and the *New England Journal of Medicine*, Merkatz inaugurated a publication trail that ensured FDA control over the narrative of women's victorious entry into clinical trials. Publishing in the major science and health journals and magazines, Merkatz told a story about an internal shift at the agency that revealed its overly protectionist attitudes towards women.[105] Sometimes Merkatz briefly narrated the role of the women's health lobby. But neither AIDS activists nor women with HIV/AIDS were anywhere to be found in the many accounts Merkatz authored.

Without fail, Merkatz's version of the story reminded readers that the 1977 guideline contained an exception for life-threatening illness. Wholesale exclusion of women had never been the FDA's policy. Instead, Merkatz clarified that "women with conditions such as cancer, and, more recently, AIDS have been included in the earliest phases of drug trials . . . the potential risk to the fetus was balanced by the compelling possibility of prolonging the life of the mother."[106] With Merkatz at the helm, and with Mary Lucey, the other women excluded from trials, and their advocates neatly clipped from history, the FDA righted itself to emerge unsullied by the paternalism that had characterized biomedicine in the past. Reproductive capacity—that "problem unique to women in the traditional sense"—would no longer keep the benefits of biomedical research and treatment out of women's grasp.[107]

Mary Lucey's case and the coalition that urgently framed the FDA guideline as a "matter of life and death" make clear that this story was far too neat. So too, did AIDS activists' demands. An aspect of the guideline vitally important to women like Lucey was women's exclusion from phase 1 and 2 trials, where drugs were tested for safety and efficacy, respectively. If women with HIV/AIDS were going to garner any potential benefits from experimental drugs, they needed to get "drugs into bodies" as soon as possible—they needed access to the earliest phases of the trial. Like the women's health lobby, women and AIDS activists rejected putting fetal protection over women's access to treatment. But the coalition of petitioners went a step further. They also rejected any process that required women to take on the burden of reproductive risk as a condition of their participation.[108] In addition to paternalism, the petitioners accused the FDA of endangering the reproductive health of both female *and* male participants by failing to complete animal reproductive studies prior to the start of phase 1 testing. By demanding that all animal studies be completed before the testing of human subjects, the petition sought to "remedy FDA 77–3040's constitutional infirmity by distinguishing between potential trial participants based not on childbearing potential or pregnancy, but on the reproductive effects of the experimental drugs."[109] The petition proposed that experimenters first determine that drugs were safe for reproductive systems instead of simply excluding participants on an assumption about who were more likely to suffer fetal abnormalities. It was not just that the FDA and pharmaceutical companies were treating women like "vessels." It was that these powerful entities expected women to take on the labor of managing reproductive risk—in exchange for treatment. Changing the structures of experimental research would allow this risk to be shared.

HLP was unimpressed with the FDA's 1993 announcement, and understandably so. For starters, Merkatz made it clear that the reversal lacked regulatory force and stated that the FDA did not "abrogate its responsibility to the fetus, nor did it specify what the community must do," but instead entrusted such decisions "to internal review boards, patients, and their physicians."[110] At a meeting with FDA representatives and AIDS organizations held shortly after the guideline had been reversed, the director of the Division of Antivirals in the Center for Drug Evaluation and Research—an agency housed with the FDA—reiterated this point, telling attendees that the FDA had no authority to tell drug companies which populations to study.[111] In a widely circulated memorandum, petitioners criticized the new guideline for failing to "address the FDA's overall failure to monitor the conduct or results of animal reproduction studies or to halt trials which unnecessarily restrict women of childbearing potential." Not satisfied with a mere reversal, and refusing to accept the FDA's disempowered posturing, the memorandum explained that "because in the past, the FDA had a policy mandating gender discrimination, the FDA must now act affirmatively and aggressively to eradicate such discrimination. The FDA must do more than recommend the inclusion of women and a by-gender analysis of drug response, the FDA must mandate this approach."[112]

Two years after the initial petition had been submitted, the petitioners received a response from the FDA. While the agency expressed great concern about the low numbers of women in AIDS-related trials, it also refused to accept responsibility. Conveniently, there was a paper trail to help them do so. Petitioners were informed of Merkatz's story. "This underrepresentation cannot be attributed to FDA restrictions because FDA has never recommended gender-based restrictions in clinical trials of drugs intended to treat life-threatening illnesses." The response further explained that "a routine requirement for completion of all reproductive studies before Phase 1 likely would hinder rather than promote drug development."[113]

While HLP continued to press FDA officials, members of ACT UP New York continued monitoring the numbers of women enrolled in federally funded trials nationwide, as well as trials sponsored by drug companies being conducted in New York and New Jersey. A report issued in September 1994 reported that women's enrollment in the ACTG program had improved, with women making up 11.1 percent of all adult participants. But celebration over this improvement was tempered by a number of caveats. The ACTG offered no information on the racial breakdown of the 11.1 percent women enrolled, a cause for concern considering women of color were overrepresented in the city's cases. Women were also greatly underrepresented in trials testing treatment for adult opportunistic infections, accounting for only 8 percent of participants. Lastly, women's past underrepresentation was starting to have an effect on women's willingness to utilize the few approved anti-HIV drugs, none of which had been tested for efficacy and safety in women during the trial period.[114]

In addition to the reproductive risk women were being asked to manage as a condition of trial participation came a number of other barriers women had to overcome if they wished to access experimental treatment. Advocates concerned about what women's inclusion in experimental research meant for women of color argued that past abuses had caused a deep mistrust of medicine among minority populations and worried about how recruitment of specific research populations could be done ethically.[115] In a similar vein, authors of the petition had explicitly warned that requiring sterilization of female participants was especially harmful for low-income women of color given the history of forced sterilizations in the United States and the abuse of Black research participants.[116] Echoing the analysis of early AIDS projects focused on women, some suggested that to genuinely overcome the challenges that accompanied recruiting poor, women of color into clinical trials, research costs would have to be increased to cover meals, social services, transportation, child care, and educational materials.[117] Physicians who had extensive experience working with women of all racial backgrounds in healthcare and research settings supported these recommendations, but above all they pointed out the necessity of running trials that accommodated and shared in women's caregiving responsibilities—lack of child care, inflexible appointment times, and poor transportation access were repeatedly cited as immense barriers to entry.[118]

In response to continued pressure from the women's health lobby that trial outcomes be analyzed for possible gender effects, the FDA attempted to put more force behind the guidelines. In 1995, the FDA proposed a rule that required researchers submitting new drug applications to analyze subgroup differences. However, the rule would only require sponsors to analyze *existing* data rather than requiring researchers to include representative numbers of women. Founder of HLP and legal advocate Theresa M. McGovern described the rule as "a retreat for the reluctant trial sponsor who is unwilling to analyze gender differences" and argued that it would "not cure the egregious lack of knowledge about how drugs affect women." Her letter replied to the proposal by invoking more than a decade of activism around women and AIDS. "Advocates for women have grown tired of fighting with the FDA over these basic principles of drug testing. If the FDA continues to answer the reasonable demands of the Task Force and countless advocacy groups with meaningless regulations, we will reasonably question the 'good faith' of the FDA on the subject of women. We will not tolerate more years of 'lip service' to women's health."[119]

Ultimately, the FDA proposed a "clinical hold" rule in 1997—which it took another three years to put into effect.[120] Modeled after the proposal McGovern authored while serving on the Presidential Advisory Council on HIV/AIDS, the rule promised that studies testing new drugs would be put on clinical hold if they barred persons with a life-threatening illness solely because of potential reproductive risk.[121] Given FDA representatives' common line that the agency was not responsible for the low numbers of women in AIDS-related trials because of the life-threatening-illness exception, this was especially significant.[122] Nearly twenty years into the AIDS epidemic, the FDA finally summoned the regulatory power that activists had argued was necessary to save lives. Having stuck with the issue until its resolution in 2000, those working at HLP celebrated the regulation.[123] Pharmaceutical companies were less enthused. Indeed, the FDA reported that two comments from sponsors regarding the proposed rule expressed continued concerns about liability, while another comment claimed that this use of the clinical hold rule turned it into a "punitive measure." Still, the agency amplified another comment pointing out how little progress had been made in terms of opening enrollment to women of childbearing age.[124] This acknowledgement implicitly conceded petitioners' earlier demand that regulatory power was necessary to counter the FDA's past "policy mandating gender discrimination." Despite being a far cry from the original demands of women and AIDS activists, the clinical hold rule represented a significant challenge to the continued practice of excluding women from trials.

CONCLUSION

In their proposed clinical hold rule published in 1997, the FDA outlined the projected costs associated with implementation of the new policy. "Implementation of this proposed rule could impart additional direct costs to the industry in one area—the cost associated with testing for pregnancy in women with reproductive potential who volunteer to participate in clinical trials that would have previously excluded them."[125] The FDA estimated that pregnancy tests for the total number of women that had been excluded from trials concerned with life-threatening illnesses would not exceed $42,000. Of the forty-three protocols analyzed, only six entailed costs exceeding $1,000. The FDA was firm in its assertion that the "societal benefits more than outweigh the potential minimal additional costs."[126]

A value system that can only see monetary costs is a value system that produces death, often through neglect. AIDS activists made this clear in their efforts to force a humane response to the epidemic *and* the unequal conditions that fueled its spread. They were equally clear about the costs of failing to mount such a response. "The government's indifference toward the actual lives of affected women helps explain the fact that women with AIDS die as much as six times faster after diagnosis than do men."[127] Accounting for women's "actual lives" required far more than a cost analysis of pregnancy tests. Instead, their reality already entailed the invisible, devalued labor of family making in the midst of racism, poverty, homelessness, and drug addiction. When AIDS arrived, managing risk alongside illness and the fear of death for their loved ones and themselves became yet another task in their "labor of love." Under the AIDS epidemic, the reproductive labor of managing risk and disease largely took place in the spaces where women were surviving their already precarious conditions: in homeless shelters, motels, prisons, hospitals, and potentially unsafe housing. Illness introduced new spaces—clinical drug trials, ASOs, support groups, activist demonstrations—that families and their advocates built or utilized in an effort to more equally share the work. The expansion of labor necessitated by the epidemic blended into the labors of family making that women were repeatedly made to shoulder alone.

What might a nonmonetary cost analysis of state neglect capture? There are, in fact, a number of ways to account for the toll. Epidemiological trends for HIV and AIDS incidence provide one measure. Despite the fact that in 1997 AIDS fell from the top ten causes of death in the United States for the first time in seven years, from 1999 through 2001 it remained the leading cause of death for black women aged 25–34.[128] As both affected women and early AIDS projects pointed out, the spread of AIDS has been fueled by preexisting forms of neglect. This is made clear by the fact that Southern states have experienced the greatest proportional increases in HIV/AIDS rates each year since 1990, where one-third of new HIV infections occur in women. This region has some of the highest levels of poverty, unemployment, and uninsured individuals in the United States, which means it also has some of the highest death rates from AIDS. The "dire need of financial assistance," echoing WAN's information session that resulted in "survival subsidies," means that providers in Southern states are confronted with meeting basic needs in addition to needs caused by the disease.[129] And Black women living in communities across the country with high rates of poverty and HIV have roughly six times the HIV incidence estimated for their similarly aged counterparts. In one of the first national multisite, multilevel studies to qualitatively examine the intersecting factors that increase women's risk for HIV, participants reported that "challenges related to acquiring food, housing, and other necessary provisions for themselves and their children" drove their participation in high-risk behaviors.[130] The systematic devaluation of this necessary work—literally keeping oneself and one's children alive— combined with the devaluation of Black mothering, continues to keep poor, Black women more vulnerable to a disease that will inevitably make such work even harder.

The current state of biomedical research on disease and treatment in women provides another measure. The logic driving the clinical trials debate—in which women were expected to manage their own reproductive risk—continues to have detrimental impacts on women's health. Women's overall representation in clinical trials has risen since 1993, but they continue to be underrepresented in phase 1 trials.[131] Women also remain underrepresented in HIV-related trials (despite the aforementioned numbers).[132] The decision to outsource the management of reproductive risk to trial participants has had the additional effect of keeping pregnant women out of experimental treatments. Only within the last decade have the FDA and other federal health agencies begun examining potential protocols for increasing medical knowledge of disease progression and treatment during pregnancy.[133]

And there are yet more ways to measure the toll. The costs of the Reagan administration's nonresponse to the epidemic are most often and most starkly represented by those who lost their lives—by the end of his term the number standing in for this incalculable cost was almost 100,000, though even that figure is likely far too low given the deaths that were unattributed to the disease.[134] While researching this chapter, I came across AIDS and women's health activist Marion Bhanzaf's 1993 planner. It was not unusual for her entries recording those she lost to the disease to appear weekly, sometimes with loved ones and comrades passing days apart. While such constant loss with no clear end in sight no longer defines the AIDS crisis in the United States, profit continues to drive pharmaceutical and healthcare industries, which keeps effective treatment out of reach for many. In 2010, women comprised a quarter of deaths among people with an HIV diagnosis in the United States.[135] Women and AIDS activists had warned that this would be the cost of an epidemic that did not take women's risk seriously, risk that was heightened by and then folded into the labor of maintaining family in the face of state neglect.

By the early 1990s, those agitating for systemic solutions to myriad forms of inequality were all too familiar with the effects of neglect: the need always exceeded the available aid, public officials all too often abdicated responsibility and doled out blame, even wins had built-in limits, and grassroots service initiatives increasingly served as the last remaining lifeline in the wasteland of neglect. But those who created "networks of compassion" in this political context were not uniformly motivated. Some, like pro-life emergency pregnancy service volunteers, were driven to act not by concern for structural inequality but by what they perceived to be the greatest threat to family—legal abortion. The "networks of compassion" developed by emergency pregnancy service volunteers comprised a service-based response to legal abortion that unfolded against the conditions documented thus far and served as a resource to struggling pregnant women and families. Lifelines that come with strings attached comprise the final cost of family making under state neglect.

5 The Labor of "Choice"

NAVIGATING THE ABORTION DEBATE AND
LIFELINES OF LAST RESORT

They call you and say, "Do you need any stuff?" I love
this place.

Cindy R., mother of two, about her local crisis pregnancy
center, 1995

In 2015, the National Abortion Rights Action League (NARAL) published a report titled *Crisis Pregnancy Centers Lie: The Insidious Threat
to Reproductive Freedom.* The report compiled numerous NARAL state
affiliates' undercover investigations into crisis pregnancy center (CPC)
operations. NARAL investigators posing as pregnant women recorded the
various tactics used by CPCs to deter women from abortion: billboards
advertising pregnancy services were put up near high schools and low-
income neighborhoods in order to draw in those most likely to be in need
of free services; CPC volunteers provided women with inaccurate medical
information regarding the health risks associated with abortion and birth
control; major coordinating organizations developed manipulative campaigns targeting African American women that compared abortion to
slavery; and centers were deliberately located near Planned Parenthood
clinics and in medical suites—what NARAL called the "co-location" strategy. Deception, the report found, was activists' most favored and powerful
weapon against abortion rights. "The American anti-choice movement
has built thousands of outposts across the country with the sole purpose
of preventing women from accessing abortion (through lies and coercion),
and they're hiding in plain sight." Systematically documenting and

exposing the movement's lies was the surest route to weakening this strategy of deception. "It is time," the report warned readers, "to recognize CPCs for what they are: a grave threat to a woman's right to choose."[1]

Forty years before NARAL published its investigative report, Eleanor Zehala telephoned Women's Health Services in Pittsburgh to make an appointment with an abortion counselor. Zehala, a volunteer at a local crisis pregnancy center called Lifeline, had recently talked with a pregnant seventeen-year-old who was afraid to tell her parents about her pregnancy (Zehala called the girl "Terry"). Despite the fact that Terry left her conversation with Zehala "armed with determination and the names and phone numbers of three pro-life doctors, maternity homes, and two social service agencies," Zehala found out three days later that the girl's family had pressured Terry into having an abortion. This news prompted Zehala to imagine Terry at an abortion clinic, and she wondered "how the abortion clinic personnel would respond to a tearful and shivering young girl. Would they hug her or would they hustle her through with impersonal precision?" Zehala's appointment with Women's Health Services was an attempt to find out. Posing as a pregnant married mother, Zehala told the abortion counselor she was very concerned because her doctor had said the "baby's heart was already pumping blood." According to Zehala, the counselor "retorted" that "we ALL know that you can't hear a heartbeat until the fetus is 24 weeks old." When Zehala pressed the counselor on whether or not the procedure would cause her pain, the counselor "became exasperated." She told Zehala that the abortion could stay a secret because "it takes 3 minutes at most to empty the uterus" and was an outpatient procedure. Zehala confided to readers of *Heartbeat Magazine,* the publication that ran her exposé of Women's Health Services, "when I reflect upon my episode at the clinic I shudder. It is painful for me to think of Terry and other girls like her."[2]

"Terry and other girls like her" have long animated the abortion debate in the United States, and not only through the angle taken by Zehala. Depending on one's perspective, pregnant women seeking an abortion are victimized by the lack of choice, by anti-abortion efforts to undermine choice, or by the high stakes of the debate itself, which often silences complex realities in the name of political expediency. This third perspective contains "the things we cannot say" about abortion for fear of emboldening anti-abortion activists or losing onlookers' support should they learn of ostensibly unsympathetic abortion stories.[3] It is also here that the historical and ongoing battle between abortion rights advocates and the CPC movement has played out, though to see it requires looking beyond Zehala's description of Terry. The anti-abortion strategy of combatting legal abortion through service provision, which pro-life, emergency pregnancy services (EPS) advocates like Zehala set out to do before the *Roe* decision, has drawn far more impoverished pregnant women and single mothers in need of support to CPCs than it has those undecided about their pregnancy.[4] Quite simply, CPCs provided at no monetary cost some of the things such women needed for family making. And as structural inequality increased over the final decades of the twentieth century, there were more families headed by mothers struggling to make ends meet.[5] While "Terry and other girls like her" no doubt strengthened *Heartbeat Magazine* subscribers' convictions, those working as EPS volunteers were more likely to encounter single mothers "setting out on a difficult path . . . with little support for their efforts."[6]

By now, readers should be quite familiar with this "difficult path," one shaped thoroughly by different forms of neglect. Like the other advocacy efforts documented in these pages, the EPS movement grew up in the shadow of this "path," but their history has largely been overlooked for one that more closely adheres to the standard terms of the abortion debate. The NARAL report, and numerous investigations published from the 1980s on, make clear that the EPS movement has pulled out all the stops, no matter how deceptive, in their efforts to reach girls like Terry. It is also clear that these efforts *did* ensnare some women seeking an abortion, and that such encounters had incredibly harmful effects.[7] But just as Zehala's interrogation of the Pittsburgh Women's Health Services set out to confirm what she already believed to be true about abortion counseling, investigations into CPCs have been singularly focused on exposing the movement's anti-abortion propaganda, thereby missing one of CPCs' most important functions. A movement that has, since 1971, promised to make abortion obsolete by providing emotional and material support to pregnant women on a "path" shaped by state neglect will necessarily be a resource, even of last resort, simply because precious few others exist. And it will mostly attract those who need what it provides—material support for pregnancy and family making, even in the limited ways it is doled out by many contemporary EPS centers. In the post-*Roe* era, as readers now know all too well, increasing numbers of women could not come by this support on their own. EPS volunteers picked up the slack created by state neglect not because they believed in building a more robust public infrastructure of support for family making, but because they believed no woman would choose abortion if shown that she would not have to face motherhood alone. Unlike other service-based advocacy that considered a significant redistribution of resources and power to be the solution to inequalities, the EPS movement relied on pro-life networks of donors and professionals that made it resilient in the face of state retrenchment. Furthermore, it garnered institutional support when abstinence-only education and marriage promotion became official goals of the country's welfare program. What began as a marginalized and largely ignored arm of the pro-life movement in the early 1970s steadily gained a role in the patchwork of public and private aid that impoverished families partially rely on to get by.

In sum, the broader conditions of state neglect documented in the preceding chapters are what made it possible for pro-life counselors like Zehala to offer both a necessary lifeline ("armed with names and phone numbers of three pro-life doctors, maternity homes, and two social service agencies") *and* a threat to choice. To better understand this history of the EPS movement, the role of CPCs as resources for family making, however limited, needs to be taken seriously. Pro-choice investigations going back to the 1980s are largely based on undercover volunteers pretending to need abortion care, not pregnancy support, and while it is true that CPCs have mostly lies to offer on this front, it reveals little about their treatment of women in need of pregnancy services. By and large, scholars have also dismissed the role of legitimate "lifelines" by lumping CPCs in with the more militant tactics of clinic blockades and die-ins that were popularized by a new, radical, and often violent wing of the pro-life movement in the 1980s.[8] The association between militant pro-life activists and the EPS movement is echoed in both popular and academic accounts describing the origins of CPCs, most of which cite Rob Pearson, a pro-life activist who believed that women seeking abortions were "killers," as the man behind the movement.[9]

Pearson's ruthless quest to save babies from the women he held in such great contempt has overshadowed the fact that combating legal abortion through service provision was just as much if not more the brainchild of the largely Catholic, white, middle-class women who started EPS centers across the country.[10] They were drawn to the movement by a more complicated belief than Pearson was apparently capable of: that legal abortion signaled the state's abandonment of single, pregnant women. In contrast to the prominent, male-led, ultimately futile effort to pass a Human Life Amendment in the years immediately following *Roe*, early EPS volunteers believed no woman would actually choose abortion if given another option. Making that other option available—providing "alternatives to abortion"—was key. If they could intervene at the moment a woman learned she was pregnant and show her that motherhood was within her reach, then the legal standing of abortion would be irrelevant. Supportive, pro-life pregnancy services would make abortion obsolete.

This strategy was immediately complicated by the same conditions that brought women to CPCs for much needed services: combating abortion through service provision necessarily meant confronting the dearth of public support available to women and families on the margins of society. In their early years, EPS centers relied on a mix of public and private resources and networks, such as Zehala's mix of pro-life doctors and social services. Any woman served, including women who did not intend to end their pregnancies but needed support, was considered by most volunteers a win in the fight against abortion. But as worsening economic circumstances drove more and more women to EPS centers' doorsteps for support, and as volunteers began reporting on the need for more and different types of pregnancy services, some leaders in the movement began to worry that centers were seeing too many "services-only clients" and too few "Terrys"—pregnant women seeking, or "at risk" for, abortion. While many center directors pursued more expansive services in an effort to meet the growing need, leadership also urged the uptake of tactics aimed at garnering more "at-risk" clients. The problem with this dual strategy, however, was that the tactic of service provision proved to be far more effective in attracting clients than was targeted outreach, particularly when CPCs had the resources to provide services other strapped agencies could not. State retrenchment, growing inequality, and private networks of support made CPCs a resilient resource, capable of securing a foothold in service provision to families in need. The widely cited quote from pro-life activist Abby Johnson—that "the best client you ever get is one who thinks they're walking into an abortion clinic"—illustrates how the movement still relies on women experiencing an unintended pregnancy in search of abortion care to strengthen their supporters' convictions.[11] But movement leaders' continued anxiety about a surfeit of services-only clients reveals just how infrequently this "ideal" client actually shows up at a CPC. This anxiety is no secret. By the movement's own admission, less than 20 percent of women served by a CPC are undecided about or actively seeking abortion services, with scholarship on the movement putting the actual number much lower. The "best" client is also the rarest one.[12]

The history of the EPS movement, told against the backdrop of state neglect, allows an alternative assessment of this decades-long experiment in combatting abortion through service provision. Anti-abortion propaganda is most certainly one cost posed by CPCs, but it is the women and families made to rely on a lifeline of last resort who encounter this reality most intimately. Those forced to piece together resources so that they might support their families are the ones who will receive aid *alongside* anti-abortion propaganda and appeals to religious conversion. The lack of public support for family making ensures the movement's continued relevance because families in need have few other places to turn. By foregrounding the increasing inequality and state retrenchment that defined the conditions in which the EPS movement attempted to make abortion obsolete, it is possible to see CPCs as an *effect* of the stubborn idea that having children is a choice that one should bear the costs of alone. Anyone who fails to adhere to such an often unattainable standard—well, how much their family making is valued can be measured by the outside care they are made to rely on. Since 1971, the EPS movement has been providing compromised resources to pregnant women and families in "plain sight." Such a reality demands an assessment of what factors ensured that "alternatives to abortion" would become a lifeline for struggling families despite the tightly attached strings. The following history is offered in service of the urgent need to imagine a new, less costly arrangement.

CREATING A "WORLD FEDERATION" OF EMERGENCY
PREGNANCY SERVICES

Zehala's undercover investigation of Women's Health Services reflected what many pro-life activists believed to be true about abortion providers during the early 1970s—they were clinical, callous, and all too eager to convince women that the decision to end a pregnancy was a casual one.[13] EPS advocates contrasted the character of the uncaring, coercive abortion provider with their own, supposedly more compassionate approach. Nearly fifteen years before the pro-life movement fully embraced the strategy of framing abortion as a threat to women, early EPS advocates proposed that legalization signified society's abandonment of women who became pregnant outside of marriage.[14] By the early 1970s, the clandestine maternity home was an increasingly irrelevant solution for the largely middle-class white women that such operations had been designed to shield from view during their pregnancies. Indeed, sex and parenting outside of marriage was becoming more commonplace even before *Roe*. In the minds of early EPS advocates, these shifting social mores made the situation of the young, unmarried, white women they envisioned helping (those vulnerable to an unexpected pregnancy and subsequent male abandonment) all the more precarious—and urgent—by legal abortion. The availability of abortion as the "solution" to an unwanted pregnancy threatened to eradicate the possibility of motherhood entirely.[15] Louise Summerhill, the founder of the EPS movement in Canada, stated in 1970 that "very few women want to destroy their babies if they see another way out. But our society gives a woman little choice but abortion or a forced marriage. Otherwise she is socially ostracized and receives little support from the community."[16] In a society that stigmatized mothers who failed to keep family making within the confines of an economically self-reliant marital partnership, legal abortion was both a logical and a harmful option. This analysis contained both a criticism of the white, middle-class nuclear family that had always been more myth than reality *and* a belief that motherhood was an essential, even compulsory, feature of women's lives.

Early EPS advocates believed that the surest way to counter legal abortion was to show pregnant women that they would not have to face single motherhood alone, that they could become mothers—even if the traditional arrangement was out of reach.[17] They were spurred to action by what they perceived to be the increasing acceptance and availability of abortion. The speed at which popular sentiment on abortion shifted and prompted legal changes at the state level confirmed advocates' belief that an unintended pregnancy constituted a crisis in need of intervention, especially as abortion referral services grew in number.[18] After Washington State legalized abortion in 1970, for example, Seattle-based feminists founded the Abortion and Birth Control Referral Service to help direct women to compassionate and well-qualified physicians.[19] Referral services also formed in states that had not yet changed their abortion law but were in close proximity to states where the procedure was legally available. After New York State legalized abortion, the Boston-based Pregnancy Counseling Service counseled 6,000 women during its first year of operation, with 64 percent of clients successfully terminating their pregnancies in neighboring New York.[20]

In response, early EPS operations replicated the tactics of abortion referral services, and hotlines became a popular first step for pro-life advocates hoping to reach pregnant women. Early attempts at outreach demonstrate the urgency advocates felt, especially when such efforts failed to connect eager volunteers with the women they believed were most vulnerable to abortion services. Unlike the Pregnancy Counseling Service, which reported that from 600 to 800 women a month sought their services "without overt publicity," Value of Life Committee's (VOLCOM) Pregnancy Guidance hotline number received only thirty calls from Boston residents in its first four and a half months of operation.[21] Lifelines of Western Massachusetts, which operated a similar referral system, was also underutilized.[22] These early attempts led members of VOLCOM to conclude that pro-life agencies were failing to "make even the initial point of contact with the overwhelming majority of these pregnant and troubled girls." They urged the Massachusetts Conference of Bishops to increase support for "a positive well-advertised and well-packaged program of care for women in pregnancy as a sound alternative to abortion."[23] Others were more suspicious about phones that remained stubbornly silent. When a reporter for the *Catholic Bulletin* went undercover as a pregnant woman undecided about what to do next, she reported that every agency she called for help in the Twin Cities referred her to an abortion provider. A volunteer at the local EPS center concluded that the "refusal to mention Birthright cannot be the result of ignorance. This one-year-old agency has been well publicized." The investigation proved to EPS advocates that women in the Twin Cities would "be advised to get an abortion, and she will be told the fastest, most efficient way to do it."[24]

Not all early hotline operations reported failure, however. Margaret Nemecek, a longtime resident of Whittier, CA, was moved to action by the state's abortion reform bill.[25] With the help of Catholic social workers, Nemecek and other concerned women received training in the principles of "non-judgment and client determination" and began to train other interested volunteers.[26] On April 5, 1971, Nemecek and a group of volunteers opened the first hotline in Southern California, one of the earliest EPS services in the country.[27] The group established a second hotline serving the San Fernando Valley a couple of months later, and the network of volunteers eventually reached even further across Southern California. What had by then become the Right to Life League of Southern California reported that "the growing use of the lines and the increasing acceptance of the referrals offered by the trained listener to the person in trouble is heartening reassurance to the volunteers. They indeed are responding to community needs as well as saving a baby's life."[28] During these early and critical years, hotlines were considered the first line of defense in the race to reach pregnant women before they found their way to an abortion clinic.[29]

Hotlines and centers that formed in the early days of the EPS movement either operated in isolation or forged connections to cover a particular region, and some advocates soon realized that broader coordination could make their endeavors more powerful. In 1970, activists who believed that abortion was best fought with pregnancy support met in Chicago. Dr. John Hillabrand, an obstetrician who boasted of delivering 8,000 infants without a single maternal death, Lorie Maier, a Holocaust survivor turned pro-life activist, and Sister Paula Vandegaer, a social worker for Catholic Charities who had trained the women in Whittier, CA in crisis intervention counseling, founded Alternatives to Abortion, International (AAI).[30] The organization dedicated itself to coordinating EPS operations that were forming in all regions of the United States. Hillabrand, Maier, and Vandegaer envisioned a "world federation of emergency pregnancy services" that would one day make abortion obsolete. Maier believed this "federation" would eventually gain worldwide recognition. "In a way, I envision AAI and EPS centers as a global entity, much like the Red Cross. While Red Cross enters in where there are catastrophic natural plights, wars, or other man-caused mishaps that affect often the multitudes, AAI in contrast deals with individual and personal crisis where the life of the unborn and the health and well-being of women and families are at stake."[31]

While the infrastructure AAI aspired to create was significant, the EPS operations that existed upon the organization's founding in 1971 were scattered and piecemeal, ranging from rudimentary to highly professionalized. A 1973 issue of AAI's newsletter, *Heartbeat Bulletin,* reported on an EPS effort in Montana that established a hotline using the switchboard of a local motel in the town of Malta, while volunteers that formed Heartbeat of Central Ohio to serve the towns of Marion, Green Camp, La Rue, New Bloomington, Prospect, and Waldo found a retired woman willing to answer the phone "24 hours a day." The Marion Chamber of Commerce allowed Heartbeat of Central Ohio to hold meetings there, free of charge.[32] In contrast, Marie Gonzalez of Birthright Pregnancy Aid in Garden City, MI told bulletin readers how EPS operations could get the most out of their board of directors if they selected members carefully. "Have on your board people who will *help*. The doctor on our board arranged for free pregnancy testing and pays half of our phone bill. The judge on our board spoke on legal concerns at our initial training seminar and is available for advice at all times."[33]

AAI got to work coordinating these scattered and varied efforts in order to fulfill its role as a clearinghouse for the burgeoning movement of EPS volunteers. In addition to circulating the newsletter, it attempted to harness the energies of existing or fledgling centers by requesting their affiliation. In return for affiliation dues, AAI provided centers with advice on how to counsel women facing unintended pregnancies, a copy of the annual AAI directory that listed all of AAI's affiliates, and connected those in the emerging field by hosting an annual academy on abortion alternatives. These resources were designed to help volunteers sort out the pragmatics of running EPS operations, but just as importantly they established the significance of the EPS movement—and AAI's role within it—in the fight against abortion. Following the passage of *Roe,* for example, *Heartbeat Bulletin* told affiliates:

> Pro-abortion activists after achieving the legality of induced abortion, frequently set about promoting these procedures on a grand scale. Phone books are usually replete with local and toll free numbers disclosing the availability of abortion counseling services, referral agencies, free standing clinics, and numerous abortion centers. On the face of it, the pro-life EPS centers were faced with a most unequal contest. There was a crying need for integration, cooperation, and communication between these centers so their efforts could be more effective and so that expanded service could be developed to deal with the growing problem.[34]

The number of EPS operations affiliated with AAI more than doubled between August of 1972 and December of 1973, a seventeen-month period that spanned both the months leading up to and those following the Supreme Court's January 1973 decision in *Roe v. Wade*.[35] By 1975, AAI boasted of having over 700 EPS affiliates in the United States, made possible by the "more than 50,000 unpaid volunteer workers" that had been drawn into the movement.[36]

Those who decided that legal abortion was best countered with pregnancy services were driven by a short-term goal, propped up by an assumption: EPS volunteers would support women through the crisis of an unintended pregnancy so that she could realize her true desire of motherhood. AAI's founders played a major role in formalizing and popularizing an approach that contained both elements. For example, AAI advised affiliates on the importance of partnering with local public and private service providers, thereby acknowledging that any "alternative" to abortion required material support. Maier instructed affiliates that community networks were essential to presenting clients with "available alternatives. Whether they are personal or practical in nature, they usually involve a wide range of workable solutions and are necessarily different with each individual client. Here are some of them: Medical care, legal aid, various types of social assistance, education, job training, housing (maternal homes), adoption services, special counseling by professionals, maternity clothes, baby layettes, etc. Community services are indispensable to the EPS centers with and without resources."[37]

But it was the so-called crisis of being unexpectedly pregnant in a society that deemed abortion the best solution to such a situation that especially shaped the movement's other key strategy: pro-life counseling. Just as she had done for women in Southern California, Vandegaer drew on her expertise in social work to put the principles of crisis intervention counseling to pro-life ends. She instructed AAI affiliates on the attitudes of the professional counselor, which included "acceptance," a "non-judgmental attitude," and "listening." "As easy as it sounds, this [listening] is one of the most difficult jobs for a volunteer. We must give the girl the feeling that she may say anything she wants to us, and she will be heard. She will not be interrupted or judged. A girl does not come to us to be told what to do. She comes to sort out her own feelings and attitudes."[38] The "girl's" situation was urgent because her future and the life of her future child were on the line. AAI's "counseling tips" made such urgency clear. "The goal of the counsellor is to provide an emergency service, often centering around the decision to abort the baby or bring the baby to term."[39]

Community networks that could turn up necessary resources and pro-life counseling that could help those facing a "crisis" pregnancy were both essential for EPS operations, but only their counseling enabled the movement to distinguish itself from other pro-life services. Writing in *Heartbeat Magazine* a decade after AAI's founding, Vandegaer reflected on the relationship between "professional" and "paraprofessional" pro-life services:

> When anti-abortion laws began to break down in 1968 and 1969, there were many professional pro-life agencies who would not refer for abortions. *The problem was that they did not find themselves competitive with the short-term abortion clinics and hot lines. Therefore, although they were ready and waiting to give pro-life counseling, girls did not come to them. The EPS movement grew up in response to this need.* We have created a new type of social service agency and a new force in our society. Ideal situations are set up when the pro-life service center is physically close to the pro-life professional center. . . . In some cities the EPS center is close to a local pro-life professional agency such as Catholic Social Service, Evangelical Welfare, Latter Day Saints Services, etc.[40]

The special service role that EPS volunteers filled was key to rectifying the imbalance in abortion and pro-life services that Vandegaer explained in her article. The feeling of always being one step behind the availability of abortion services, a sentiment that further stoked advocates' sense of urgency, was also expressed by Maier. She pointed out that while "most abortion referral agencies and most abortion-performing centers appear to be well advertised . . . EPS centers, conversely, have not been well advertised."[41] The most unique service EPS volunteers had to offer, then, was pro-life counseling. Referrals and material support were important, but only the trained pro-life counselor could ensure that any woman who called a hotline or walked through a center's door would "be heard" during that vital encounter.

These key aspects—the belief that no women would choose abortion if given another option, that such alternatives were not readily available, and that EPS services should target pregnant women with short-term crisis intervention—fundamentally shaped the strategies adopted by the EPS movement in the United States. During its first decade, the movement emphasized pro-life counseling and community services to counter the cultural shift among some segments of American society that deemed abortion an acceptable form of medical care. But the legalization of abortion did not comprise the entirety of the movement's origins even if it largely consumed participants' field of vision. That society made it so difficult for single pregnant women to raise and provide for their children directly impacted both EPS operations and the movement's broader strategies. As EPS volunteers began to realize that many of the women they saw were not threatened by abortion but were instead women struggling to keep their families afloat, the movement was forced to reckon with structural inequities that increasingly drove women to the doorsteps of EPS centers. While EPS participants did not respond to these changes uniformly, state neglect nevertheless drove both a steady stream of need and widened the movement's relevance.

STATE NEGLECT AND FAMILY VALUES

In 1979, Ritaellen B. wrote AAI in hopes of finding "moral and financial support" from a local EPS center. Seventeen years old with a six-month-old son, Ritaellen B. told AAI, "My son's father left me when I became pregnant. And not having no one to turn to besides my parents I was in a sense of the word forced to have and keep my child. . . . Please don't get me wrong I love my son very much and far from regretting having and keeping him." Vandegaer instructed the Friends of Life center in West Palm Beach to get in touch with Ritaellen B. and "give her whatever encouragement and support you can."[42]

The EPS movement had formed with women like Ritaellen B. in mind. Despite the fact that Ritaellen B. described having her child as "forced" rather than the reverse scenario imagined by many pro-lifers, her situation nevertheless confirmed the abandonment the movement was trying to mitigate. The fact that Ritaellen B. had "no one to turn to" was why EPS volunteers were so urgently needed on the front lines. Vandegaer's insistence that Friends of Life do all they could to help her also illustrates the broad brush with which the movement tended to depict women in need of EPS services. It did not matter that Ritaellen B. was already a mother and not facing the "crisis" of a possible abortion. During its first fifteen years, the volunteers that powered the EPS movement considered helping any woman who sought their services a step towards reversing the culture created by legal abortion. For example, Beth Golden from Birthright of Siouxland wrote AAI in 1973 to report that of their 130 calls in the first six months of operation "about a third were pregnant women looking for help. Another third were requests for information, many asking for abortion information. . . . We have worked with two mothers and babies through their hospital stay and offering further encouragement. Have referred some to agencies for help, given clothes to others, pregnancy tests, etc. And, of course, we will never really know how many we have helped."[43] Similarly, Sally Pinchok from Heartbeat of Central Ohio reported, "since February 1974 we have helped 75 girls. Five have had abortions, but we tried. And the calls keep pouring in."[44] Rita Marker, the director of Pregnancy Aid in Everett, WA even went so far as to shame those EPS volunteers who made distinctions like Pinchok's. "I believe our particular type of organization must be a positive type of endeavor! Please, let's not get bogged down in counting how many abortions we've avoided, in fighting the 'battle,' in strategic maneuvering in the 'war for life.' If we were to take a direct anti-abortion stand . . . we would be saying that we do not respect each woman as an individual, as a person who has the right to make her own choices."[45]

While many EPS volunteers took an "anti-abortion stand" that may have been too "direct" for Marker, these reports make clear that the movement had a broad metric for assessing success. Any woman that the movement helped, even if such help did not directly entail "avoiding" abortion, was evidence that advocates were doing their job. In this way, EPS volunteers could move easily between their dual roles as pro-life counselors and service providers without making too much of a distinction between the two—both were necessary to make "alternatives to abortion" a reality. But as the movement entered its second decade, it underwent two significant changes. First, centers were seeing more and more women who felt the strain of growing economic insecurity, and in their search for support they brought a crisis of structural inequality to EPS centers' doorsteps. This forced many EPS centers to expand their list of services in order to meet clients' needs. Most did so happily, though some also began to reflect on how additional pregnancy services were unlikely to attract more pregnant clients considering abortion. Second, two major affiliate organizations, Heartbeat International (formerly AAI) and Care Net, assumed leadership of the movement, and those at the helm attempted to steer it away from new mothers like Ritaellen B. in hopes of reaching those actually considering abortion. These two realities ultimately caused a significant shift in approach, and for the first time since the movement's founding, some EPS operations began distinguishing between *types* of clients: those seeking abortion services and those seeking pregnancy-related support.

In the summer of 1985, *Heartbeat* featured a guest article on client outreach written by Julie Huband, the director of the Women's Pregnancy Center in Ocala, FL. Huband explained, "When our center opened four years ago, we unconsciously chose an image of service to pregnant women who need practical help and support. We saw few clients who were considering abortion as our promotional efforts were not geared to reach them. Upon reevaluating our promotions plan, I decided I wanted to add another audience—women who were intent upon or considering an abortion." Huband's experience taught her that "the woman considering abortion rarely perceives herself as being in a crisis and therefore is not particularly interested in counseling or pregnancy support services." In response to this realization, Huband's center separated pregnancy-related support from the free pregnancy testing "with results while you wait" geared towards clients considering abortion.[46]

Huband did not do away with pregnancy support services altogether. In fact, she revamped these services, which included "prenatal care, clothing, housing, adoption referral, and childbirth classes," and emphasized the "equal importance" of both audiences.[47] The fact that pregnant women managed to find Huband's center even before she rebranded the pregnancy support program "New Beginnings" is consistent with other center updates from this time period. In a 1984 issue of *Heartbeat Magazine,* Vandegaer informed readers about the demand for additional types of pregnancy services. "One of the greatest needs in the U.S. right now is for housing for pregnant women. Many groups all over the country are starting short-term and long-term housing. Another growth area is after-delivery services. Many pro-life groups are now in a position to consider after-delivery services and are offering group counseling, day care centers, residence, and other after-delivery supportive services for women and children."[48]

The "greatest need" that Vandegaer highlighted in *Heartbeat* was fueled by the same political and economic changes that have been explored in prior chapters. Incarceration, unemployment or underemployment, homelessness, poverty, inaccessible healthcare, disease, lack of child care, and cuts to social welfare programs comprised the conditions confronting the EPS movement in its second decade. But while Reagan's cuts to social spending imperiled many local organizations that combined aid with advocacy, such as women's health clinics, EPS centers perfectly articulated the administration's vision of reining in the supposed largesse of government: social problems would be addressed by charitable networks of volunteers.[49] The volunteer base of EPS advocates and their pro-life connections that pulled together medical care, housing, maternity clothes, and referrals free of charge easily weathered the storm that decimated agencies more reliant on federal funds. EPS centers were able to continue their efforts in earnest, and while their services may have not been comprehensive, they nevertheless became more visible and sought after as a result of other agencies' limited capacity.

As a result, even though (as one center director put it), "the economy tanked several times" since the movement's founding in 1971, EPS operations enjoyed relative stability amidst the insecurities that produced more and different clients. One center reported that while it had largely seen pregnant teenagers during its first years of operation in the early to mid-1970s, as economic circumstances worsened into the early 1980s, volunteers saw more married women coming for help because there "was basically no other place to go."[50] Many centers actively responded to the resource gaps their clients were facing. In 1987, the Johnson Family Memorial Fund run by EPS Pregnancy Services in Omaha, NE started providing pregnant women and families with cash grants for "problems ranging from utility shutoffs to possible eviction to emergency food assistance."[51] A.L.F.A. Pregnancy Services played a similar role in Philadelphia for a Maternity Care Coalition (MCC) client who could not afford a breast pump after giving birth—having exhausted all public options, an MCC client advocate arranged for A.L.F.A. to provide the necessary cash.[52] When volunteers at a center in Washington State learned that the county would no longer provide funding for prenatal vitamins due to budget cuts, the center added vitamins to its list of services.[53] Through donations to their Prenatal Partners Program, Matrix Lifeline in Lafayette, IA hoped to cover the cost of prenatal care for immigrant clients ineligible for Medicaid coverage due to citizenship restrictions.[54] By the early 1990s, Heartbeat of Monroe, MI, had implemented a housing grant program for homeless clients that were pregnant or had a child under the age of one year. And when volunteers learned that childbirth preparation classes at the nearby hospital were consistently over capacity, limiting clients' ability to have a support person present at their delivery, the EPS center started offering classes in order to "fill the gap."[55]

EPS centers' reliance on and cooperation with public aid programs varied just as widely. For example, volunteers that founded a network of centers on the West Coast also served as Women and Infant Care (WIC) service stations—the centers saw 10,000 WIC clients a month.[56] Bethlehem Home, an affiliate of Heartbeat International in Columbia, MI, stood in stark contrast. The EPS operation had successfully received a state license to open a home for pregnant teens and women, and the State Division of Family Services frequently referred pregnant girls from foster care homes. Despite this admittedly limited form of cooperation, Bethlehem Home did not allow women staying there to use food stamps or WIC. Instead, the maternity home frequented food banks and relied on community donations because staff running the maternity home believed it was modeling for its clients a "new attitude, away from the second and third generation of welfare mentality."[57] And still other EPS operations fell somewhere in between. Expectant Mother Care in New York City, for example, praised the city's "generous" prenatal care assistance program that covered both immigrant women and those living up to 85 percent above the poverty level while teenagers at the Harbor House Home for Unwed Mothers in Celina, OH received health insurance through the state's Medicaid program.[58]

As evidenced by these various arrangements, EPS centers' ability to provide a combination of services depended not only on the community relationships volunteers had cultivated, but also on advocates' beliefs about the terms that should accompany aid. The broader political context also shaped how advocates narrated women's needs. Whereas AAI counseled affiliates to "arrive at a reciprocal working relationship" with community agencies as long as they did not recommend abortion to any EPS clients, by the early 1990s well-worn conservative arguments about "welfare dependency" and the dissolution of family values were also motivating movement participants. An influx of evangelical donors, volunteers, and leaders helped ensure that such views were increasingly well represented in the service response to abortion.[59] Primary among such influences was the decision by Christian Action Council (CAC), a pro-life lobbying group, to prioritize its "crisis pregnancy center ministry" in earnest in 1980. The CAC had established over a hundred centers by the mid-1980s, and would eventually become Care Net, one of the two leading affiliate organizations in the movement.[60] AAI also underwent significant changes during this period, emerging as Heartbeat International in the early 1990s. The rebranded organization no longer described itself as nonsectarian, emphasized conservative Christian values, and eventually established a close partnership with Care Net as the two organizations made a concerted effort to professionalize the movement.[61] Whereas AAI had emphasized the need for EPS centers to be nonjudgmental so that they might reach as many women as possible, the new leadership undertook the difficult task of threading a needle between judgment-free support and the promotion of conservative Christian values.[62] Like Bethlehem Home, some EPS centers began combining material support with services meant to shape clients' values beyond abortion. Slippery Rock Crisis Pregnancy Support Center in Butler County, PA, for example, merged typical services like pregnancy tests, community referrals, and material aid with classes on single parenthood.[63]

These forays into explicitly faith-based programming such as parenting classes and abstinence-only education did little to stem the tide of "anecdotal reports" that EPS centers were seeing more and more services-only clients, reports that greatly concerned the new leadership.[64] Their anxieties were fueled by more than just the availability of abortion. Instead, combating what the director of Bethlehem Home described as a "welfare mentality" also became a movement goal. By the early 1990s, "years of anti-poor, anti-welfare rhetoric beamed across the country," instilling welfare myths—such as the idea that women have children in order to obtain more aid—in the minds of a public who increasingly found poor mothers to be irredeemable as a result.[65] As states eagerly sought to place limits on welfare aid through punitive mechanisms like the family cap (which denied benefits to families that had additional children while receiving AFDC payments), and as conservative researchers and politicians drew up plans for a welfare reform bill, some within the pro-life movement began to wonder if EPS centers might be playing too large a role in cultivating "dependency."[66] Pro-life activist Frederica Mathewes-Green profiled an EPS volunteer who described her typical client: "She probably gets $225 a month on welfare, and there's food stamps, WIC, and medical assistance. . . . In all these years, I've seen less than a half-dozen find a way to work. . . . We do put people on welfare. We do create single-parent homes, but at least the baby is alive." Drawing on the long-standing racist and sexist trope that poor mothers had children in order to get more aid, Mathewes-Green used the EPS volunteer's admission to argue that "welfare causes more crisis pregnancies" because "welfare dollars remove the stigma of sex and pregnancy outside marriage" by "making single-parent households possible."[67] *Time* magazine aired the movement's internal debates to a public eager for shocking commentary on welfare when it described the supposedly ironic scenario. "The volunteers at roughly 3,000 crisis pregnancy centers nationwide are promoting childbirth among the very women the Contract with America hopes to discourage from motherhood: unwed teens and welfare mothers having additional children." The *Time* piece profiled a client of a Care Net affiliate in Poughkeepsie, NY that no doubt secretly pleased Mathewes-Green, though from the vantage point of the movement's original aims, it was hardly remarkable. Cindy R., a twenty-two-year-old mother of two, told *Time*, "They call you and say, 'Do you need any stuff?' I love this place."[68]

Cindy R.'s experience hardly indicated that EPS centers had somehow diverged from their standard practices, but the debate over welfare reform brought attention to the movement that new leadership found undesirable. Curt Young, then president of Care Net, decided to do something about reports that centers were seeing more and more services-only clients. The Christian fundamentalist Family Research Council provided Young with funds to conduct a center assessment report, which Young presented to movement leaders at a Focus on the Family conference in 1998. Anecdotal reports had indicated both an increase in women looking for services and a decrease in women seeking abortion care. The study confirmed this anecdotal evidence. Researchers reportedly found that a select sample of CPCs showed a 7 percent increase of "services-only clients" compared to a 1 percent increase of "clients at risk" between 1994 and 1996. An editor's note amended the finding that rising numbers of women "desire only material assistance" and reminded readers that "it is of importance to serve these women well also, since they will spread the word to possible women at risk for abortion." But how to "serve these women well" was not the primary research objective. In fact, such findings threatened "the primary mission of Centers to reach women at risk by shifting CPCs off-center from at least two of their core values—to save children from abortion and to show compassion to women confronted with abortion."[69] If EPS centers failed to foreground these core values, they risked providing a service that reinforced the very culture leaders hoped to combat.

The distinction that Julie Huband had discovered at her EPS center in Ocala, FL over a decade prior was cemented with Young's report. But whereas Huband stressed the "importance of both populations," Young directed leaders to a single question: "How do we increase the number of Clients at Risk?" Echoing the center director who reported an increase in older, married women seeking support due to economic downturns, the report highlighted a decline since 1980 in women aged 15–29 visiting the centers. It also attributed the lower numbers of "at risk" clients to an increased acceptance of single parenthood, demonstrating how the movement's original aim of ensuring single pregnant women would not be abandoned had contributed to the culture shift that now so concerned the new leaders. Despite the fact that focus groups indicated money would be a woman's primary concern if faced with an unintended pregnancy—the material concerns that drew "services-only" clients to EPS centers—the report suggested that the movement could attract more "at-risk" clients by framing its services as "empowering a woman to make healthy choices for her life."[70] With proper image management and targeted advertising that avoided the framework of "crisis pregnancy," the movement might be able to re-center its core values.

REACHING "AT-RISK" CLIENTS

While focus groups orchestrated by Young's research initiative may have indicated a preference for images of capable, self-assured, happy clients, it would ultimately prove quite challenging for the movement to overcome its originating beliefs: that legal abortion posed a threat to vulnerable women and that EPS services were necessary to intervene in the crisis of an unplanned pregnancy. Around the same time Care Net began looking into anecdotal reports about "services-only" clients, Heartbeat International began investigating one of its own informal observations. Upon trying to schedule a regional outreach meeting for EPS volunteers in the Northeast in the early 1990s, Heartbeat International staff realized that there were very few EPS centers they could send an invitation to. At the same time, staff understood places like New York City to have high rates of abortion. Heartbeat staff began developing a theory. Perhaps there were higher numbers of abortions in places where abortion providers outnumbered EPS centers, as was the case in both Boston and New York City. Following numerous meetings with EPS directors in each city, Heartbeat initiated Project REACH in 1999 in order to provide direct support to the beleaguered centers.[71] Support included training center volunteers in Heartbeat's Volunteer Certification Program and funding advertisements for the centers. But Project REACH also initiated research aimed at testing the theory. The initiative got to work developing "detailed maps showing abortion statistics by zip code to identify neighborhoods in crisis and assist pregnancy centers in their expansion strategies."[72]

The "detailed maps" developed by Project REACH ultimately became the Abortion Hub Study, launched by Heartbeat in the early 2000s. The Abortion Hub Study completed the work started by Project REACH in that it mapped the distance between abortion clinics and EPS centers in every state. The greater the distance between an EPS center and an abortion clinic, the more an area was determined to be "in need" of the movement's attention and resources. Leaders at Heartbeat International shared their findings with Care Net and other pro-life organizations. Collectively, the groups settled on the theory that abortion clinics were not only overrepresented in major cities, but were specifically located in neighborhoods that were predominately African American or Latino. (The Guttmacher Institute debunked this conclusion in 2014 with its finding that the majority of abortion providers are located in neighborhoods where more than half of the residents were white).[73] The movement connected the unfounded claim about geographic concentration of abortion providers to statistics showing higher rates of abortion among Black and Latina women as compared to white women, decontexuatlized from the structural inequalities—such as lack of access to contraception—that help explain those differences. Heartbeat International's research provided an alternative explanation to why EPS centers were seeing fewer at-risk clients—EPS volunteers had overlooked what Heartbeat dubbed "areas of greatest need." Failing to be located in areas where abortion services were supposedly widely available exacerbated women's vulnerability to abortion, vulnerability that—according to the study—disproportionately impacted women of color living in urban areas.[74]

These claims provided rationale for the Urban Initiatives and Underserved Outreach campaigns, which depicted Black and Latina women as victims of predatory pro-choice organizations, and helped CPCs move from predominantly white, suburban and rural areas into larger cities. Care Net first set its sights on Atlanta, while Heartbeat sent John Ensor to Miami, based on his success expanding centers throughout the Boston area during the 1990s.[75] According to Heartbeat and its pilot project Heartbeat of Miami, Florida was targeted because it showed up as one of four states with the highest rates of abortion. When the study further determined that Miami had thirty-seven abortion facilities, the city became Heartbeat's testing grounds for its Urban Initiatives campaign.[76] The first center was established in Hialeah, a city with a predominately conservative, Catholic, Cuban American population, followed by a center in the predominately Black area of North Dade.[77] Care Net began projects in Atlanta, Chicago, Dallas, Houston, and Indianapolis, with Atlanta being subject to especially rapid growth with four new centers opening in just three years. By 2006, Care Net claimed that 20 percent of CPCs were serving populations with 500,000 or more people.[78]

As these initiatives demonstrate, the collapsing of demographic differences in abortion rates with EPS center scarcity not only provided an explanation for why the movement was failing to reach at-risk women. It also created an opportunity to direct center growth. Whereas AAI had endeavored to coordinate and support centers that were by and large homegrown initiatives, Heartbeat International and Care Net intended for their respective campaigns to drive center expansion. They did so by blowing fresh air into well-worn sails. While the new campaign sometimes mentioned Latina women, it especially focused on the idea that Black, urban neighborhoods were targeted by abortion clinics, drawing on long-standing claims that pro-choice organizations like Planned Parenthood were invested in a project of population control at best and modern-day Black genocide at worst. Such arguments predated *Roe* and were mobilized by both white and Black pro-lifers to argue against abortion rights. In her work as president of the National Right to Life Committee, Dr. Mildred Jefferson, one of the organization's few African American members, compared fetuses' legal status under *Roe* to that of the enslaved and warned that "the people who are fewer will disappear faster."[79] Jefferson herself drew on debates among African Americans, many of them prominent civil rights and Black liberation activists, who likened abortion and birth control to state-sponsored genocide, all of which helped popularize what activist and scholar Loretta Ross has described as "race-based attacks on abortion rights."[80] For the purpose of arguing against the right to abortion, such claims exploited the histories of reproductive coercion exercised against Black women under slavery and against poor, Black, Latina, and Indigenous women who were involuntarily sterilized during the twentieth century.[81]

In addition to driving center growth, the race-based strategy employed by Care Net and Heartbeat International also allowed the movement to channel internal concerns about services-only clients into an anti-abortion argument exposing the supposed eugenicist aims of pro-choice organizations. Pro-choice organizations defended themselves against such charges by exposing these outreach initiatives as yet more evidence of the movement's deception—this time aimed directly at barring women of color from accessing abortion.[82] But there is reason to stay focused on the internal concerns that originally motivated movement leaders to pursue such campaigns. The outreach initiatives relied heavily on a narrative that EPS centers successfully helped pregnant women "choose life" rather than falling prey to abortion providers. Such initiatives gained traction from the idea that operations needed only to bring their successful approach to areas where women were made especially vulnerable to predatory abortion clinics.

However, the historical evidence suggests that this narrative oversimplifies and even inaccurately describes EPS centers' role in women's lives. EPS operations that continue to report on the difficulty of getting "at-risk" clients to walk through their doors, for many years did not even bother to make such distinctions about their clients. Instead, since 1971, EPS centers have provided varying degrees of material and emotional support to poor and low-income pregnant women and families.[83] Scholarship examining the movement's current operations bears this out as well, reporting that "families seeking material aid for children who have already been born" comprised a "notable share of clientele."[84] It is *these* clients who have borne the costs of much needed support. Depending on the period in which they sought help and the center they ended up at, they had to navigate the evolving and diverse strings attached to far from comprehensive EPS aid. These strings may include anti-abortion propaganda, proselytizing, and even requirements that clients enroll in classes before they receive certain items. But in a landscape of neglect, enduring strings in exchange for much needed support is yet another reality of making ends meet. And yet, the automatic sorting of CPCs into the entrenched framework of the abortion debate renders such troubling realities invisible. Instead, the idea that the greatest threat EPS centers pose is to abortion access—or, alternatively, that EPS operations do, in fact, "save" women contemplating abortion from the procedure —persists. What are the costs of allowing such narratives to go unchallenged?

For starters, the rigid pro-life versus pro-choice framework of the abortion debate distracts from a simple fact documented repeatedly throughout *Reproduction Reconceived:* state neglect necessitates that far too many families must scrape together resources in order to make ends meet. State neglect in the post-*Roe* era has produced a situation in which compromised and insufficient services nonetheless have a role to play in the spotty patchwork of available support For example, when the Maternity Care Coalition (MCC) attempted to connect new mothers with much needed resources as part of the fight against infant mortality, they leaned on an EPS center because no funds were forthcoming from any other organization in Philadelphia. A.L.F.A. Pregnancy Services also stepped in when one of MCC's clients, a pregnant teenager who "did not have anywhere to stay," wished to carry her pregnancy to term and give her child up for adoption. MCC helped set up the appointment, and she enrolled in the A.L.F.A. program until the birth of her child. MCC's notes make clear that the organization considered pro-life service providers just one of many resources they might utilize in order to meet their clients' needs.[85] Such collaborations are not altogether surprising when one considers that pro-life services expanded during the same period city officials were largely refusing to put additional public resources towards improving their track record of poor birth outcomes.[86] Scholarship on current-day EPS centers confirms the persistence of such collaborations. Researchers have found that "centers often responded to social workers' requests for emergency aid for specific people," with one center reporting that it provided "material help on a virtually daily basis to women referred by the local department of social services."[87] And it is not just public agencies that EPS centers collaborate with. MCC, now serving the suburbs of Philadelphia as well as the city itself, still sends clients of their child development program to EPS centers for material items, and they in turn send pregnant women to MCC to enroll in its early childhood parenting classes.[88] EPS centers are so deeply ensconced in the patchwork of public and private agencies serving low-income families that one pro-life critic derided them as "social welfare agencies" rather than "cutting edge forces to reduce abortion."[89]

The narrative that EPS centers successfully deter women from abortion has also proven incredibly beneficial to pro-life initiatives that seek to restrict access to the procedure. Whereas the movement was originally ignored by male clergy and politicians pushing for a Human Life Amendment in the years following *Roe,* by the late 1980s some officials saw the political potential of "alternatives to abortion." Pennsylvania's Abortion Control Act, first passed in 1988 before being partially upheld by the Supreme Court in 1992, included a counseling provision that women be informed of agencies that provided "alternatives to abortion" in the state. Subsequently, Pennsylvania became the first state to allocate a portion of its budget to agencies that provided said "alternatives." At least thirteen states have drawn from Pennsylvania's playbook since it unveiled Project Women In Need in 1996.[90] While these initiatives rely heavily on the idea that EPS centers actually convince women not to obtain an abortion, the funneling of federal monies to EPS centers through Temporary Assistance to Needy Families (TANF) funds depend on movement leaders' explicit adherence to conservative family values (and the idea that volunteers successfully instill such values in their clients). Both Care Net and Heartbeat International instruct affiliates to counsel single pregnant women towards either marriage or adoption so as to not fuel the so-called culture of single parenthood that is then blamed for struggling families' circumstances.[91] Such counseling meets TANF's funding criteria for initiatives aimed at reducing non-marital pregnancies. Those concerned about taxpayer dollars going to unregulated EPS centers highlight how diverting funds meant to aid low-income families to "anti-choice" operations is simply more evidence that pro-lifers only care about life when it is in the womb.[92]

Such criticisms remain locked in the abortion debate framework. Would it not be more effective to take the legs out from under the entire act? Scholarship on current-day EPS operations and the volunteers who carry them out shows not only that clients by and large choose single parenthood over marriage and adoption, but that counselors do not push the values that emanate so loudly from movement leaders. The volunteer who in 1996 admitted to Frederica Mathewes-Green that "we do create single-parent homes" appears to share much with the counselors who "do not rank unhappy marriages above single motherhood." This suggests a through-line of the animating concerns that first motivated women to join the service-based response to abortion—advocates believe that helping the pregnant woman see that motherhood is a viable path is the surest way to render the procedure obsolete.[93] Research showing that pregnant women who seek services from EPS centers were not considering abortion, and that families seek services as well, suggests another through-line in terms of client *type*. The client that has relied most heavily on services provided by pro-life volunteers has not usually been, in the words of Abby Johnson, the "best client." Despite the movement's reliance on various types of anti-abortion propaganda and conservative Christian values, and despite the animating impulse to reach out to newly pregnant, undecided women, EPS centers largely have disseminated their views, along with much needed aid, to those building family on the economic and racial margins of society. Since the passage of the Clinton administration's Personal Responsibility and Work Opportunity Reconciliation Act, they have done so with an explicit mandate from the federal government "to make moral education a central focus of [its own] welfare programs." And they have provided services that "manage," but do not "eradicate," families' social problems.[94] Despite all of this, as long as state neglect is a fixture of family making in the United States, there will be a place and a need for EPS centers, no matter if their deception is as great as their services are insufficient to meet families' needs.

CONCLUSION

A 2004 report published by Care Net showed that 90 percent of the more than 110,000 women who visited Care Net affiliates that year carried their pregnancies to term. While applauding the results of Care Net's venture into producing statistical reports on its affiliate operations, then-president Melinda Delahoyde offered a caveat. "These are encouraging statistics; however, a majority of the women who are currently visiting pregnancy centers are likely to carry their babies to term, but need resources and emotional support that may not be found elsewhere in the community. While this is a valuable service, pregnancy centers want the majority of women who visit their centers to be those who are actually considering, or at risk of, having an abortion. Analysis of annual statistics helps Care Net know what is needed to help pregnancy centers better reach the population most at risk."[95]

Delahoyde's comment illustrates that some in the EPS movement are still plagued by the broader conditions which challenged its central tactic from the start: combating abortion by providing services has meant confronting state neglect of family making in the United States. Delahoyde and other movement leaders have concluded that EPS centers are consistently drawing the wrong kind of client. "Services-only" clients, many of whom are single mothers or pregnant women, rely on the aid offered by EPS centers in their fight against legal abortion but, as a result, distract the movement from reaching women who are undecided about their pregnancies. Yet, for many past and current participants in the EPS movement, particularly those providing direct services, such parsing of clients makes little sense. While motivated first and foremost by the belief that legal abortion poses an urgent threat to pregnant women, many EPS volunteers consider *any* woman helped a win in the fight against legal abortion. In this way, the very neglect that plagued and frustrated Delahoyde—due to a constant stream of services-only clients—also buoys volunteers' roles as support people and services providers. State neglect necessarily strains any political strategy rooted in service provision even as it ensures its continued relevance. This paradox certainly characterizes the EPS movement, though it is the movement's more recent leaders who are most likely to consider this a problem.

Abortion rights supporters point out that comments like Delahoyde's are proof of the movement's prioritization of fetuses over women in need, and they dismiss claims about EPS centers serving as legitimate resources. The problem with this assessment is that it too ignores the broader conditions that have enabled the movement to aid struggling families. As state neglect and inequality have worsened during the course of the movement's existence, many centers attempted to meet the proliferating needs identified by their clients. And unlike some of the other service-based projects documented in prior chapters, they had an easier time navigating austerity because services had always been made possible by volunteer and donor-based networks. This ensured that the support EPS centers could provide was far from comprehensive and was subject to volunteers' terms, but it also made them resilient. Broader conditions of neglect made them necessary, particularly as other resources reliant on public funding scaled back or were forced to close altogether. State neglect in the post-*Roe* era has meant that EPS centers play a dual role: they provide pregnancy services at the same time that they undermine choice through anti-abortion propaganda. Another important lesson demonstrated repeatedly in *Reproduction Reconceived* is that neglect does not produce an abundance of choice, an insight illustrated forcefully by the service-based approach to combating abortion.

Political and economic shifts placed new demands on the movement, at least from the perspective of some leaders. Not only were there too many "services-only" clients (albeit clients that many volunteers still considered signs of the movement's success), but by the late 1980s and 1990s, such clients made the movement vulnerable to charges that it fueled so-called "welfare dependency." Made anxious by these realities, leaders hoped to provide an alternative explanation for the abundance of "service-only" clients, and refocus the movement on those women supposedly most vulnerable to abortion providers. Care Net and Heartbeat International unveiled outreach campaigns that recycled race-based anti-abortion narratives and especially targeted Black women in urban centers as most in need of EPS services. Ironically, the movement's blatant targeting of Black women was justified by the claim that racist abortion providers, especially Planned Parenthood, were the actual threat to Black pregnant women. Through appeals to "race-based attacks on abortion," such campaigns successfully spurred some growth of centers in so-called underserved areas defined as poor, Black neighborhoods overserved by abortion providers and in need of pro-life interventions.[96] At the same time, pro-life lawmakers began to make "alternatives to abortion" a piece of their legislative strategy to limit abortion access, and found ways to fund EPS centers with taxpayer dollars. By 2013, the *New York Times* was reporting that CPCs were "the darlings of the pro-life movement."[97]

Such strategies and admiration are only possible when pregnant women considering abortion occupy the frame, and when EPS centers are imagined as such clients' first line of defense against the procedure. My own and other research demonstrates that this focus misses those most impacted by the practices at EPS centers. By holding the abortion debate at bay, pregnant women and mothers forced to piece together pregnancy support can enter the frame. These clients, reliant on free services they hope will mitigate their impoverished circumstances, must navigate the variety of strings attached to much needed resources: misinformation that is central to EPS volunteers' beliefs about abortion; attempts at religious conversion which motivates many volunteers' participation; race-based anti-abortion propaganda that positions Black women as dupes and stigmatizes their reproductive decision-making; and the withholding of needed items and services unless clients participate in center activities. These are some of the same families navigating the various constraints documented in previous chapters, and EPS centers' deceptive tactics are but one of many impediments they must overcome to survive under state neglect—only this time support and constraint go hand in hand. This reality is made clear by a recent study examining women's experiences of visiting EPS centers. Women reported that they appreciated the support they encountered, so much that they said they would refer friends to the center they had visited. At the same time, researchers concluded that the constraints placed on aid were significant enough that centers should not be considered "a reliable system of care and support."[98]

Under state neglect, it is precisely the absence of such a reliable system that ensures EPS centers remain relevant in families' lives despite their significant constraints. And we might go one step further still. It is reasonable to suggest that the movement has long been bolstered by society's investment in a key ideology greatly aided by *Roe* and fleshed out through decades of state neglect—having children is a choice, the costs and labors of which individuals should meet on their own. How labor intensive this family-making is, both inherently and made more so by different constraints, and how many costs pile up when the work becomes too much, is not a public concern but an individual and private responsibility. As a result, when systemic harm, neglect, and inequality create intolerable circumstances, the conditions families face are transformed into their own personal failings. To those on the margins suffering the consequences of such delusions, the lifelines of last resort provided by EPS centers are but another reminder of how far we have to go before family making is accessible to all.

Epilogue

Beginning in 2010, researchers with Advancing New Standards in Reproductive Health at the University of California, San Francisco started interviewing women who had been "turned away" from abortion care because they were past the state gestational limit as well as women who successfully accessed the procedure. The researchers repeatedly interviewed study participants over a period of five years about everything from relationship status to their emotional states to employment to the health of the children born to those who had initially tried to end their pregnancies. The longitudinal study, based on nearly 8,000 interviews and titled the "Turnaway Study," found that women had multiple reasons for seeking abortion, including finances, issues with a partner, and the demands of caring for their children. Researchers also found that women who were denied access to abortion, "the turnaways," experienced an increase in household poverty lasting at least four years as compared to those who received an abortion. They were also more likely not to have enough money to cover basic living expenses like food, housing, and transportation, resulting in increased debt and evictions.[1]

Scholarship on reproduction, abortion rights activism, and the sheer number of restrictions on abortion care enacted at the state level since

2011 have made the aforementioned results a familiar story. Legally sanctioned choice is meaningless without access, and there are serious consequences for those who are kept from obtaining abortions they want. Indeed, the Turnaway Study was at least partially conceived to put to rest once and for all the anti-abortion claims that "abortion harms women." The study makes clear that the reverse is true: being denied an abortion harms not just women but their children, too.[2] Research like this demonstrates that while *Roe* might still be standing, this fact counts for very little when it comes to the question of whether or not one can access abortion care. Increasingly, thanks in large part to abortion rights activists working within a reproductive justice framework, wide swaths of the public understand that "choice" is a fairly meaningless concept when it comes to abortion.

There is, however, another story contained in the results of the Turnaway Study, one about women's ability to have and raise children they want. It is worth asking if the women who sought an abortion due to finances were driven by the low-grade coercion of being out of options. Even this possibility should alert us to the fact that the invisible half of the choice equation, where "choice = motherhood," is also fatally flawed. Both for families who want children but cannot imagine how they would manage, and for families who are raising children where constraints vastly outnumber options, choice is fairly meaningless. And yet, the ways that choice fails to accurately describe the ability to make family is still poorly misunderstood by many. This is in part due to decades of defining reproductive choice as solely concerned with one's ability not to have children, for which the hyper-visible and entrenched abortion debate is in many ways responsible. It is tempting, for example, to see the Turnaway Study's findings about women's economic insecurity following a child's birth *solely* as evidence of the necessity of accessible abortion. It most certainly is this, but the study is also evidence of just how resource- and labor-intensive having and raising children is as a rule, and of the costs that befall families who cannot meet the demands of parenting on their own. *Reproduction Reconceived* has endeavored to tell a version of this other story, to make clear just how few options and just how many constraints have defined family making since the 1970s.

As I was finishing this book, COVID-19 and the ensuing economic devastation forced the American public to confront the myth of choice and the costs of neglect on an unprecedented scale. The pandemic both exposed and exacerbated long-standing inequalities of race, gender, class, and location, including a phenomenon central to this book: the devaluation of caring labor performed overwhelmingly by women both as unpaid workers in the home and as paid workers in the racially stratified care economy. For the first time in an economic recession, women lost more jobs than men, an outcome fueled both by the fact that women of color are concentrated in the low-wage service jobs hit hardest by public health lockdowns and by women's disproportionate child care responsibilities. (When schools closed, single mothers of all racial backgrounds were forced to choose between their two jobs, and the one that kept their kid alive won out over the one that brought in a paycheck.) Partnered women who did not lose their jobs but who, like their single counterparts, did lose the child care function of in-person schooling outside of the home reported doing far more domestic tasks and childrearing than their male partners who were also working from home.[3]

The idea that COVID-19 merely cracked open preexisting fault lines with regard to the persistent devaluation of reproductive labor is illustrated by the Spring 2021 issue of *Ms. Magazine*. The feminist magazine reprised the iconic illustration that had graced the cover of its first issue, published in 1972. A Kali-inspired woman with eight arms irons, drives, answers the phone, cooks, sweeps, types, and holds up a mirror and a clock while a baby glows from her mid-section. The illustration was a message to all housewives that society's expectations for middle-class wives and mothers were untenable, and that women deserved more. In the 2021 version, a Black woman with eight arms represents the frontline healthcare workers called "essential" but treated as expendable (two hands are gloved and hold a mask and syringe) as well as the child care and domestic labor tasks (hands hold an infant, a broom, laundry detergent, and groceries) that middle-class women could no longer outsource to low-waged women of color during the initial months of the pandemic. One hand types on a computer while another video-conferences with elderly family members on an iPad, and a young child sits at the table, learning remotely. Instead of a wake-up call to housewives, the Spring 2021 issue puts government and elected officials on notice. The heading above the illustration reads "Do We Care? The Nation's Moment of Truth."

Feminist economists have especially seized this moment to make the case for the necessity of human or care "infrastructure," a framework popularized by National Domestic Workers Alliance founder and labor activist Ai-jen Poo.[4] The Biden administration has responded to the numerous crises it inherited with a willingness to spend so uncharacteristic of the Democratic party that commentators have had to reach back sixty years to find a comparison in Lyndon B. Johnson. Making history as the first president to say the word "caregiving" in a pubic speech, Biden has also made a point of addressing the care crisis.[5] The administration's proposal targeting the issue allocates trillions for paid family leave, universal pre-K (beginning at age three), and child care, though the fate of both the American Jobs Plan and the American Families Plan remains to be seen. The United States has long been infamous for being the only industrialized country without paid family leave, not to mention other crucial programs, so such legislation actually making it through Congress without being gutted would begin to bring the country in line with its peers. This would certainly be a welcome development, but I also want to pay attention to the arguments being marshalled in the name of righting our denigration of care and to the benefits such a correction will supposedly bring. As the White House's own press release for the American Families Plan states, a major component of "build back better" is ensuring that the "approximately two million women who left [the workforce] due to COVID" can "rejoin and stay in the workforce."[6] Many feminist economists have a similar line. Those who authored the feature article for the Spring 2021 *Ms. Magazine* wrote, "In this moment of relief and recovery, if we settle for benching half the population because of a care crisis, there is no way we will enjoy a sustainable, inclusive economy going forward."[7] And as the *New York Times* recently wrote in a piece highlighting the scholarship and activism of those who are pressing the Biden administration to prioritize care, "a system where working parents do not have reliable, affordable child care is one where they cannot reliably build a career."[8]

With the exception of labor activism that has used this moment to highlight the exploitation of care workers and demand that these jobs be paid a living wage, it seems we are in the midst of a conversation about how valuing care is good for capital, obscured only slightly by a Trojan horse of liberal feminism. Here, it is instructive to reflect on the demands of a social movement mentioned at the very start of this book, one that had a different analysis of and solution to the devaluation of care. The National Welfare Rights Organization, in its push for a guaranteed annual income, popularized the idea that motherhood itself was work and that the state should pay welfare mothers a living wage for raising their children. In the 1970s, Marxist feminists would build on this political insight to form the Wages for Housework campaign in an effort to further expose the gendered and racialized exploitation of reproductive labor under capitalism. The current terms of debate over the care crisis leave very little room for such an analysis. There is even less space to consider how truly centering and valuing care would require an entirely new set of relations, where making sure children, the elderly, and those who fall ill are cared for is not first subject to a cost–benefit analysis meant to assess whether the economy's health could tolerate ensuring the health of humans.

Still, it is my hope that this history creates a little more room to think differently, both about the political obstacles that stand between us and meaningful reproductive freedom, and possible strategies for overcoming what stands in our way. The current debate over the care crisis holds promise because the pandemic has made it impossible to treat the dual demands of productive and reproductive labor as a problem of "work-life balance." However, even this round of the debate over who is doing too much of the work is centered around the familiar plot points of home, work, and child care. As this book shows, significant political and social developments in the final decades of the twentieth century created numerous constraints for families, ensuring that reproductive labor both proliferated and extended far beyond work and the home. Providing the life-sustaining care that happens within families is harder and often impossible when that essential work is forced to the precarious, neglected margins by epidemics whose impacts on women and their families are ignored, by a system of for-profit healthcare tied to employment, by imprisonment, and by insufficient legal recognition. Along the way, family caregivers are made to rely on piecemeal, moralizing aid.

State neglect is painstakingly documented in this book in an attempt to expose it for the lethal force that it has become in so many families' lives. Which is another way of saying that it will take much more than paid family leave to counter the historical and systemic neglect that makes it so hard to be with, care for, and ensure the health and safety of one's loved ones—all so that we might actually take joy in family, in all of its varied forms. Just last week, a local newspaper in D.C., where I live, reported on pregnant women's and mothers' struggle to find stable housing, health-care, and other services during the pandemic.[9] The story investigated reports that, despite the city's claim that it had paused terminations of participants' enrollment in the affordable housing program for the dura-tion of the pandemic, women unexpectedly lost their housing vouchers, informed by a notice posted on their door. While some women reported that their landlords were letting them stay while they worked out admin-istrative problems with the program, the eviction moratorium put in place for the duration of the pandemic ends on July 20. This is the reality of family making under state harm and neglect.

To bring about a different reality will take more people first realizing that exploitation-fueled inequalities of race, gender, class, and sexuality are not of families' own making, and then following in the footsteps of those who, upon their own realization of this fact, have been moved to act by the belief that things can and must be better. Reproduction—and its value—can be reconceived, again.

Acknowledgments

I have found it very difficult to let this book out into the world, unsure if I had done the subject matter justice, which made it hard to know if it was ever really complete. Thankfully, numerous people lent their invaluable care to me and this project in different, but always generous, ways. Each one of them saw in *Reproduction Reconceived* a book that could not only be done, but that needed to be out in the world. My heart is full of gratitude for those who lit the path by which this book took shape, was refined, and would eventually be free.

Numerous people generously shared their time, expertise, and experiences with me at various stages of this project. This book would simply not exist were it not for the individuals who opened their personal records to me and spoke with me about their life's work. I personally find archival research to be a lonely process, but spending time with the people who helped make the history documented in these pages has been one of the most rewarding aspects of this experience.

Celine Parreñas Shimizu first taught me that motherhood was a deeply political project and saw in me the urgent curiosity that is necessary to complete a PhD program. She, more than anyone, showed me a career that seemed truly worth my while when I was a junior in college with bad grades and little interest in my professional future.

I was fortunate to find yet more, generous mentors at Brown University, where I spent eight years working on this project. Tricia Rose helped me cultivate my voice at a critical moment in my graduate career, provided expert guidance on writing (and getting through) the dissertation, and gave me the gift of the awesome title for this book. Robert O. Self showed me the political necessity of history. I am, first and foremost, a historian because of his teaching, scholarship, and mentorship. Saida Hodžić agreed to serve as my field advisor even though she was on a temporary, two-year postdoctoral fellowship—a truly selfless act—and it is the kindness she showed me during exam prep that I now pass onto my own students. Both she and Sherine Hamdy taught me how to think like an anthropologist, a perspective that helped me see new questions in topics seemingly done to death. Laura Briggs saw potential in and got excited about the project even though we were at different universities. She generously mentored me and guided my scholarly thinking from afar, and she continues to serve as a model for how scholarship can help create radical change. Gail Cohee not only offered me a job that was a welcome reprieve from my dissertation, but also showed me how to navigate the politics of higher education and put the university's resources towards social justice ends. The work I did with her, Felicia Salinas-Moniz, and the rest of the Sarah Doyle Women's Center staff quite honestly made it possible for me to stay in graduate school, as they kept me focused on what questions and concerns really mattered. It was through the Sarah Doyle Women's Center that I was fortunate enough to meet the feminist artist Meredith Stern when her series "This Is an Emergency! A Reproductive Rights and Gender Justice Portfolio" was featured in the art gallery. I brought my class to listen to her artist talk long before I knew what this book would become, and I am humbled that she also thought her beautiful piece, "Sustainable Growth," belonged on the cover.

Moving across the country is a hard thing to do, but it is especially hard for Californians who tend to have a superiority complex about their beloved "best coast." I was lucky to meet amazing people during my eight years in Providence, Rhode Island, who made that trip more than worthwhile. I remain grateful for their love, support, and good humor. Colleen Trip, Alessa Dominguez, Jessica Johnson, Heather Lee, and Sean Dinces did much to shape my understanding of American Studies. Sasha Berkoff, Jessica Johnson, Colleen Tripp, Alessa Dominguez, and Sean Dinces made me feel at home. Lindsay Goss and Kate Diedrick inspired me with their unfailing convictions and continue to teach me much about organizing. Stand Up for Graduate Student Employees (SUGSE) made me an organizer. I am especially proud of everything we—and those who are still organizing at Brown—have done since a protest in front of President Christina Paxson's house in 2014 gave rise to our scrappy crew. Katy Roth literally kept me sane and continues to show me the way. Majida Kargbo, Elizabeth Wolfson, Robyn Schroeder, and Sarah Brown made sure my grad school days were filled with laughter. Dan Platt and Anne Gray Fischer encouraged me to think deeply about history when I was tired of my project. Majida Kargbo, Elizabeth Searcy, John Rosenberg, Brooke Lamperd, Sam Franklin, Virginia Thomas, Anne Gray Fischer, Oddný Helgadóttir, and Elizabeth Wolfson loved me unconditionally, caught me when it mattered most, and continue to bring so much wisdom, joy, and love into my life. Ben Holtzman introduced me to a world full of people, past and present, courageous enough to believe that the conditions under which we live can be changed for the better. From Providence to DC to Durham, he caught me most of all.

Beyond graduate school at Brown, Emily Thuma, Nicole Burrowes, Rana Jaleel, Emily Owens, Katrina Kimport, Deborah Dinner, Melinda Chateauvert, and Risa Cromer have nurtured me as a scholar and been generous collaborators in different ways over the last ten years. Given that I have tended to keep the ideas that ultimately formed this book to myself, I am especially appreciative to them for sharing space in which we could think together.

My colleagues in the History Department and the Women's, Gender, and Sexuality Studies Program at George Washington University not only hired me, but have also proven to be an amazingly talented, kind, and supportive community of scholars. In a hollowed-out job market comprised largely of temporary gigs that pay poverty wages, it is easy to say that one is grateful for the tenure-track job they were able to land with luck on their side. In my case, my gratitude for my colleagues is genuine rather than scarcity-induced. I am especially grateful to Andi Zimmerman, Johanna Bockman, Erin Chapman, Ivy Ken, Samantha Pinto, Dara Orenstein, Tyler Anbinder, Vanessa Wills, Abbey Agresta, and Leah Richardson for their fast friendship.

The Brocher Foundation generously supported a writing retreat that came at a critical juncture in the project. I was lucky enough to share that retreat with a cohort full of brilliant, welcoming, and jovial scholars who taught me a lot in a very short amount of time. Joan McCarthy and Helen Kohlen have one of the most beautiful friendships I have ever witnessed, and taught me that deep connections are easily forged when you go through the world with an open heart. I am grateful for the time I get to spend with them. Nichole Smith, Madeline Brown, Nora Cavanaugh, and Sarah-Anne Gresham provided invaluable research support, with Sarah-Anne Gresham lending critical help at the final hour.

This project would not be a book were it not for everyone at UC Press who believed *Reproduction Reconceived* should be published. I remember learning about the then new Reproductive Justice series during my fourth year of graduate school and thinking that my project belonged there. I remain thrilled that the series editors agreed. I am especially grateful to Rickie Solinger, whose enthusiasm for this project from the very beginning, along with her attentive engagement with some of its core ideas along the way, were invaluable contributions throughout the writing process. The attentive and sharp feedback provided by two careful readers, as well as thorough editorial feedback from Kathleen MacDougall and Julie Van Pelt, made this a far better, more enjoyable book to read. Naomi Schneider and Summer Farah made sure I stayed on track and helped bring out the best of the book.

My new home in DC has brought yet more magical people into my life. Trevor Jackson and Beki Cohen are the best Californians in DC. Together, we make it feel like home. Melinda Chateauvert and Mary Frances Berry have shown me more generosity than I knew was possible, and I am grateful to them for bringing me into the fold. Nell Geiser has been a source of political wisdom and quick, easy friendship. Patrick Young and Katie Donnelly are forever teaching me about the depths of joyful, sustaining friendship. The amazing folks in and around Shut-DownDC inspire me weekly if not daily, and I am constantly learning from all of them. I am grateful for an organizing home full of solidarity, creativity, friendship, and the bravery demanded by direct action.

Cari Ham, Alyise Temores, Carrie Scobee, Bryan Fauth, Ian Aragon, Chris Revay, Molly Mayer, Alvaro Bernal, and Peggy Lee have given me more years of friendship than I'd like to admit. Cari Ham especially has been my biggest fan and provided her legal expertise to this project free of charge more times than I can count. I hope someday to be as self-possessed as she has been since the day we met at age five. These friends have stood by me through immense change, geographical distance, and my unflattering quality of being really hard to get hold of. I have the deepest admiration for what each of them has become—being a part of their journeys is one of my greatest joys. Sandra Hemsworth and Kim Lerch took me in as their own, while Ariel Buck continues to shower me with best cousin love.

I am incredibly lucky to have a family that has always loved me, been proud of me, and told me so, repeatedly. It is rare that family members are able to do all of those things for most of one's life. They more than anyone supported my initial decision to pursue graduate school and saw me through the hardest parts of this professional journey, not to mention others that inevitably unfolded along the way. Leaving them remains one of the hardest things I have ever done, and I am grateful that they have never once begrudged me doing so. Even from so far away, they have offered respite, reassurance, and unconditional love at every turn. I am especially lucky that my brother is also my best friend. I know they never expected anything in return for believing in me, but this book is dedicated to them.

I do not know if the final stages of writing a book are always the hardest, or if they were made so by the fact that the last of my deadlines coincided with life under a global pandemic that revealed a willingness of those in power to tolerate mass death alongside the steady march of violence and neglect that also evidences such willingness, though in varied ways and at different scales. Regardless, it has not been easy. A key group of people offered their varying talents, time, and wisdom to make sure I got to the other side. Thank you to Emily Thuma, Anne Gray Fischer, Will Meyers, Majida Kargbo, Katie Donnelly, Ben Holtzman, and Laura Beth Pelner. Anne Gray Fischer in particular provided brilliant feedback whenever I asked her to read something, not to mention unconditional support. Ben Holtzman has especially seen this project through from beginning to end.

More importantly, he has believed in me from the very start, and I remain forever grateful to him for all that we learned, explored, and built together.

This book was well under way by the time I met Laura Beth Pelner, and she has supported it and me in ways too numerous to count. More so than anyone, Laura has urged me to let the book go so that it can do what it is meant to do in the world. She has done so with the incomparable kindness, patience, and compassion that she brings to those lucky enough to know her. Mostly, she has made life sweeter and more joyful than I could have ever imagined. It is her light that shines brightest on my path.

Notes

INTRODUCTION

1. Claire Cain Miller, "The Costs of Motherhood Are Rising, and Catching Women Off Guard," *New York Times*, Aug. 18, 2018.

2. Ilyana Kuziemko, Jessica Pan, Jenny Shen, and Ebonya Washington, "The Mommy Effect: Do Women Anticipate the Employment Effects of Motherhood?" (Cambridge, MA: National Bureau of Economic Research (NBER), Working Paper no. 24740 (June 2019), 1–2.

3. Sharon Hays, *The Cultural Contradictions of Motherhood* (New Haven, CT: Yale University Press, 1996).

4. Kuziemko et al., "The Mommy Effect," 1.

5. Adrienne Rich, *Of Woman Born: Motherhood as Experience and Institution* (New York: W. W. Norton, 1986), xiv (emphasis mine).

6. Cynthia Hess and Ariane Hegewisch, *The Future of Care Work: Improving the Quality of America's Fastest-Growing Jobs* (Washington, DC: Institute for Women's Policy Research, 2019); Eileen Boris and Jennifer Klein, *Caring for America: Home Health Workers in the Shadow of the Welfare State* (New York: Oxford University Press, 2012); Evelyn Nakano Glenn, *Forced to Care: Coercion and Caregiving in America* (Cambridge, MA: Harvard University Press, 2012); Gabriel Winant, *The Next Shift: The Fall of Industry and the Rise of Health Care in Rust Belt America* (Cambridge, MA: Harvard University Press, 2021).

7. Elise Gould, *State of Working America: Wages 2019* (Washington, DC: Economic Policy Institute, Feb. 2020); Estelle Sommeiller and Mark Price, *The New Gilded Age: Income Inequality in the U.S. by State, Metropolitan Area, and County* (Washington, DC: Economic Policy Institute, July 2018); Irene Padavic, Robin J. Ely, and Erin M. Reid, "Explaining the Persistence of Gender Inequality: The Work-Family Narrative as a Social Defense against the 24/7 Work Culture," *Administrative Science Quarterly* 65, no. 1 (2020). For the period 2017-18, Emmanuel Saez reported modest income growth for all groups, a minor correction to the disparity in wage growth. Discussion of 2009–12 income disparity on p. 3 of Emmanuel Saez, "Striking It Richer: The Evolution of Top Incomes in the United States (Updated with 2018 Estimates)," https://eml .berkeley.edu/~saez/saez-UStopincomes-2018.pdf (accessed Feb. 3, 2020); Annelise Orleck, *"We Are All Fast-Food Workers Now": The Global Uprising against Poverty Wages* (Boston: Beacon Press, 2018), 7.

8. Mark Lino, Kevin Kuczynski, Nestor Rodriguez, and TusaRebecca Schap, *Expenditures on Children by Families, 2015*, Miscellaneous Publication No. 1528-2015 (U.S. Department of Agriculture, Center for Nutrition Policy and Promotion, 2017); Orleck, *"We Are All Fast-Food Workers Now,"* 7.

9. Ilyana Kuziemko et al., "The Mommy Effect," 36.

10. Foundational texts outlining the necessity of an alternative value system that can prioritize care over profit include Angela Y. Davis, *Women, Race and Class* (New York: Vintage Books, 1981), ch. 3; Heidi I. Hartmann, "The Family as the Locus of Gender, Class, and Political Struggle: The Example of Housework," *Signs* 6, no. 3 (1981): 366–94; Combahee River Collective, *The Combahee River Collective Statement: Black Feminist Organizing in the Seventies and Eighties* (Albany, NY: Kitchen Table Women of Color Press, 1986); Mariarosa Dalla Costa, *Women and the Subversion of the Community: A Mariarosa Dalla Costa Reader,* ed. Camille Barbagallo (Oakland: PM Press, 2019); Leopoldina Fortunati, *The Arcane of Reproduction: Housework, Prostitution, Labor and Capital* (Brooklyn: Autonomedia, 1995); Silvia Federici, *Revolution at Point Zero: Housework, Reproduction, and Feminist Struggle* (Oakland: PM Press, 2012). For scholarship examining the continued devaluation of care work and the persistence of racial and gendered hierarchies within the care economy domestically as well as globally, see Barbara Ehrenreich and Arlie Hochschild, eds., *Global Woman: Nannies, Maids, and Sex Workers in the New Economy* (New York: Henry Holt, 2002); Melissa W. Wright, *Disposable Women and Other Myths of Global Capitalism* (New York: Routledge, 2006); Eileen Boris and Jennifer Klein, *Caring for America;* Evelyn Nakano Glenn, *Forced to Care;* Nancy Fraser, "Crisis of Care? On the Social-Reproductive Contradictions of Contemporary Capitalism," in *Social Reproduction Theory: Remapping Class, Recentering Oppression,* ed. Tithi Bhattacharya (London: Pluto Press, 2017); Mignon Duffy, "Doing the Dirty Work: Gender, Race, and Reproductive Labor in Historical Per-

spective," *Gender and Society* 21, no. 3 (2007); Grace Chang, *Disposable Domestics: Immigrant Women Workers in the Global Economy* (Chicago: Haymarket Books, 2016); Rhacel Parrenas, *The Force of Domesticity: Filipina Migrants and Globalization* (New York: NYU Press, 2008). Nancy Folbre, "'Holding Hands at Midnight': The Paradox of Caring Labor," *Feminist Economics* 1, no. 1 (1995).

11. On "life-making," see Tithi Bhattacharya's work profiled by Sarah Jaffe, "Social Reproduction and the Pandemic, with Tithi Bhattacharya," *Dissent*, Apr. 2, 2020; Tithi Bhattacharya, "Introduction: Mapping Social Reproduction Theory," in *Social Reproduction Theory: Remapping Class, Recentering Oppression*, ed. Tithi Bhattacharya (London: Pluto Press, 2017).

12. On reproductive justice, see Loretta Ross and Rickie Solinger, *Reproductive Justice: An Introduction* (Berkeley: University of California Press, 2017); Loretta Ross, Elena Gutierrez, Marlene Gerber Fried, and Jael Silliman, *Undivided Rights: Women of Color Organize for Reproductive Justice* (Boston: South End Press, 2004); Marlene Gerber Fried, ed., *From Abortion to Reproductive Freedom: Transforming a Movement* (Boston: South End Press, 1990); Jennifer Nelson, *More Than Medicine: A History of the Feminist Women's Health Movement* (New York: NYU Press, 2015); Melissa Murray, Katherine Shaw, and Reva B. Siegel, eds., *Reproductive Rights and Justice Stories* (St. Paul, MN: Foundation Press, 2019); Zakiya Luna, *Reproductive Rights as Human Rights: Women of Color and the Fight for Reproductive Justice* (New York: NYU Press, 2020).

13. For scholarship that complicates this neat narrative, see Mary Ziegler, *After Roe: The Lost History of the Abortion Debate* (Cambridge, MA: Harvard University Press, 2015) and *Beyond Abortion: Roe v. Wade and the Fight for Privacy* (Cambridge, MA: Harvard University Press, 2018); Kristin Luker, *Abortion and the Politics of Motherhood* (Berkeley: University of California Press, 1984); Linda Greenhouse and Reva B. Siegel, "The Unfinished Story of *Roe v. Wade*," in *Reproductive Rights and Justice Stories*, ed. Melissa Murray, Katherine Shaw, and Reva B. Siegel (St. Paul, MN: Foundation Press, 2019).

14. The ways in which abortion access was inherently limited by the legal architecture of *Roe* (secured by the negative right to privacy) and the subsequent rhetoric of choice have been widely discussed. Scholars have argued that choice is a meaningless concept for women who lack the resources and autonomy necessary to exercise this newfound right. For a legal discussion of the limitations of the right to privacy, see Rhonda Copelon, "From Privacy to Autonomy: The Conditions for Sexual and Reproductive Freedom," in *From Abortion to Reproductive Freedom: Transforming a Movement*, ed. Marlene Gerber Fried (Boston: South End Press, 1990) (Gerber Fried's anthology was an important contribution to feminist discussions on reproductive rights looking to move beyond choice). For a broader discussion of negative versus positive liberty in relation to reproductive freedom, see Dorothy E. Roberts, *Killing the Black Body: Race, Reproduction, and the Meaning of Liberty* (New York: Vintage Books, 1997), 294–312. Scholars

have also shown how choice ensured abortion would be subject to market forces, available only to those with sufficient resources. See Rickie Solinger, *Beggars and Choosers: How the Politics of Choice Shapes Adoption, Abortion, and Welfare in the United States* (New York: Hill and Wang, 2001); Robert O. Self, *All in the Family: The Realignment of American Democracy since the 1960s* (New York: Hill and Wang, 2012), 159–60; Rosalind P. Petchesky, *Abortion and Woman's Choice: The State, Sexuality and Reproductive Freedom* (Boston: Northeastern University Press, 1985). In commenting on the outpouring of support for abortion in anticipation of the 1989 Supreme Court decision in *Webster v. Reproductive Health Services*, Gerber Fried asked then if choice was even worth fighting for: "Freedom of choice circumscribed by race and class, removed from feminist demands about women's autonomy, and shrouded in 'privacy'?" Gerber Fried, *From Abortion to Reproductive Freedom*, ix.

15. For a discussion on this point in relation to attacks on welfare recipients in the 1980s see Solinger, *Beggars and Choosers*, 146.

16. Changing views on abortion, contraception, and premarital sex during this period, as well as the rise of premarital sex, co-habitation, and single motherhood are documented by Kristen Luker in *When Sex Goes to School: Warring Views on Sex—and Sex Education—since the Sixties* (New York: W. W. Norton, 2006), ch. 3. See also Elizabeth Pleck, *Not Just Roommates: Cohabitation after the Sexual Revolution* (Chicago: University of Chicago Press, 2012).

17. Specifically, women of color and feminists' analyses that legal abortion was but one piece of what was required for liberation in a white supremacist, capitalist, imperialist society stood in contrast to and, in some cases, deeply influenced the predominately white abortion rights movement's belief that legalization represented a panacea for women's liberation. See Davis, *Women, Race, and Class*, ch. 12; Jennifer Nelson, *Women of Color and the Reproductive Rights Movement* (New York: NYU Press, 2003); Sherrie M. Randolph, *Florynce "Flo" Kennedy: The Life of a Black Feminist Radical* (Chapel Hill: University of North Carolina Press, 2015), ch. 8; Ashley Farmer, *Remaking Black Power: How Black Women Transformed an Era* (Chapel Hill: University of North Carolina Press, 2017), ch. 5. For an overview examining how these analyses stemmed in part from the mothering responsibilities of predominately poor, women of color, see Annelise Orleck, *Rethinking American Women's Activism* (New York: Routledge, 2015), ch. 6.

18. During the 1960s and 1970s, the National Welfare Rights Organization did more than any other group to popularize the idea that child-rearing was a job. On the history of the NWRO, see Premilla Nadasen, *Welfare Warriors: The Welfare Rights Movement in the United States* (New York: Routledge, 2005). See also Annelise Orleck, *Storming Cesar's Palace: How Black Mothers Fought Their Own War on Poverty* (Boston: Beacon Press, 2005); Felicia Kornbluh, *The Battle for Welfare Rights: Politics and Poverty in Modern America* (Philadelphia: University of Pennsylvania Press, 2007).

19. Self, *All in the Family,* 7.

20. On feminism, sexuality, and the family, see Self, *All in the Family.* On urban rebellions and law and order politics, see Elizabeth Hinton, *From the War on Poverty to the War on Crime: The Making of Mass Incarceration* (Cambridge, MA: Harvard University Press, 2016). On civil rights and race, see Dan T. Carter, *The Politics of Rage: George Wallace, the Origins of the New Conservatism, and the Transformation of American Politics* (New York: Simon and Schuster, 1995).

21. Scholarship on the influence of "choice" after *Roe* that has been especially influential to my own formulation comes from Angela Y. Davis, Dorothy Roberts, Rickie Solinger, and Robin West. In her now seminal essay, "Racism, Birth Control, and Reproductive Rights," Davis warned that reproductive choice could become reproductive coercion for poor, women of color whose procreation was discouraged through explicit attacks such as forced sterilization and through the low-grade coercion of racial and economic exploitation. Davis, *Women, Race and Class,* ch. 12. In 1997, Roberts extended critiques of privacy rights typically applied to abortion to the full spectrum of Black women's reproductive experiences in her groundbreaking *Killing the Black Body.* Solinger charted the political changes that made some mothers "beggars" and some mothers "choosers" in relation to abortion, adoption, and welfare post-*Roe* in 2001. Solinger, *Beggars and Choosers.* In 2009, West argued that "by giving pregnant women the choice to opt *out* of parenting by purchasing an abortion, we render parenting a market commodity, and thereby legitimate, systematically, the various baselines to which she agrees when she opts *in* . . . by giving her the choice, her consent legitimates the parental burden to which *she* has consented." Robin West, "From Choice to Reproductive Justice: De-Constitutionalizing Abortion Rights," *Yale Law Journal* 118 (2009): 1411 (emphasis in original).

22. This is Judith Stein's contribution. She points out that what economists called the Age of Compression officially ended in 1973 when wages first stagnated, the same year *Roe* was decided. See Judith Stein, *Pivotal Decade: How the United States Traded Factories for Finance in the Seventies* (New Haven, CT: Yale University Press, 2010), xi.

23. Jefferson Cowie, *Capital Moves: RCA's Seventy-Year Quest for Cheap Labor* (New York: The New Press, 2001). See also Stein, *Pivotal Decade.*

24. All women's participation in the labor force had been increasing since 1955, but married women's participation rose most dramatically between 1955 and 1999. See Kristie M. Engemann and Michael T. Owyang, "Social Changes Lead Married Women into Labor Force," *The Regional Economist,* Apr. 2006.

25. Kristen Swinth, "Post–Family Wage, Postindustrial Society: Reframing the Gender and Family Order through Working Mothers in Reagan's America," *Journal of American History* 105, no. 2 (Sept. 2018).

26. Stein, *Pivotal Decade,* xi.

27. Welfare rolls rose 214 percent in the 1960s, with the majority of the growth at the end of the decade. Marisa Chappell, "Rethinking Women's Politics in the 1970s: The League of Women Voters and the National Organization for Women Confront Poverty," *Journal of Women's History* 13 (2002): 161. As Premilla Nadasen and others have shown, the welfare rolls were increasing even before the 1960s, and it was the rise of recipients who had divorced, had children born out of wedlock, or were nonwhite who joined the rolls between 1950 and 1960 that would help ensure that "the politics of welfare converged on the stereotypical image of a Black unmarried welfare mother with a child born of out of wedlock." See Nadasen, *Welfare Warriors*, 7. On the turn to self-support in welfare policy of the 1960s, and how this planted the seeds for "personal responsibility" that enabled welfare's demise by the end of the twentieth century, see Jennifer Mittlestadt, *From Welfare to Workfare: The Unintended Consequences of Liberal Reform, 1945–1965* (Chapel Hill: University of North Carolina Press, 2005).

28. Diane Pearce is credited with coining "feminization of poverty." The statistic comes from the article where she introduced the term, "The Feminization of Poverty: Women, Work and Welfare," *Urban and Social Change Review* 11, no. 28 (1978): 28. Jennifer Mittlestadt suggests that the feminization of poverty may very well be dated to prior to 1978. "In 1960, 70 percent of African American female-headed households were below the poverty line, as were 42 percent of white female-headed households." Mittlestadt, *From Welfare to Workfare*, 152–53.

29. Davis, *Women, Race, and Class*, 204–6.

30. Self, *All in the Family*; Stacie Taranto, *Kitchen-Table Politics: Conservative Women and Family Values in New York* (Philadelphia: University of Pennsylvania Press, 2017); Lisa Duggan, *The Twilight of Equality: Neoliberalism, Cultural Politics, and the Attack on Democracy* (Boston: Beacon Press, 2004); Melinda Cooper, *Family Values: Between Neoliberalism and the New Social Conservatism* (New York: Zone Books, 2017); Laura Briggs, *How All Politics Became Reproductive Politics: From Welfare Reform to Foreclosure to Trump* (Berkeley: University of California Press, 2017).

31. For commentary on using the end of the family, or breadwinner, wage as scholarly points of departure, see Nancy Fraser, *Fortunes of Feminism: From State-Managed Capitalism to Neoliberal Crisis* (New York: Verso Books, 2013), 111–35; Nancy Maclean, "Postwar Women's History: The 'Second Wave' or the End of the Family Wage?" in *A Companion to Post-45 America*, ed. Jean-Christophe Agnew and Roy Rosenzweig (Malden, MA: Blackwell, 2002).

32. Self, *All in the Family*, 9.

33. On welfare see Marisa Chappell, *The War on Welfare: Family, Poverty, and Politics in Modern America* (Philadelphia: University of Pennsylvania Press, 2009); Gwendolyn Mink, *Welfare's End* (Ithaca, NY: Cornell University Press, 1998); Ange-Marie Hancock, *The Politics of Disgust: The Public Identity of the*

Welfare Queen (New York: NYU Press, 2004); Felicia Kornbluh and Gwendolyn Mink, *Ensuring Poverty: Welfare Reform in Feminist Perspective* (Philadelphia: University of Pennsylvania Press, 2019); Nancy Fraser and Linda Gordon, "A Genealogy of 'Dependency': Tracing a Keyword of the American Welfare State," *Signs* 19, no. 2 (Winter 1994); Briggs, *How All Politics Became Reproductive Politics*, 47–74; Susan Douglas and Meredith Michaels, *The Mommy Myth: The Idealization of Motherhood and How It Has Undermined Women* (New York: The Free Press, 2004), 173–202. On the many limitations baked into welfare, see Mittlestadt, *From Welfare to Workfare;* Jill Quadagno, *The Color of Welfare: How Racism Undermined the War on Poverty* (New York: Oxford University Press, 1994); Linda Gordon, *Pitied but Not Entitled: Single Mothers and the History of Welfare, 1890–1935* (New York: The Free Press, 1994). On women's entry into the labor market and the problem of reproductive labor, see Kristen Swinth, *Feminism's Forgotten Fight: The Unfinished Struggle for Work and Family* (Cambridge, MA: Harvard University Press, 2018); Katherine Turk, *Equality on Trial: Gender and Rights in the Modern American Workplace* (Philadelphia: University of Pennsylvania Press, 2016), 174–202; Douglas and Michaels, *The Mommy Myth*, 236–67; Arlie Hochschild, *The Second Shift: Working Families and the Revolution at Home* (New York: Penguin Press, 1989). For a more popular treatment of this problem, see Ann Crittenden, *The Price of Motherhood: Why the Most Important Job in the World Is Still the Least Valued* (New York: Owl Books, 2001). For an analysis that keeps home and work in view at the same time, see Susan Thistle, *From Marriage to the Market: The Transformation of Women's Lives and Work* (Berkeley: University of California Press, 2006). For a recent history that brings these two plot points together and adds other examples of neoliberalism's impact on the family see Briggs, *How All Politics Became Reproductive Politics*. Another recent work that extends beyond these examples is Cooper, *Family Values*.

34. MacLean, "Postwar Women's History," 238.

35. Swinth, *Feminism's Forgotten Fight*, 248.

36. In addition to the aforementioned work on caring labor, here I am benefitting from and building off of feminist activism and scholarship that has theorized the value of reproductive labor in a variety of contexts. On activism see Silvia Federici, *Wages against Housework* (Bristol and London: Power of Women Collective; Falling Wall Press, 1975); Nadasen, *Welfare Warriors*. On the disciplining of women's labor and knowledge in the transition to capitalism, see Silvia Federici, *Caliban and the Witch: Women, the Body, and Primitive Accumulation* (Brooklyn, NY: Autonomedia, 2004). On the integral role of enslaved women's reproductive labor to the system of slavery, see Jennifer Morgan, *Laboring Women: Reproduction and Gender in New World Slavery* (Philadelphia: University of Pennsylvania Press, 2004). On the recent historical origins of the devaluation of reproductive labor, see Gwendolyn Mink, *Wages of Motherhood: Inequality in the*

Welfare State, 1917–1942 (Ithaca, NY: Cornell University Press, 1996). On feminist interventions into Marxism, see Heidi Hartmann, "The Unhappy Marriage of Marxism and Feminism: Towards a More Progressive Union," *Capital and Class* 3 (1979). On the link between reproductive labor, racial hierarchies in the United States, and citizenship, see Evelyn Nakano Glenn, *Unequal Freedom: How Race and Gender Shaped American Citizenship and Labor* (Cambridge, MA: Harvard University Press, 2002). My aim to follow the labors and costs of family making beyond the home and wage system is also informed by Sarah Haley's recent work on Black, incarcerated women's domestic labor in the homes of white families as a condition of their parole in early twentieth-century Jim Crow Georgia. Haley illustrates how the historically specific constraints of the chain gang, its legal codes, and the gendered racial hierarchy of the Jim Crow South made it possible to extract Black women's reproductive labor in an altogether new context—the "domestic carceral sphere." My book aims to highlight a set of historically specific constraints that added new labors and costs to the project of family making, thereby expanding our view of why the devaluation of reproductive labor produces so much gendered and racialized economic inequality. Sarah Hayley, *No Mercy Here: Gender, Punishment, and the Making of Jim Crow Modernity* (Chapel Hill: University of North Carolina Press, 2016).

37. Briggs, *How All Politics Became Reproductive Politics*, 8.

38. Lisa Duggan has helpfully described these collective efforts as "cultures of downward distribution" aimed at redistributing "money, political power, cultural capital, pleasure, and freedom." She contends that these efforts were, in the early 1970s, met by a pro-business movement organized around a "culture of upward (re)distribution." Duggan, *The Twilight of Equality?*, xvii.

39. Alice Kessler-Harris, *In Pursuit of Equity: Women, Men, and the Quest for Economic Citizenship in 20th-Century America* (New York: Oxford University Press, 2001).

40. Gordon, *Pitied but Not Entitled*; Mittlestadt, *From Welfare to Workfare*; Quadagno, *The Color of Welfare*; Nadasen, *Welfare Warriors*.

41. This literature is particularly intent on putting to rest once and for all the false divide between economics and so-called cultural values. See especially Cooper, *Family Values*; Duggan, *The Twilight of Equality?*; Self, *All in the Family*; Briggs, *How All Politics Became Reproductive Politics*; Clare Daniel, *Mediating Morality: The Politics of Teen Pregnancy in the Post-Welfare Era* (Amherst: University of Massachusetts Press, 2017); Anne Marie Smith, *Welfare Reform and Sexual Regulation* (New York: Cambridge University Press, 2007).

42. Following Michel Foucault, Wendy Brown and others have demonstrated how the logic of neoliberalism—obsessed with personal responsibility, safeguarding the private, and enhancing profitability in every corner of life—has reached into the very "soul of the citizen-subject." Wendy Brown, "Neo-Liberalism and the End of Liberal Democracy," *Theory and Event* 7, no. 1 (2003): 39.

This literature has been concerned especially with how neoliberalism altered conceptions of citizenship and shaped self-governance. See especially Lauren Berlant, *The Queen of America Goes to Washington City: Essays on Sex and Citizenship* (Durham, NC: Duke University Press, 1997); Aihwa Ong, *Neoliberalism as Exception* (Durham, NC: Duke University Press, 2006).

43. As Melinda Cooper writes, "Personal responsibility was invoked nowhere more forcefully than at the margins." Cooper, *Family Values*, 193.

44. On the history of the control and exploitation of enslaved women's reproduction, see Roberts, *Killing the Black Body;* Morgan, *Laboring Women;* Davis, *Women, Race, and Class,* ch. 1; Diedre Cooper Owens, *Medical Bondage: Race, Gender, and the Origins of American Gynecology* (Athens: University of Georgia Press, 2017); Marie Jenkins Schwartz, *Birthing a Slave: Motherhood and Medicine in the Antebellum South* (Cambridge, MA: Harvard University Press, 2010). On the history of the ways eugenics projects moved from racial hierarchies to gender and sex roles in the first half of the twentieth century, see Alexandra Minna Stern, *Eugenic Nation: Faults and Frontiers of Better Breeding in Modern America* (Berkeley: University of California Press, 2005). On the history of the interrelated experiences of sterilization for white women and women of color during the second half of the twentieth century, see Rebecca Kluchin, *Fit to Be Tied: Sterilization and Reproductive Rights in America, 1950–1980* (New Brunswick, NJ: Rutgers University Press, 2009). On efforts to control Indigenous families and women's reproduction since the late nineteenth century and Indigenous women's resistance to colonialism, see Brianna Theobald, *Reproduction on the Reservation: Pregnancy, Childbirth, and Colonialism in the Long Twentieth Century* (Chapel Hill: University of North Carolina Press, 2019). On how sterilization, abortion, and birth control created both choice and coercion during the twentieth century, see Johanna Schoen, *Choice and Coercion: Birth Control, Sterilization, and Abortion in Public Health and Welfare* (Chapel Hill: University of North Carolina Press, 2005). On the history of activism against forced sterilization during the 1960 and 1970s, see Jennifer Nelson, *Women of Color and the Reproductive Rights Movement* (New York: NYU Press, 2003). On the coercion many unmarried mothers faced to give up their children, and the disparate treatment afforded white and Black unmarried pregnant women before *Roe*, see Rickie Solinger, *Wake Up Little Susie: Single Pregnancy and Race before Roe v. Wade* (New York: Routledge, 1992). On the coercive forces that drove transnational and transracial adoption in the second half of the twentieth century, see Laura Briggs, *Somebody's Children: The Politics of Transracial and Transnational Adoption* (Durham, NC: Duke University Press, 2012). For the long-standing practice of child removal in the United States see Laura Briggs, *Taking Children: A History of American Terror* (Berkeley: University of California Press, 2020). On the history of the criminalization of abortion, see Leslie Reagan, *When Abortion Was a Crime: Women, Medicine, and Law* (Berkeley:

University of California Press, 1996). On the role of reproduction in shoring up citizenship through the regulation of immigrant women's reproduction, see Elena R. Gutiérrez, *Fertile Matters: The Politics of Mexican-Origin Women's Reproduction* (Austin: University of Texas Press, 2008). On the role of reproduction in maintaining U.S. imperial power, see Laura Briggs, *Reproducing Empire: Race, Sex, Science, and U.S. Imperialism in Puerto Rico* (Berkeley: University of California Press, 2003). On curtailing abortion as fundamental to the New Right's agenda to restore traditional gender roles, see Petchesky, *Abortion and Woman's Choice;* Linda Gordon, "Who Is Frightened of Reproductive Freedom for Women and Why? Some Historical Answers," *Frontiers: A Journal of Women's Studies* 9, no. 1 (1986). On the use of the fetus in the pro-life/anti-abortion movement, see Sara Dubow, *Ourselves Unborn: A History of the Fetus in Modern America* (New York: Oxford University Press, 2011), 112–83.

45. On the ways the ascendance of the fetus post-*Roe* has been instrumental in constraining women's reproductive rights, see Rachel Roth, *Making Women Pay: The Hidden Cost of Fetal Rights* (Ithaca, NY: Cornell University Press, 2003); Janelle Taylor, *The Public Life of the Fetal Sonogram: Technology, Consumption, and the Politics of Reproduction* (New Brunswick, NJ: Rutgers University Press, 2008). On appeals to the legacy of slavery to advance personhood arguments for embryos, see Risa Cromer, "Racial Politics of Frozen Embryo Personhood in the U.S. Antiabortion Movement," *Transforming Anthropology* 27, no. 1 (Apr. 2019). On the ways reproductive healthcare available to Native women serves the interests settler colonialism, see Barbara Gurr, *Reproductive Justice: The Politics of Health Care for Native American Women* (New Brunswick, NJ: Rutgers University Press, 2014). On connections between past and present reproductive rights abuses of Black women in the United States, see Roberts, *Killing the Black Body.* On the criminalization of women's reproduction, see Jeanne Flavin, *Our Bodies, Our Crimes: The Policing of Women's Reproduction in America* (New York: NYU Press, 2009). On the systemic racism of the child welfare system in the United States, see Dorothy Roberts, *Shattered Bonds: The Color of Child Welfare* (New York: Basic *Civitas* Books, 2002).

46. Rayna Rapp and Faye Ginsburg summarize Shelle Colen's term "stratified reproduction" as "the power relations by which some categories of people are empowered to nurture and reproduce, while others are disempowered." Ginsburg and Rapp, *Conceiving the New World Order: The Global Politics of Reproduction* (Berkeley: University of California Press, 1995), 3.

47. For example, a 2018 roundtable published in *Dissent* posed this question about the explicative value of the term "neoliberalism." See "The Uses and Abuses of Neoliberalism," *Dissent*, Jan. 22, 2018. Aihwa Ong, one of the foremost scholars of neoliberalism put it in a slightly different vein in 2006 when she wrote, "Neoliberalism seems to mean many different things depending on one's vantage point." Ong, *Neoliberalism as Exception,* 1. I also find Daniel Rodgers's recent

argument that neoliberalism is not the sort of word that has "experientially graspable legs" compelling, and this too has motivated my desire to describe the forces documented in *Reproduction Reconceived* as "state neglect." See Rodgers, "Reply: Fault Lines," *Dissent*, Jan. 22, 2018.

48. Davis, *Women, Race, and Class*, 204.

49. On Ruth Wilson Gilmore's "organized abandonment," which she pairs with "organized violence," see Ruth Wilson Gilmore, "Organized Abandonment and Organized Violence: Devolution and the Police," Nov. 9, 2015, lecture at the Humanities Institute, University of California, Santa Cruz, available at https://vimeo.com/146450686. On the pairing of "care" and "responsibility" with neglect" in what Barbara Gurr calls the "double discourse" to describe colonization and subsequent medical management of Indigenous peoples in the United States, see Gurr, *Reproductive Justice*. On "privatization and punishment" in the context of reproductive technologies, see Dorothy Roberts, "Privatization and Punishment in the New Age of Reprogenetics," *Emory Law Journal* 54 (2005).

50. Cooper, *Family Values*, 22.

51. The idea that constraints set the limits of one's choices is central to the reproductive justice framework. The spirit of this sentiment is described by Loretta Ross and Rickie Solinger as "individual choices have only been as capacious and empowering as the resources any woman can turn to in her community." Ross and Solinger, *Reproductive Justice*, 16.

52. Zakiya Luna, *Reproductive Rights as Human Rights: Women of Color and the Fight for Reproductive Justice* (New York: NYU Press, 2020).

53. Ross and Solinger, *Reproductive Justice*, 65.

54. Tressie McMillan Cottom, "Trickle-Down Feminism, Revisited," *Dissent*, Apr. 21, 2016; Catherine Rottenberg, *The Rise of Neoliberal Feminism* (New York: Oxford University Press, 2018); Fraser, "Crisis of Care?"

55. First quote in Evelyn Nakano Glenn, "Creating a Caring Society," *Contemporary Sociology* 29, no. 1 (Jan. 2000): 86, second quote references Glenn's classic "From Servitude to Service Work: Historical Continuities in the Racial Division of Paid Reproductive Labor," *Signs* 18, no. 1 (1992).

56. Thomas J. Sugrue, *The Origins of the Urban Crisis: Race and Inequality in Postwar Detroit* (Princeton, NJ: Princeton University Press, 1996), 5.

57. West, "From Choice to Reproductive Justice," 1412.

CHAPTER 1. THE LABOR OF ILLEGIBILITY

Epigraph: "Lesbians Choosing Children: A Legal, Social, and Medical Look at Conception by Donor Insemination," Feb. 11, 1984, Folder "LCP Legal Workshop Group, 1983," Box CTN 1, Cheri Pies Papers, GLBT Historical Society, San Francisco.

1. For photo and references to key descriptors, see Stephen Vider, "Picturing a Lesbian Feminist Household: Cathy Cade Interviewed by Stephen Vider," *OutHistory*, June 25, 2015, http://outhistory.org/exhibits/show/cathy-cade /introduction-and-interview. If, as Shawn Michelle Smith has argued, family photography circulates as visual evidence of "ancestry and inheritance," Cade's staging disrupts this logic by refusing to provide the viewer any clear route by which to trace this family's genealogy. Shawn Michelle Smith, *American Archives: Gender, Race, and Class in Visual Culture.* (Princeton, NJ: Princeton University Press, 1999), 113–35.

2. Gina Kolata, "Lesbian Partners Find the Means to Be Parents," *New York Times*, Jan. 30, 1989.

3. This trend began in the 1960s, and between 1964 and 1975 the divorce rate doubled. Divorce increased across all ages and educational levels, with men just as disillusioned with marriage as were the feminists who issued strong critiques of the institution. At the same time, so-called shotgun weddings greatly declined as social mores around pregnancy outside of marriage shifted. By the end of the 1970s, less than one-third of women who conceived out of wedlock married by the time their infant was born. These trends—along with persistent racial and gender discrimination in employment and an overall increase in economic precarity for working people—helped fuel the growth of female-headed households living in poverty, which grew from 26 percent of poor adults in 1959 to 50 percent by 1973. Thistle, *From Marriage to the Market*, 47, 50, 212n6. See also Elizabeth Pleck, *Not Just Roommates: Cohabitation after the Sexual Revolution* (Chicago: University of Chicago Press, 2012), 142.

4. Courts ordered all sorts of conditions, including keeping lesbian and gay parents from living with their lovers, barring them from participation in gay rights activism, and even undergoing regular psychiatric examinations that could attest they had repudiated their same-sex desires. See Self, *All in the Family*, 230; Daniel Rivers, *Radical Relations: Lesbian Mothers, Gay Fathers, and Their Children in the United States since World War II* (Chapel Hill: University of North Carolina Press, 2015), 63. For a thorough overview of lesbian mother and gay father custody cases stemming from divorce during this period, how courts used "the legal doctrine of 'the best interests of the child'" as a "smokescreen for judicial bias against homosexuality," and the political mobilizations that ultimately slowed the tide of gay parents losing their children, see Rivers, *Radical Relations*, ch. 3, quote on p. 57.

5. As Rivers notes in his history of gay and lesbian activism regarding custody cases, "The threat of losing one's children in a custody battle affected a whole generation of lesbian mothers and gay fathers who may have never seen the inside of a family court." Lesbians who looked to artificial insemination as a pathway to motherhood may have "come of age in the wake of lesbian and gay pride" and were therefore "less likely to think of themselves as pathologically

perverse or to regard their desires and relations as inherently dangerous to children," but they nevertheless remained profoundly aware that their sexuality could cost them their (future) children. See quote from Rivers, *Radical Relations*, 72; subsequent quotes reference Liz Montegary, *Familiar Perversions: The Racial, Sexual, and Economic Politics of LGBT Families* (New Brunswick, NJ: Rutgers University Press, 2018), 43.

6. Karen Sharpe, "Making Babies (Doing What Comes Artificially)," *San Francisco Chronicle*, Nov. 14, 1982, p. 14, Folder "Making Babies—Doing What Comes Artificially, SF Chronicle 1982," Box CTN 1, Cheri Pies Papers, GLBT Historical Society, San Francisco.

7. Klausner and Chasnoff had a gay friend serve as the donor so "the child's roots could be known." Gina Kolata, "Lesbian Partners Find the Means to Be Parents," *New York Times*, Jan. 30, 1989.

8. Many DIY guides and how-to articles used the language of "alternative fertilization" to move away from the idea that insemination was unnatural or "artificial." See, for example, Mary O'Donnell, Val Leoffler, Kater Pollock, and Ziesel Saunders, *Lesbian Health Matters!* (Santa Cruz: Santa Cruz Women's Health Center, 1979).

9. For more on the ties between self-insemination and the women's and gay health movements during this period, see Katie Batza, "From Sperm Runners to Sperm Banks: Lesbians, Assisted Conception, and Challenging the Fertility Industry, 1971–1983," *Journal of Women's History* 28, no. 2 (2016).

10. For especially thorough overviews of how family values took center stage in both liberal and conservative politics during this period, see Swinth, *Feminism's Forgotten Fight*; Self, *All in the Family*; Montegary, *Familiar Perversions*.

11. Quoted phrase is from Francie Hornstein, who described the feminist health movement's foray into do-it-yourself (DIY) insemination this way: "It seemed particularly fitting that the same women who developed the practice of menstrual extraction, a procedure which could be used for early abortion, also were among the pioneers in the practice of self-help donor insemination. We figured if we could safely help a woman end her pregnancy without the help of physicians and patriarchal laws, we could certainly help women get pregnant." Rita Arditti, Renate Klein, and Shelley Minden, *Test Tube Women: What Future for Motherhood?* (London: Pandora Press, 1984), 374.

12. Sarah and Mary Anonymous, *Woman Controlled Conception* (Grants Pass, OR: Womanshare Books, 1979), 23.

13. While the series of Supreme Court cases discussed in this chapter are often described as representing a "revolution" in illegitimacy law, legal scholars, like the attorneys fighting these laws in the 1960s and 1970s, have explained that this language mischaracterizes the legal reasoning used to strike down illegitimacy. See especially Melissa Murray, "What's So New about the New Illegitimacy?" *American University Journal of Gender, Social Policy, and the Law* 20,

no. 387 (2011). Also see Serena Mayeri, "Intersectionality and the Constitution of Family Status," *Constitutional Commentary* 32 (2017), and "Marital Supremacy and the Constitution of the Nonmarital Family," *California Law Review* 103 (2015).

14. Indeed, the history presented here suggests that feminist scholarship on assisted reproductive technologies (ARTs), which attributes lesbians' paradoxical participation in fertility treatment beginning in the 1990s to the biomedicalization of—and market in reproductive life, largely misses how *legal* concerns about a woman's right to her child convinced many women to trade in their turkey basters for expert insemination. This literature focuses on the rise of "Fertility Inc.," the collision of innovations in reproductive science to assist reproduction with a market in which to sell such technologies to the patient-consumer. Scholars agree that this biomedical market, while not ubiquitous nor monolithic, has nevertheless come to play a significant role in people's reproductive lives. Technological advances shape more and more individuals' experiences of procreative reproduction by providing more and more "choices" in which reproduction can be achieved, manipulated, and directed. Despite the ease with which insemination can be performed, the buying and selling of sperm that is a defining feature of this market's enabling of consumer choice has ensured the procedure gets cast as one of many ARTs on offer. As women turn to sperm banks to purchase sperm, they often become embroiled in "Fertility Inc." despite the fact that their only infertility "symptom" is a lack of semen. The following history argues that women's concern about custody of children conceived through AID was an equal if not greater motivator than the ascendance of a market in ARTs. For more on "Fertility Inc." and its specific impact on lesbians' and queers' reproductive practices, see Laura Mamo, *Queering Reproduction: Achieving Pregnancy in the Age of Technoscience* (Durham, NC: Duke University Press, 2007); Laura Mamo, "Fertility Inc.: Consumption and Subjectification in U.S. Lesbian Reproductive Practices," in *Biomedicalization: Technoscience, Health, and Illness in the U.S.*, ed. A. E. Clarke, L. Mamo, J. R. Fosket, J. R. Fishman and J. K. Shim (Durham, NC: Duke University Press, 2010); Diane Tober, *Romancing the Sperm: Shifting Biopolitics and the Making of Modern Families* (New Brunswick, NJ: Rutgers University Press, 2018); Laura Mamo and Eli Alston-Stepnitz, "Queer Intimacies and Structural Inequalities: New Directions in Stratified Reproduction," *Journal of Family Issues* 36, no. 4 (2015; Amy Agigian, *Baby Steps: How Lesbian Alternative Insemination Is Changing the World* (Middletown, CT: Wesleyan University Press, 2004). "Fertility Inc." comes from Gina Kolata, "Fertility Inc.: Clinics Race to Lure Clients," *New York Times,* Jan. 1, 2002. For additional works that have helped foreground biomedicine as an alluring market that often reinforces race, gender, and class hierarchies, see Rene Almeling, *Sex Cells: The Medical Market for Eggs and Sperm* (Berkeley: University of California Press, 2011); Michelle Goodwin, *Baby Markets: Money and the New Politics of Creating Fami-*

lies (Cambridge: Cambridge University Press, 2010); Lisa Jean Moore, *Sperm Counts: Overcome by Man's Most Precious Fluid* (New York: NYU Press, 2007), ch. 5; Debora Spar, *The Baby Business: How Money, Science, and Politics Drive the Commerce of Conception* (Cambridge, MA: Harvard Business School Press, 2006); France Winndance Twine, *Outsourcing the Womb: Race, Class and Gestational Surrogacy in a Global Market* (New York: Routledge, 2011); Charis Thompson, *Making Parents: The Ontological Choreography of Reproductive Technologies* (Boston: MIT Press, 2005); Laura Harrison, *Brown Bodies, White Babies: The Politics of Cross-Racial Surrogacy* (New York: NYU Press, 2016). More popular accounts also center the biomedical market in narratives of reproduction: see Harlyn Aizley, *Buying Dad: One Woman's Search for the Perfect Sperm Donor* (New York: Alyson Books, 2003). For a similar observation about the importance of the law in determining lesbians' fertility practices, one that suggests such a history is waiting to be written, see Laura Briggs, "Of Lesbians and Technosperm," *GLQ* 15, no. 2 (2009).

15. As Jennifer Nash has argued, in contrast to some feminist analyses theorizing the private sphere as a site of harm and violence, "the private can function as a radical site for culturally marginalized subjects," particularly those subject to racist state surveillance and intervention that has made such privacy precarious at best and unattainable at worst. Jennifer Nash, "From Lavender to Purple: Privacy, Black Women, and Feminist Legal Theory," *Cardozo Women's Law Journal* 11 (2005): 305.

16. Wilfred Finegold, *Artificial Insemination,* 1st ed. (Charles C. Thomas, 1964), 64.

17. This included efforts to criminalize the procedure, efforts to make children conceived through artificial insemination legitimate, and efforts to criminalize the procedure while declaring as legitimate those children who were conceived through artificial insemination. Finegold, *Artificial Insemination,* 68. For a discussion of legal concerns about the procedure leading up to the Georgia law, see Kara Swanson, *Banking on the Body: The Market in Blood, Milk, and Sperm in Modern America* (Cambridge, MA: Harvard University Press, 2014), 209–17.

18. For an extended discussion of one of the more well-known cases in which the mother was declared an adulteress and the child illegitimate, thereby confirming the fears long noted by physicians as partial justification for their secrecy, see Swanson, *Banking on the Body,* 216–17.

19. Finegold, *Artificial Insemination,* 69.

20. Gursky v. Gursky, 39 Misc.2d 1083 (1963).

21. Dr. Alan Guttmacher, for example, referred to this thinking as "balderdash." Quoted in Swanson, *Banking on the Body,* 210.

22. Finegold, *Artificial Insemination,* 75.

23. Kara Swanson has shown how this secrecy, well established by the 1940s, delayed the arrival of sperm banks or registries due to the belief that such

institutions would make the procedure far too visible. For this and an extended discussion of what steps were taken to ensure anonymity, see Swanson, *Banking on the Body*, 206–10.

24. Finegold, *Artificial Insemination*, 29.

25. Ibid., 29–31.

26. See Anders Walker, *The Ghost of Jim Crow: How Southern Moderates Used Brown v. Board of Education to Stall Civil Rights* (New York: Oxford University Press, 2009).

27. For a thorough discussion of the evolution in legal strategy surrounding illegitimacy, see Mayeri, "Marital Supremacy." Mayeri attributes the idea to attack illegitimacy laws on the basis of racial discrimination to a young lawyer named Melvin Wulf who in 1960 informed the Department of Health, Education, and Welfare that Louisiana's "suitable home" law was racially motivated. Wulf also borrowed from *Brown v. Board of Education* (1954) to argue, "We believe that any differential treatment to which out-of-wedlock children are subjected is invidious and likely unconstitutional." Quoted in Mayeri, "Marital Supremacy," 1287. Mayeri's article argues for an expansion of what are typically considered the core illegitimacy cases decided in the 1960s and 1970s, which include *Levy* and *Glona*, followed by *Perez* and *Trimble*. Mayeri considers laws that disadvantaged nonmarital families, such as the well-known "suitable home" law, as evidence of the persistence of what she calls "marital supremacy" through changes to laws governing sexual behavior during this period. In particular, she shows how appeals to protecting children from the harms of their parents' actions enjoyed greater support than the claims to sexual privacy and racial and economic discrimination forwarded by civil rights and feminist attorneys.

28. Trimble v. Gordon, 430 U.S. 762 at 766. Quoted in Mayeri, "Marital Supremacy," 1326. Mayeri argues that what truly solidified the "child-focused account of illegitimacy's harm" was the decision in *Weber v. Aetna* (1973), which found a Louisiana law prohibiting nonmarital children from recovering workmen's compensation to be in violation of the Equal Protection Clause of the Fourteenth Amendment on the basis that "legal burdens should bear some relationship to individual responsibility or wrongdoing"; the decision continued, "no child is responsible for his birth and penalizing the illegitimate child is an ineffectual—as well as unjust—way of deterring the parent." Quoted in Mayeri, "Marital Supremacy," 1308.

29. Harry Krause, "Bringing the Bastard into the Great Society—A Proposed Uniform Act on Legitimacy," *Texas Law Review* 44, no. 5 (1966): 829. Krause also helped bolster the legal argument that illegitimacy laws were racially discriminatory. At the request of the NAACP Legal Defense and Education Fund, he authored amicus briefs outlining illegitimacy law's discriminatory intent for the *Levy* case. See Mayeri, "Marital Supremacy," 1291. See also Harry Krause,

"Legitimate and Illegitimate Offspring of *Levy v. Louisiana*—First Decisions on Equal Protection and Paternity," *University of Chicago Law Review* 36, no. 2 (1969). The 1960s liberal ideal that access to a male breadwinner was the best solution to the so-called "culture of poverty" within African American families headed by single mothers is perhaps best represented by the infamous Moynihan Report, which further cemented the link between illegitimacy and blackness fueled by the very morals regulations that came under scrutiny during this period.

30. For example, Krause wrote: "There is no question that the state may properly regulate many aspects of sexual conduct. Our society holds that intercourse outside of marriage is undesirable, and thus the discouragement of 'illicit' intercourse is considered a proper end of legislation." Krause suggested that if the state wanted to regulate nonmarital sex it should do so directly. Krause, quoted in Mayeri, "Marital Supremacy," 1289.

31. Krause, "Bringing the Bastard into the Great Society," 831.

32. Mayeri, "Marital Supremacy."

33. Harry Krause, "The Uniform Parentage Act," *Family Law Quarterly* 8, no. 1 (Spring 1974): 8.

34. For the full text of Krause's first attempt at proposed legislation, see "Bringing the Bastard into the Great Society." There is also an updated draft in his 1971 book, *Illegitimacy: Law and Social Policy* (Indianapolis, IN: Bobbs-Merrill, 1971). For the full text and discussion of the Uniform Parentage Act, see Krause, "The Uniform Parentage Act."

35. Krause, "The Uniform Parentage Act," 1.

36. Uniform Law Commission, "Parentage Act Summary," http://www.uniformlaws.org/ActSummary.aspx?title=Parentage%20Act.

37. Krause himself acknowledged this in his review of *Levy* (1968) when he wrote, "In their immediate extension, these decisions should eliminate all other legal distinctions between legitimate and illegitimate children in their relation to their mother. If this were the only meaning of these cases, they would not be important. In most states, the illegitimate child's relationship with its mother today is all but equal to that of the legitimate child." Krause, "Legitimate and Illegitimate Offspring of *Levy v. Louisiana*," 338.

38. Krause, "Bringing the Bastard into the Great Society," 832–33.

39. Krause, "The Uniform Parentage Act," 17–18.

40. Patricia Tenoso and Aleta Wallach, "Book Review," *UCLA Law Review* 19 (1972): 865.

41. Quoted in Mayeri, "Marital Supremacy," 1312.

42. Or, as Douglas NeJaime recently put it, "biological connection served as an explicit basis for constitutional protection, for both mother-child and father-child relationships." NeJaime, "The Nature of Parenthood," *Yale Law Journal* 126, no. 8 (2017): 2267.

43. It should also be noted that the second part of the clause made sure to nullify biology and make clear that the nonparental donor had no rights or obligations to a child thereby conceived.

44. Quoted in Mayeri, "Marital Supremacy," 1312.

45. Tenoso and Wallach, "Book Review," 859. For an extended discussion of the failure of these arguments to penetrate Supreme Court decisions on illegitimacy cases, see Mayeri, "Marital Supremacy," 1310–40.

46. Finegold, *Artificial Insemination*, 49.

47. For an in-depth discussion of this guiding principle and its varied meanings during this period, see Michelle Murphy's book by the same name, *Seizing the Means of Reproduction: Entanglements of Feminism, Health, and Technoscience* (Durham, NC: Duke University Press, 2012). Also *Our Bodies, Ourselves*, 1st ed. (1971). The reference to "pregnancy without men" is taken from the name of a workshop on artificial insemination held at a Women and Health Conference in Boston, MA, in 1975. See Marcia Durfee and Dorie Ellzey, "Conference on Women and Health," *off our backs* 5, no. 6 (1975): 24.

48. Laurel Galana, "Radical Reproduction," *Amazon Quarterly*, 2, no. 3 (1974): 6–7.

49. The lesbian separatist group The Furies helped to popularize the goals of reproducing without men and ensuring that such endeavors did not produce more men. See for example, "Cloning," *The Furies*, May 1972. For more on the promise of parthenogenesis in lesbian separatist communities during this period, see Greta Rensenbrink, "Parthenogenesis and Lesbian Separatism: Regenerating Women's Community through Virgin Birth in the United States in the 1970s and 1980s," *Journal of the History of Sexuality* 19, no. 2 (May 2010). See also Kara Swanson, "The End of Men, Again," *Boston University Law Review Annex* 93 (2013): 26–36, 31–33. Daniel Rivers argues that lesbians who became mothers during the 1970s represent one way that lesbian feminist nationalism survived the 1970s, with mothers raising their children in a "resistance culture." Rivers, *Radical Relations*, 171.

50. For an extended discussion of debates within lesbian communities regarding male children and motherhood more generally, see Rivers, *Radical Relations*, ch. 6.

51. Jeanne Cordova, "Cutting the Patriarchal Umbilical Cord," *Lesbian Tide* 6, no. 4 (Jan./Feb., 1977): 3, 15.

52. Ibid., 15.

53. Marcia Durfee and Dorie Ellzey, "Conference on Women and Health," *off our backs* 5, no. 6 (1975): 24.

54. Cordova, "Cutting the Patriarchal Umbilical Cord," 15.

55. Arditti et al., *Test Tube Women*, 374.

56. For example, an article by Martha Heath published in *Lesbian Tide* described how "Corrine and Joyce . . . were told that only married (heterosexual)

women were accepted as patients." Martha Heath, "Do It Yourself Lesbian Insemination," *Lesbian Tide* 8, no. 2 (Sept./Oct. 1978): 26.

57. Marcia Durfee and Dorie Ellzey, "Conference on Women and Health," *off our backs* 5, no. 6 (1975); Martha Heath, "Do It Yourself Lesbian Insemination," *Lesbian Tide* 8, no. 2 (Sept./Oct. 1978); Marie Ahmed, "Artificial Insemination for Lesbians," *Seattle Gay News* 6, no. 4 (1979); Susan Stern, "A Different Type of Baby Boom in S.F.: Artificial Insemination for Lesbians," *Synapse* (1979), and "Amateur Insemination," *Whole Earth Catalog* (n.d.). Prior to written circulation, self-insemination networks traded information, resources, and support via in-person meetings/groups. By the mid-1970s, networks were operating in Boston, New York City, Burlington, VT, and Oakland, CA. See Rivers, *Radical Relations,* 169–71.

58. Mary Wings, *Conception Comix!* (1978), printed in Mary O'Donnell, Val Leoffler, Kater Pollock, and Ziesel Saunders, *Lesbian Health Matters!* (Santa Cruz: Santa Cruz Women's Health Center, 1979).

59. Quoted in *Artificial Insemination: An Alternative Conception for the Lesbian and Gay Community* (Lesbian Health Information Project, 1979). Another anonymous pamphlet was Sarah and Mary Anonymous, *Woman Controlled Conception.* See also O'Donnell et al., *Lesbian Health Matters!,* which contains a chapter dedicated to artificial insemination.

60. Sarah and Mary Anonymous, *Woman Controlled Conception,* 1.

61. For a thorough overview of the labor involved in making AID accessible to lesbians, see Batza, "From Sperm Runners to Sperm Banks."

62. Martha Heath, "Do It Yourself Lesbian Insemination," *Lesbian Tide* 8, no. 2 (Sept./Oct. 1978): 26.

63. For example, one of the anonymous authors of *Woman Controlled Conception* procured sperm through a private physician. Sarah and Mary Anonymous, *Woman Controlled Conception,* 2–3. Furthermore, a 1979 article surveying the practice of AID reported that of all physicians surveyed, 9.5 percent reported that they had provided treatment to women without male partners. See Martin Curie-Cohen, Lesleigh Luttrell, and Sander Shapiro, "Current Practice of Artificial Insemination by Donor in the United States," *New England Journal of Medicine* 300, no. 11 (1979): 589. There is also evidence that at least some women threatened to sue or did sue clinics who denied them on the basis of marital status. See "A Single Woman Sues for Artificial Insemination," *Seattle Times,* July 17, 1980, detailing a lawsuit brought by Mary Ann Smedes against Wayne State University; and George Dullea, "Artificial Insemination of Single Women Poses Difficult Questions," *New York Times,* Mar. 9, 1979, mentioning a lesbian who threatened to sue a Philadelphia doctor, with the help of the ACLU.

64. These clinics were the Feminist Women's Health Center in Los Angeles, CA and the Vermont Women's Health Center in Burlington, VA. Rivers, *Radical Relations,* 179.

65. For example, one profile of midwife Christmas Leubrie reported that whereas physicians could charge from 25 to 80 dollars for each round of insemination, Leubrie only charged 12 dollars. See Susan Stern, "Artificial Insemination for Lesbians." While it is possible individual physicians may have charged within this range, other documents suggest this is an underestimation. An informational sheet on the AID program at UC Davis from this same period listed a charge of 500 dollars for the first visit, with an additional 200 dollars for each monthly insemination. A private physician in San Francisco was not much of an improvement. A woman he helped reported that he charged a 400-dollar one-time lab fee and 75 dollars for each insemination. See "Information Concerning the Artificial Insemination Program of the University of California, Davis," n.d., in Folder "Originals," and "Unsigned Questionnaire" in Folder "Returned Questionnaires," both in Box CTN 1, Cheri Pies Papers, GLBT Historical Society, San Francisco.

66. Wings, *Conception Comix!*

67. Susan Stern, "Lesbian Insemination," *CoEvolution Quarterly*, Summer 1980, p. 111.

68. Karen Sharpe, "Making Babies," p. 14, Folder "Making Babies—Doing What Comes Artificially, SF Chronicle 1982," Box CTN 1, Cheri Pies Papers, GLBT Historical Society, San Francisco.

69. Wings, *Conception Comix!*

70. National Association of Black Social Workers, "Position Statement on Trans-Racial Adoptions," Sept. 1972, https://cdn.ymaws.com/www.nabsw.org /resource/collection/E1582D77-E4CD-4104-996A-D42D08F9CA7D/NABSW _Trans-Racial_Adoption_1972_Position_(b).pdf (accessed Aug. 21, 2019). For a discussion of transracial adoption during the mid-twentieth century and the impact of the NABSW's statement, see Ellen Herman, *Kinship by Design: A History of Modern Adoption in the United States* (Chicago: Chicago University Press), ch. 7.

71. Sue Zemel, "Choosing to Parent," *The Advocate*, Apr. 30, 1981, p. 19.

72. Sarah and Mary Anonymous, *Woman Controlled Conception*, 25.

73. Ibid. The couple's speech was reprinted in a 1979 issue of *off our backs*, which is where the "contradiction" quote can be found. See Maria Pena and Barbara Carey, "A Big Contradiction?" *off our backs* 9, no. 6 (June 1979): 19.

74. The practice of using a "lover's brother" is referenced in the 1983 profile on "Toby's Mothers" in *West*, commenting that this was a route being pursued by "many lesbian mothers" for the purposes of "creating more than just the romantic bond between lovers. Genes are kept in the family and the baby has a chance of looking like both 'parents.'" Jill Wolfson, "Toby's Mothers," *West*, Dec. 1983. It is also referenced in a 1982 profile published in the *San Jose Mercury News* quoting a psychologist with numerous lesbian clients: "A common story is that the lover's brother becomes the donor. . . . If it's your lover's brother, there's a bond

between you and your lover and her family." See Susan Ager, "Gay Parenting: Can Love Conquer All?" *San Jose Mercury News*, Nov. 28, 1982.

75. While my historical discussion largely concerns women who were made to rely on informal routes to sourcing semen, both Laura Mamo and Sandra Patton-Imani have documented how these desires continue to inform couples' choices, even those who obtain sperm through donor registries rather than relatives. Patton-Imani has described this as the "as if model, matching races, ethnicities, and physical characteristics of the non-birth mother in order to make a family that reflected the identities of both parents." Sandra Patton-Imani, *Queering Family Trees: Race, Reproductive Justice, and Lesbian Motherhood* (New York: NYU Press, 2020), 91. Mamo has described the practice of selecting and consuming sperm via commercialized sperm banks as engaging in the construction of what she calls "affinity-ties." See Laura Mamo, "Biomedicalizing Kinship: Sperm Banks and the Creation of Affinity-Ties," *Science as Culture* 14, no. 3 (2005): 237.

76. This meaning of "real"—where the notion of a "real family" is as much fiction as it is *real* legally, phenotypically, and affectively—is borrowed from Emily A. Owens's exploration of interracial lesbian parenthood and alternative insemination. Owens points out that one way the law demarcated family was through nineteenth-century prohibitions on interracial marriage, which effectively "undid racial intimacies" and placed mixed-race children "outside of the family." In this instance, racial categories produced by the law outweighed the association between family and "blood." See Emily A. Owens, "Reproducing Racial Fictions: Critical Meditations on (a) Lesbian Pregnancy," *Signs* 44, no. 4 (2019): 869.

77. "Lesbian Mothers," *Newsweek*, Feb. 12, 1979.

78. These are the names used in the *Newsweek* article, and which I use throughout the chapter, but court documents show that "Lynn" was actually Linda L. and "Bobbi" was actually Mary F. See Donald Shapiro and Lisa Schultz, "Single-Sex Families: The Impact of Birth Innovations upon Traditional Family Notions," *Journal of Family Law* 24, no. 2 (1985): 271–81.

79. "Lesbian Mothers," *Newsweek*, Feb. 12, 1979. As Cheryl D. Hicks and Siobhan Somerville have shown, interracial lesbian sex was not immune to charges of miscegenation, and Somerville in particular has discussed how racial difference and sexual difference preoccupied early twentieth-century sexologists and eugenicists, who saw these topics as closely related projects. While both of their observations are specific to the first decades of the twentieth century, Hicks's return to Somerville's question, "Did the girls' intimacy trouble the authorities because it was homosexual or because it was interracial?" is relevant to both *Newsweek*'s coverage of Bobbi and Lynn and other documented cases of interracial lesbian couples who sought to build families through insemination, which are discussed later in the chapter. For Hicks's general discussion, see

Cheryl D. Hicks, "'Bright and Good Looking Colored Girl': Black Women's Sexuality and 'Harmful Intimacy' in Early-Twentieth-Century New York," *Journal of the History of Sexuality* 18, no. 3 (Sept. 2009) (Hicks quotes Somerville on p. 449). For Somerville's general discussion, see Siobhan Somerville, "Scientific Racism and the Emergence of the Homosexual Body," *Journal of the History of Sexuality* 5, no. 2 (Oct. 1994). Melissa Murray has shown that despite the landmark Supreme Court decision *Loving v. Virginia* (1967), which decriminalized interracial unions, the state's willingness to punish such couplings through other means persisted long after the decision, helping to fuel the continued stigmatization of interracial sex and marriage. See Melissa Murray, "Loving's Legacy: Decriminalization and the Regulation of Sex and Sexuality," *Fordham Law Review* 86, no. 6 (2018).

80. "Lesbian Mothers," *Newsweek*, Feb. 12, 1979. In addition to undermining both Lynn's claims to biological motherhood and the couple's claims to family via shared genetic offspring, the reference to "her baby" also draws on the "the visual logic of race" to emphasize the relation between the Black child and her Black mother. As Emily A. Owens has written, this reference is not innocent but instead "surfaces an insidious thread of history" in which the "ironclad 'one-drop rule'" ensured that a Black woman could never be the mother of a white child—a reality constituted by law to justify the enslavement of human beings through attendant racial hierarchies. Within this logic, the legacy told readers that no matter Lynn's (brother's) blood, the baby would always be Bobbi's because "whiteness could only ever be absorbed by blackness." See Owens, "Reproducing Racial Fictions," 870–74.

81. Sue Zemel, "Choosing to Parent," *The Advocate*, Apr. 30, 1981, p. 22.

82. As a member of a support group in the Bay Area put it, "Then there are some of us who are struggling to introduce the concept of donor friend to our children." Ibid.

83. Fran Moira, "Lesbian Self-Insemination: Life without Father?" *off our backs*, Jan. 1982, pp. 12–13.

84. For more on "go-betweens," or what were also called "sperm-runners" during the mid-1970s to early 1980s, see Batza, "From Sperm Runners to Sperm Banks."

85. Martha Heath, "Do It Yourself Lesbian Insemination," *Lesbian Tide* 8, no. 2 (Sept./Oct. 1978): 26.

86. Author correspondence.

87. Leubrie is profiled as "Lily" in *CoEvolution Quarterly*, Summer 1980. Author interview.

88. Marie Ahmed, "Artificial Insemination for Lesbians," *Seattle Gay News* 6, no. 4 (1979). While my concern here is with the motivations for maintaining anonymity, it should be noted that especially in the early years of informal arrangements women used a variety of avenues to obtain sperm. One of the how-

to pamphlets sums this up: "It's important for each woman to figure out how she'll be most comfortable finding a donor. Potential sources are American Medical Association-type doctors, friendship ties, women's self-help groups, alternative health services and other movement connections, each of which has various advantages and disadvantages." Sarah and Mary Anonymous, *Woman Controlled Conception*, 2.

89. Martha Heath, "Artificial Insemination, Pt. II," *Lesbian Tide*, n.d., p. 32.

90. Wings, *Conception Comix!*

91. Fran Moira, "Lesbian Self-Insemination: Life without Father?" *off our backs*, Jan. 1982, pp. 12–13.

92. For an extensive discussion of these court rulings and the groups that fought for gay parents' rights, see Rivers, *Radical Relations*, ch. 3.

93. Susan Stern, "Lesbian Insemination," *CoEvolution Quarterly*, Summer 1980, p. 111.

94. Petra Liljesfraund, "Children without Fathers," *Out/Look*, Fall 1988, p. 24.

95. "He Makes Babies for Lesbians," *In Times of India*, Jan. 8, 1978.

96. Melanie Phillips, "Babies Are Born with Lesbians' AID to Motherhood," *Guardian*, Jan. 6, 1978.

97. One of the anonymous how-to pamphlets also made the link between both the events in London and increasing media coverage in the United States and the possibility of repressive legislation. While encouraged by the British Medical Association's vote that it was not unethical to inseminate single women, the authors pointed out that "political climate changes rapidly and England is not Amerika." *Artificial Insemination: An Alternative Conception* (Lesbian Health Information Project, 1979), 2.

98. "Lesbians Having Babies by AID," *The Advocate*, Feb. 22 1978, p. 6. This fear of exposure is also evidenced by articles where both mothers-to-be and sperm runners/midwives remained anonymous, and where other mothers declined to be interviewed. See for example Susan Stern, "Lesbian Insemination," *CoEvolution Quarterly*, Summer 1980, p. 111.

99. "Rights and Referendums," *Lesbian Tide*, n.d., p. 12.

100. Lesbian publications dedicated to the rights of lesbian mothers also reported on the case. See, for example, the Sept. 1977 issue of the Lesbian Mothers National Defense Fund newsletter, *Mom's Apple Pie*, p. 5, Folder "Cartoons and Illustrations," Box CTN 1, Cheri Pies Papers, GLBT Historical Society, San Francisco.

101. George Dullea, "Artificial Insemination of Single Women Poses Difficult Questions." *New York Times*, Mar. 9, 1979.

102. *Lesbian Tide* continued to provide updates. The British Medical Association's decision was printed in the Nov./Dec. 1979 issue. Quote taken from article by Fran Moira, "Lesbian Self-Insemination: Life without Father?" *off our backs*, Jan. 1982, p. 12.

103. C.M. v. C.C. 152 N.J. Super. 160, 377 A.2d 821 (Juvenile and Dom. Rel. Ct. 1977).

104. C.M. v. C.C. 19 Jul 1977, *The Atlantic Reporter*, 177 (1977): 824.

105. Ibid. The decision also reflected the growing recognition, on the part of the courts, of fathers' rights that followed from the increase in divorce. Legal scholar Martha Fineman has argued that this shift ultimately produced "a legal system that empowers fathers." See Martha Fineman, *The Neutered Mother, the Sexual Family and Other Twentieth Century Tragedies* (New York: Routledge, 1995), 83. For an overview of how this development largely excluded nonmarital fathers and why "the legal primacy" of marriage endured, even as rates of nonmarital cohabitation and childrearing soared, see Serena Mayeri, "Foundling Fathers: (Non-)Marriage and Parental Rights in the Age of Equality," *Yale Law Journal* 125 (2016): 2295.

106. Fran Moira, "Lesbian Self-Insemination: Life without Father?" *off our backs*, Jan. 1982, pp. 12–13. An article on lesbian insemination in *CoEvolution Quarterly* also mentions this case as a warning to women considering known donors. Susan Stern, "Lesbian Insemination," *CoEvolution Quarterly*, Summer 1980, p. 111. Johnnie Tillmon, "Welfare Is a Women's Issue," *Ms.*, Spring 1972 (emphasis in original).

107. Bryant quoted in Gil Frank, "'The Civil Rights of Parents': Race and Conservative Politics in Anita Bryant's Campaign against Gay Rights in 1970s Florida," *Journal of the History of Sexuality* 22, no. 1 (Jan. 2013): 127.

108. Falwell quoted in Self, *All in the Family*, 353.

109. On this last point, it would take nearly twenty-five more years before the Supreme Court declared sodomy laws unconstitutional in *Lawrence v. Texas* (2003). In the interim, existing sodomy laws would get a boost from the Court with *Bowers v. Hardwick* (1986). For a discussion on the significance of *Bowers* to queers' parental aspirations, see Montegary, *Familiar Perversions*, 46.

110. The Lesbian Rights Project (LRP) was instrumental in shifting the legal trend of denying women custody on the basis of same-sex sexuality, and Hitchens's work in this area undoubtedly informed her legal guidance on the use of AID. A bibliography of legal and psychological resources meant to assist legal advocates in representing lesbian mothers described the reality that Hitchens knew all too well from her legal work: "Lesbian mothers and their families live with the constant threat of having their relationships severed or severely limited because of the sexual preference of the mother." See Donna Hitchens and Ann G. Thomas, eds., "Lesbian Mothers and Their Children: An Annotated Bibliography of Legal and Psychological Materials," Lesbian Rights Project, 1980, p. i, Box CTN 1, Cheri Pies GLBT Historical Society, San Francisco.

111. See the "Advisor" column in *The Advocate*, no. 330, Nov. 12, 1981. Other representative examples include Susan Stern, "Lesbian Insemination," *CoEvolution Quarterly*, Summer 1980, p. 112: "Lesbians who know their donors often

have them sign agreements relinquishing their rights and responsibilities to the child. But if the donor has a change of heart, lesbian rights lawyers say these written agreements may not stand up in court. Consequently, many would-be mothers are using anonymous donors." Also see Susan Ager, "Gay Parenting: Can Love Conquer All?" *San Jose Mercury News,* Nov. 28, 1982, where Hitchens cites the California Uniform Parentage Age, though not by name, to make clear that "lesbian women who inseminate themselves at home are legally at risk if the donor, through a paternity action, demands custody or visitation rights to the child."

112. Jill Wolfson, "Toby's Mothers," *West,* Dec. 1983. Whether there was an increase in anonymous donors is difficult to determine. Warnings repeatedly appeared in publications on AID, but so did stories about women who deliberately chose a known donor. As I discuss later in the chapter, the only case of a donor bringing suit against a lesbian mother during the 1980s was in California. Those working on this issue did not remember an abundance of arrangements going wrong. Still, the 1983 LRP pamphlet refers to "a number of cases" where donors changed their minds after the baby was born. Author interview.

113. The pamphlet appeared on the LRP's 1984 list of materials available for purchase. Donna Hitchens, "Lesbians Choosing Motherhood: Legal Issues in Donor Insemination, 1983 Edition," Folder "Papers and Publications Legal Issues in Donor Insemination 1983, LRP," Carton 1, Donna Hitchens Papers, GLBT Historical Society, San Francisco.

114. LRP hosted the conference along with the Lyon-Martin Clinic, referenced in Nancy Langer, "Mothers by Choice," in *Lesbians Choosing Motherhood: Legal, Medical, and Social Issues,* Lambda Legal Defense and Education Fund Inc., n.d., p. 12, Folder "Lambda Legal Defense Fund, 'Lesbians Choosing Motherhood,'" Carton 1, Donna Hitchens Papers, GLBT Historical Society, San Francisco. Hitchens also appeared at the workshop "Lesbians and Motherhood" in Cambridge, MA, referenced in Carol Anne Douglas, "Lesbians and Motherhood," *off our backs,* May 1983, p. 6. LRP staff attorney Roberta Achtenberg also shared the developing guidance at a conference hosted by Lambda Legal Defense and Education Fund in New York City in 1984. See conference program, Folder "Lambda Legal Defense NYC Workshop," Box CTN 1, Cheri Pies Papers, GLBT Historical Society, San Francisco.

115. Donna Hitchens, "Lesbians Choosing Motherhood, 1984 Edition."

116. See Susan Ager, "Gay Parenting: Can Love Conquer All?" *San Jose Mercury News,* Nov. 28, 1982.

117. Sally Chew, "Lesbians Choosing Motherhood," *New York Native,* Dec. 3–16, 1984.

118. Hitchens lists seven in the pamphlet, but Carol Donovan lists nine in her 1982 article. Carol A. Donovan, "The Uniform Parentage Act and Nonmarital Motherhood-by-Choice," *NYU Review of Law and Social Change* 11 (1982): 219. According to the Uniform Law Commission, nineteen states ultimately adopted the

act prior to its revision in 2000. See "Why States Should Adopt the UPA," http://www.uniformlaws.org/Narrative.aspx?title=Why%20States%20Should%20 Adopt%20UPA. Around twenty-seven states had passed legislation specific to artificial insemination by 1984, with guidelines that varied widely. See "Cases, Law Review Articles, and a Comparison of Statutes," n.d., Folder "Legal Issues in Donor Insemination, LRP 1983," Box CTN 1, Cheri Pies Papers, GLBT Historical Society, San Francisco.

119. California's Uniform Parentage Act, adopted in 1975, stated: "The donor of semen provided a licensed physician for use in artificial insemination of a woman other than the donor's wife is treated in law as if he were not the natural father of a child thereby conceived." Quoted in Stuart A. Sutton, "The Lesbian Family: Rights in Conflict Under the California Uniform Parentage Act," *Golden Gate University Law Review* 10 (Jan. 1980): 1023.

120. Donna Hitchens, "Lesbians Choosing Motherhood: Legal Issues in Donor Insemination, 1983 Edition," p. 4, Folder "Papers and Publications: 'Legal Issues in Donor Insemination' 1983, LRP," Carton 1, Donna Hitchens Papers, GLBT Historical Society, San Francisco.

121. Ibid., 5.

122. The sperm bank would eventually split from the feminist health center and exists now as The Sperm Bank of California. Of course, the San Francisco Bay Area's long history of gay and lesbian migration, activism, and community also played a fundamental role in making the sperm bank and, more importantly, its public declarations about non-normative family making, possible. For an overview of this history prior to the period being examined here, see Nan Alamilla Boyd, *Wide-Open Town: A History of Queer San Francisco to 1965* (Berkeley: University of California Press, 2005).

123. Author interview.

124. "Feminists Have Own Sperm Banks," *Los Angeles Times,* Nov. 18, 1982.

125. Pearl Stewart, "First Bay Area Sperm Bank Opens," *San Francisco Chronicle,* Oct. 6, 1982. Catalogued in the Sperm Bank of California files.

126. "The Birth of a Feminist Sperm Bank: New Social Agendas for AID," *The Hastings Center Report* 13 (1983).

127. Sample contract from Nov. 1, 1982, provided by Alice Ruby, on file with author. A staff member who helped start the center had this to say about physician involvement: "I knew in my heart of hearts even as a feminist there was no way we were going to operate without a physician. . . . They had the credentials. We needed the credentials." This staff member also pointed out that all the physicians on staff were feminists dedicated to the project of lesbian motherhood, even as she also described the physician strategy as a "compromise." Author interview.

128. See Susan Ager, "Gay Parenting: Can Love Conquer All?" *San Jose Mercury News,* Nov. 28, 1982.

129. An appeals court upheld the ruling in 1986. Jhordan C. v. Mary K., 179 Cal. App. 3d 386 (1986). For a brief discussion of this case, see Rivers, *Radical Relations*, 187–88.

130. Susan Sklonick, "Lesbian Rights Project: Changing the System," *The Sentinel*, 1987.

131. Ibid. See also Judy Berelsen, "The Challenges of Lesbian Parenting," *Frontline*, Dec. 31, 1984. Hitchens's pamphlet was reprinted in different publications. For example, see Donna Hitchens, "Maternity," *I know you know*, 2 no. 1 (1985).

132. Case report, n.d., unmarked folder, Carton 1, Donna Hitchens Papers, GLBT Historical Society, San Francisco.

133. Achtenberg's recollection as presented at a keynote speech, quoted in Rivers, *Radical Relations*, 188. Quote from judge is in Philip Carrizosa, "Three-Way Fight Examines Rights of Sperm Donors," *Los Angeles Daily Journal*, Jan. 31, 1986.

134. Cathy Cohen, "Punks, Bulldaggers, and Welfare Queens: The Radical Potential of Queer Politics?" *GLQ* 3, no. 4 (1997): 447 (the parenthetical phrase in this section's heading refers to Cohen's title). Cohen's groundbreaking article called for an intersectional queer politics that could highlight the "*nonnormative* and *marginal* position of punks, bulldaggers, and welfare queens" as "the basis for progressive transformative work." Cohen offered this intervention into queer activism that had reinscribed yet another binary of "heterosexual and everything 'queer,'" and in doing so failed to address the different subjects whose marginalization on the basis of race, class, gender, and sexual behaviors located them outside of the white, patriarchal family (quotes from p. 438). The description of a lesbian as always "a single" in this section's heading comes from a *Seattle Times* article profiling the potential lawsuit against the Mott Clinic at Wayne State University for denying a single woman AID. "A Single Sues for Artificial Insemination," *Seattle Times*, July 17, 1980.

135. For example, a June 6, 1983, article in *New York Magazine* titled "Mommy Only: The Rise of the Middle-Class Unwed Mother," by Patricia Morrisroe, reinforced the prominent stereotype of single mothers as Black welfare recipients when it cited "a growing number of white, middle-class women who are changing the scope of the words 'unwed mother'" (p. 23). Of course, radical lesbian feminists did not need media coverage to alert them to this fact. As the Radicalesbians argued in 1970, "For a woman to be independent means she can't be a woman—she must be a dyke." "The Woman-Identified-Woman," Atlanta Lesbian Feminist Alliance Archives, Sallie Bingham Center for Women's History and Culture, Rubenstein Library, Duke University, Durham, NC.

136. Georgia Dullea, "For Women Seeking Motherhood There Is AID," *Chicago Tribune*, Mar. 25, 1979.

137. Jill Wolfson, "Toby's Mothers," *West*, Dec. 1983.

138. This observation is especially true for the early to mid-1980s, before the "lesbian baby boom" had become the sole focus of media articles. Jill Wolfson, "Toby's Mothers," *West*, Dec. 1983; Anne Taylor Fleming, "New Frontiers in Conception," *New York Times*, July 20, 1980. For another representative example of anxiety regarding evidence that procreation was increasingly leaving the confines of marriage, see Alan Otten, "Fertility Rights," *Wall Street Journal*, Aug. 7, 1984.

139. Robert Cooke, "Some Single Women Inseminating Selves Artificially," *Boston Globe*, Apr. 5, 1984.

140. George Dullea, "Artificial Insemination of Single Women Poses Difficult Questions," *New York Times*, Mar. 9, 1979.

141. The authors rested this right on the fact that AID was not strictly treating a disease or any "health-related need" in the single woman, suggesting that only *married* women were eligible patients for treating male infertility by proxy. Carson Strong and Jay S. Schinfeld, "The Single Woman and Artificial Insemination by Donor," *Journal of Reproductive Medicine* 29, no. 5 (May 1984): 293, 298.

142. Maureen McGuire and Nancy J. Alexander, "Artificial Insemination of Single Women," *Fertility and Sterility* 43, no. 2 (Feb. 1985): 182–84; "Letter to Cherry Pies from Lisa Radcliffe," Mar. 30, 1983, Folder, "Whole Birth Catalogue, 1983," Box CTN 1, Cheri Pies Papers, GLBT Historical Society, San Francisco.

143. See Gerald T. Perkoff, "Artificial Insemination in a Lesbian: A Case Analysis," *Archives of Internal Medicine* 145 (Mar. 1985): 527–31.

144. "AID and the Single Welfare Mother," *The Hastings Center Report*, Feb. 1983, pp. 22–23.

145. Carol Anne Douglas, "Lesbians and Motherhood," *off our backs*, May 1983, p. 6.

146. Cohen, "Punks, Bulldaggers, and Welfare Queens," 447.

147. For a representative example that applies this explanation to the case of Bobbi and Lynn, see Shapiro and Schultz, "Single-Sex Families." For a more general discussion of how gay and lesbian parents were forced to enter "extrajudicial agreements" due to the state's refusal to recognize homosexuals as parents, see Rivers, *Radical Relations*, 187. Douglas NeJaime's extensive legal history of same-sex couples' successes and failures with the Uniform Parentage Act (UPA) in California also omits the state's interest in returning welfare mothers to a private provider. See NeJaime, "Marriage Equality and the New Parenthood," *Harvard Law Review* 129, no. 5 (Mar. 2016).

148. Lance Williams, "Lesbian Seeks Visitation Rights to Ex-Lover's Child," *San Francisco Examiner*, Apr. 23, 1983. Shapiro and Schultz, "Single-Sex Families," 273. For a thorough overview of how courts have expressed disapproval of heterosexual, interracial unions through custodial decisions that rely on race-neutral arguments, see Murray, "Loving's Legacy."

149. Philip Carrizosa, "Three-Way Fight Examines Rights of Sperm Donors," *Los Angeles Daily Journal*, Jan. 31, 1986.

150. Feminist attorneys of the time reiterated the concerns made by their earlier counterparts, though this time those concerns were in the context of the "illegitimacy" created by lesbian insemination. See Sutton, "The Lesbian Family"; Donovan, "The Uniform Parentage Act and Nonmarital Motherhood -by-Choice."

151. For a thorough history of what the UPA did and did not deliver to lesbian families in California following this case, see NeJaime, "Marriage Equality and the New Parenthood."

152. Lesbian Rights Project (LRP) Newsletter 3, no. 1 (1986), Folder "Lesbian Parenting, 1984–1987," Box CTN 1, Cheri Pies Papers, GLBT Historical Society, San Francisco.

153. Nan Hunter and Nancy Polikoff, "Organizers Dialog," *Quest: A Feminist Quarterly*, Folder "Vol. 5(1): Organizer's Dialogue: lesbian mother cases, 1975," Box 31, Records of *Quest: A Feminist Quarterly*, 1970–1985, Schlesinger Library, Harvard University, Cambridge, MA; Cohen, "Punks, Bulldaggers, and Welfare Queens," 438.

154. Kath Weston, *Families We Choose: Lesbians, Gays, Kinship* (New York: Columbia University Press, 1997), xv.

155. For example, Sandra Patton-Imani's ethnography on lesbian mothers documents couples' ambivalence about same-sex marriage, including standard leftist critiques, even as they were desperate for legal protections that could sanction—and finally make secure—their familial ties. Patton-Imani, *Queering Families Trees*, 6. Laura Briggs has also argued that gay marriage should be seen as less a gay rights victory and more a necessary strategy for non-normative families forced—like all families—to take on caretaking and in need of a way to legally ensure access to their dependents. See Briggs, *How All Politics Became Reproductive Politics*, ch. 5. For a related and more critical discussion of same-sex marriage's role in privatizing the costs of family making, see Montegary, *Familiar Perversions*, ch. 4 (quote in text from p. 26).

156. Author interview. Economic barriers to sperm banks and fertility treatment remain today, as do reports about sperm banks offering predominantly white donors. See Patton-Imani, *Queering Family Trees*, ch. 3; Hannah E. Karpman, Emily H. Ruppel, and Maria Toress, "'It wasn't feasible for us': Queer Women of Color Navigating Family Formation," *Family Relations* 67, no. 4 (2018); Cynthia R. Daniels and Erin Heidt-Forsythe, "Gendered Eugenics and the Problematic of Free Market Reproductive Technologies: Sperm and Egg Donation in the United States," *Signs* 37, no. 3 (2012). Of course, as Mignon Moore has shown, this exclusion also means that "working class and poor lesbians are left with fewer strategies for becoming parents that do not include heterosexual intercourse," which means that while the literature on queer family formation has overwhelmingly studied "lesbians becoming mothers," families are also formed by "mothers becoming lesbians"—a process Moore traces in her

study of Black lesbians and argues is the far more common pathway by which queer families form. Mignon Moore, *Invisible Families: Gay Identities, Relationships, and Motherhood among Black Women* (Berkeley: University of California Press, 2011), 117, 218. Lastly, Laura Briggs points out that "by the 2000 census . . . gay parents were disproportionately likely to be Southern, rural, and people of color. The census found 2 million children being raised by two same-sex parents. Their families were disproportionately poor, about twice as likely to live in poverty as the children of married, heterosexual couples." Briggs, *How All Politics Became Reproductive Politics*, 175.

157. Patton-Imani, *Queering Family Trees*, 85.

158. For more on how states treat nonmarital children conceived through AID, and how marriage equality has not resolved gender and sex-based inequalities baked into parentage law more generally, see NeJaime, "The Nature of Parenthood."

CHAPTER 2. THE LABOR OF CAPTIVITY

Epigraphs: Janine Bertram and Carla Lowenberg, "Prison MATCH/PCC Advisory Board," n.d., p. 2, Denise Johnston Personal Papers; Young, "Sometimes I Feel Like a Motherless Child," *The Clarion*, July and Aug. 1974, Folder "Prisoner Writings," Carton 1 of 27, Inventory of the Nancy Stoller Papers Concerning Prison Inmate Health, 1970s–2000s, Archives and Special Collections, University of California, San Francisco.

1. Incident Report to J. J. Enomoto, DOC Director from Brook Carey, CIW Superintendent, Dec. 19, 1975, Folder "CIM, Chino Incident Report 1975, F3717:1535," Institutions—California Institution for Women, Tehachapi (CIW), 1952-54, 1956-57, 1960-61, 1967-77, Department of Corrections Records, F3717, California State Archives.

2. Incident Report to Midge Carroll, Correctional Captain, from W. S. Wolters, Correctional Lieutenant, Dec. 17, 1975, Folder "CIM, Chino Incident Report 1975, F3717:1535," Institutions—California Institution for Women, Tehachapi (CIW), 1952-54, 1956-57, 1960-61, 1967-77, Department of Corrections Records, F3717, California State Archives.

3. Incident Report to S. Greene, Lt. 3rd Watch Commander from Virginia Andrade, C.O., Dec. 17, 1975, Folder "CIM, Chino Incident Report 1975, F3717:1535," Institutions—California Institution for Women, Tehachapi (CIW), 1952-54, 1956-57, 1960-61, 1967-77, Department of Corrections Records, F3717, California State Archives.

4. Incident Report to S. Greene, Lt. 3rd Watch Commander from Frank R. Searcy, Sgt., Dec. 16, 1975, Folder "CIM, Chino Incident Report 1975, F3717:1535," Institutions—California Institution for Women, Tehachapi (CIW),

1952-54, 1956-57, 1960-61, 1967-77, Department of Corrections Records, F3717, California State Archives.

5. Incident Report to S. Greene, Lt. 3rd Watch Commander from Virginia Andrade, C.O., Dec. 17, 1975, Folder "CIM, Chino Incident Report 1975, F3717:1535," Institutions—California Institution for Women, Tehachapi (CIW), 1952-54, 1956-57, 1960-61, 1967-77, Department of Corrections Records, F3717, California State Archives.

6. Letter to Honorable John T. Knox, Assemblyman from Philip D. Guthrie, Asst. Director of Public Information, Apr. 19, 1976, Folder "CIM Tehachapi, Alternative Program Unit, 1976, F317:1533," Institutions—California Institution for Women, Tehachapi (CIW), 1952-54, 1956-57, 1960-61, 1967-77, Department of Corrections Records, F3717, California State Archives.

7. Enomoto references the proposal in his letter to Mr. John J. Cleary from Apr. 5, 1976, but the proposal itself is contained in a letter to Superintendent Kathleen Anderson, CIW from Nelson P. Kempsky, Deputy Director Policy and Planning, from Mar. 25, 1976. Both letters can be found in Folder "CIM Tehachapi, Alternative Program Unit, 1976, F317:1533," Institutions—California Institution for Women, Tehachapi (CIW), 1952-54, 1956-57, 1960-61, 1967-77, Department of Corrections Records, F3717, California State Archives. Despite the line that CIW was only *considering* an alternate unit program (APU), it seems clear from the archive that one was put in place, however limited or experimental, following the riot. The letter from Kempsky admits that his proposal needs to be more detailed, "but without coming down and becoming familiar with the unit we couldn't do that sort of thing from here." The Women's Prison Coalition reported that a petition signed by 400 women incarcerated at CIW was delivered to prison staff in January, calling for an end to the APU. And when the State Bar Committee on Corrections requested a community visit, Enomoto denied the request. See Letter to Mr. J. J. Enomoto, Director of CDC, from Laurie Hauer for the Women's Prison Coalition, May 20, 1976, and Letter to Honorable John T. Knox, Assemblyman, from J. J. Enomoto, Director of CDC, Apr. 19, 1976. Both letters can be found in Folder "CIM Tehachapi, Alternative Program Unit, 1976, F317:1533," Institutions—California Institution for Women, Tehachapi (CIW), 1952-54, 1956-57, 1960-61, 1967-77, Department of Corrections Records, F3717, California State Archives. Emily Thuma's history of anti-prison feminist activism during this period reports that by striking in 1973 incarcerated women successfully shut down a project titled the "Intensive Program Unit," which provides evidence that the APU was not CIW's first foray into behavior modification. Emily L. Thuma, *All Our Trials: Prisons, Policing, and the Feminist Fight to End Violence* (Chicago: University of Illinois Press, 2019), 61.

8. Letter to Honorable John T. Knox, Assemblyman from Philip D. Guthrie, Asst. Director of Public Information, Apr. 19, 1976, Folder "CIM Tehachapi, Alternative Program Unit, 1976, F317:1533," Institutions—California Institution

for Women, Tehachapi (CIW), 1952-54, 1956-57, 1960-61, 1967-77, Department of Corrections Records, F3717, California State Archives.

9. Letter to Honorable John T. Knox, Assemblyman from J. J. Enomoto, Director of CDC, Apr. 19, 1976, Folder "CIM Tehachapi, Alternative Program Unit, 1976, F317:1533," Institutions—California Institution for Women, Tehachapi (CIW), 1952-54, 1956-57, 1960-61, 1967-77, Department of Corrections Records, F3717, California State Archives.

10. For a helpful overview of the prison movement during this period, see Dan Berger and Toussaint Losier, *Rethinking the American Prison Movement* (New York: Routledge, 2018), chs. 3 and 4. For a history of anticarceral feminism that emerged as one part of the broader rebellions against incarceration in the 1960s and 1970s, see Thuma, *All Our Trials*.

11. Additionally, as Liat Ben-Moshe has argued, the very conditions that define incarceration makes it likely that "even if an individual enters prison without a disability or mental health diagnosis, she is likely to get one." The "disabling" nature of prisons demonstrate how even if it were somehow possible for treatments not simply to be punishments by another name, they would necessarily fail to counter the punitive and dehumanizing logics that constitute the project of incarceration in its varied settings. The solitary confinement example is also referenced in Ben-Moshe's discussion. See Liat Ben-Moshe, *Decarcerating Disability: Deinstitutionalization and Prison Abolition* (Minneapolis: University of Minnesota Press, 2020), 8, 15. For more on the shared logics of incarceration across its many "enclosed settings," see Liat Ben-Moshe, Allison Carey, and Chris Chapman, *Disability Incarcerated: Imprisonment and Disability in the United States and Canada* (New York: Palgrave Macmillan, 2014).

12. American Friends Service Committee, *Struggle for Justice: A Report on Crime and Punishment in America* (New York: Hill and Wang, 1971), 26–27.

13. Instead, AFSC joined the call for an end to indeterminate sentencing and a return to the retributive function of punishment concerned solely with the crime committed, rather than the individual's psychological tendencies. "When we punish the offender and simultaneously try to treat him, we hurt the individual more profoundly and more permanently than if we merely imprison him for a specific length of time." Ibid., 147–48. On the important role prisoners' activism played in undermining the treatment principle and especially indeterminate sentencing, see Julilly Kohler-Hausmann, *Getting Tough: Welfare and Imprisonment in 1970s America* (Princeton, NJ: Princeton University Press, 2017), ch. 5.

14. For more on the wide-ranging criticisms of indeterminate sentencing during this period, as well as subsequent analyses about how some skeptics of rehabilitation offered measured assessments rather than full-scale indictments, see this work of Marie Gottschalk, *The Prison and the Gallows: The Politics of Mass Incarceration in America* (New York: Cambridge University Press, 2006), 37–39.

15. In other words, "In the early 1970s, the future of prisons was 'up for grabs.'" Berger and Losier, *Rethinking the American Prison Movement,* 102.

16. Ruth Wilson Gilmore, *Golden Gulag: Prisons, Surplus, Crisis, and Opposition in Globalizing California* (Berkeley: University of California Press, 2007), 21. Marie Gottschalk warns against the idea that "deep public angst about crime, violence, and disorder are something relatively new" and reads the turn to law and order in the 1970s as one of many throughout American history. See Gottschalk, *The Prison and the Gallows,* 75, and more generally ch. 3.

17. Peter Wagner and Wendy Sawyer, "Mass Incarceration: The Whole Pie 2020," Mar. 24, 2020, https://www.prisonpolicy.org/factsheets/pie2020_allimages.pdf (accessed Jan. 18, 2021).

18. See Christopher Wildeman, Anna Haskins, and Christopher Muller, "Implications of Mass Imprisonment for Inequality among American Children," in *The Punitive Turn: New Approaches to Race and Incarceration,* ed. Deborah McDowell, Claudrena N. Harold, and Juan Battle (Charlottesville: University of Virginia Press, 2013), 177; Wendy Sawyer, "The Gender Divide: Tracking Women's State Prison Growth," Jan. 9, 2019, Prison Policy Initiative, https://www.prisonpolicy.org/reports/women_overtime.html (accessed Jan. 18, 2021).

19. Eric A. Stanley and Nat Smith, eds., *Captive Genders: Trans Embodiment and the Prison Industrial Complex,* 2nd ed. (Oakland: AK Press, 2015), 10.

20. For two recent histories documenting the sexual and physical abuses as well as the labor exploitation brought upon Black women incarcerated in the Jim Crow South, see Haley, *No Mercy Here;* and Talitha L. LefLouria, *Chained in Silence: Black Women and Convict Labor in the New South* (Chapel Hill: University of North Carolina Press, 2015). On the history of psychological "treatment" as torture and violence, see Thuma, *All Our Trials,* ch. 2. On the reproductive healthcare administered to pregnant incarcerated women that is both coercive and inadequate, see Flavin, *Our Bodies, Our Crimes,* ch. 6, and for the specific practice of shackling during childbirth, see Roxanne Nelson, "Laboring in Chains: Shackling Pregnant Inmates, Even during Childbirth, Still Happens," *American Journal of Nursing* 106, no. 10 (2005). On the very recent history of coercive sterilization of women incarcerated in California's correctional facilities, see Corey G. Johnson, "Female Inmates Sterilized in California Prisons without Approval," Center for Investigative Reporting, July 7, 2013, https://www.revealnews.org/article/female-inmates-sterilized-in-california-prisons-without-approval (accessed Sept. 15, 2019). On violence against transgender and gender-nonconforming people in sex-segregated prisons, see D. Morgan Bassichis, *It's War in Here: A Report on the Treatment of Transgender and Intersex People in New York State Men's Prisons* (New York: Sylvia Rivera Law Project, 2007); Lori Girshick, "Out of Compliance: Masculine-Identified People in Women's Prisons," in *Captive Genders: Trans Embodiment and the Prison Industrial Complex,* 2nd ed., ed. Eric A. Stanley and Nat Smith (Oakland: AK Press, 2015).

21. On the criminalization of Black women who are victims of abuse, see Angela Y. Davis, "Joan Little: The Dialectics of Rape," *Ms.*, June 1975, 74–77, 106–8; Beth E. Richie, *Arrested Justice: Black Women, Violence, and America's Prison Nation* (New York: NYU Press, 2012). On the legal ramifications stemming from women of color's use of self-defense, see Donna Coker, "The Story of Wanrow: The Reasonable Woman and the Law of Self-Defense," in *Criminal Law Stories*, ed. Donna Coker and Robert Weisberg (New York: Foundation Press, 2013). On police brutality against Black women and women of color, see Andrea J. Ritchie, *Invisible No More: Police Violence against Black Women and Women of Color* (Boston: Beacon Press, 2017). On the history of organizing efforts that helped produce this anticarceral feminist insight, see Thuma, *All Our Trials*.

22. "Warehousing" is a reference to Dan Berger and Toussaint Losier's description of the punitive turn' main feature: "simply warehousing people in cages." Berger and Losier, *Rethinking the American Prison Movement*, 143.

23. Letter to Judge Haberkorn from Attorney General Hirsch, Jan. 27, 1976, Ellen Barry Personal Papers.

24. "Memorandum of Points and Authorities in Support of Petition for Writ of Mandate," Jan. 22, 1976, p. 10, Ellen Barry Personal Papers (emphasis mine).

25. "Declaration of Annette Harris," Aug. 21, 1985, Ellen Barry Personal Papers.

26. See note 24 above.

27. Laura Bresler and Donald Leonard, "Women's Jail: Pretrial and Post-Conviction Alternatives, a Report on Women Arrested in San Francisco," Nov. 1978, Folder "Report on Women Arrested in San Francisco," Friends Committee on Legislation of California Records, Donald and Beverly Gerth Special Collections and University Archives, California State University, Sacramento. The idea that criminality in women was biological can be traced back to famed nineteenth-century criminologist Cesare Lombroso and his publication *La donna delinquent*. See Cesare Lombroso and Guiglielmo Ferrero, *Criminal Woman, the Prostitute, and the Normal Woman*, trans. Mary Gibson and Nicole Hahn Rafter (1893; Durham, NC: Duke University Press, 2004).

28. See "Female Offenders in the District of Columbia," *Congressional Record*, May 22, 1972, pp. E5535–5541; "From Convict to Citizen: Programs for the Woman Offender," District of Columbia Commission on the Status of Women, June 1974, Crime, Prisons, Reform Schools Collection, Folder "Prisons/Prisoners," Box 1, Sophia Smith Collection, Smith College, Northampton, MA; "Education Task Force Report: The Female Offender," Massachusetts Governor's Commission on the Status of Women, by Kay Bourne, 1972, Crime, Prisons, Reform Schools Collection, Folder "Prisons/Prisoners," Box 1, Sophia Smith Collection, Smith College; Mary Louise Cox, Judith Glazer, Sister Elaine Roulet, "Women in

Prison," *VIP Examiner*, Summer 1975. The Pennsylvania Commission on the Status of Women was supportive of Pennsylvania Program for Women and Girl Offenders' (PPWGO) efforts to produce state-funded community treatment centers as an alternative to incarceration. See PPWGO newsletter *News, Resources, and Research*, Series 1, no. 1, and *The CSW Report*, Apr. 9, 1973, Crime, Prisons, Reform Schools Collection, Folder "Penn Program for Women and Girl Offenders," Box 1, Sophia Smith Collection, Smith College.

29. Thuma, *All Our Trials*, 21.

30. *The Woman Offender Report* 1, no. 1 (Mar./Apr. 1975): 1, ACLU Prison Project Papers, Folder "Women's National Resource Center," Box 2999, Mudd Library, Princeton University, Princeton, NJ.

31. "From Convict to Citizen: Programs for the Woman Offender," District of Columbia Commission on the Status of Women, June 1974, Crime, Prisons, Reform Schools, Folder "Prisons/Prisoners," Box 1, Sophia Smith Collection, Smith College.

32. Omar Hendrix, "A Study in Neglect: A Report on Women Prisoners" (New York: Women's Prison Association, 1972), 1.

33. In the acknowledgments to their San Francisco report, authors Bresler and Leonard offered the following: "Finally, we would like to thank the network of people working in this city from within and without the system, to bring some justice into that too-large and arbitrary machine that we call, for lack of a more pungent and descriptive term, the criminal justice system. And our thanks go out particularly to the arrested women who shared some of the details of their lives with us, and from whom we learned much about anger, dignity and hope." Laura Bresler and Donald Leonard, "Women's Jail: Pretrial and Post-Conviction Alternatives, a Report on Women Arrested in San Francisco," Nov. 1978, Friends Committee on Legislation of California Records, Donald and Beverly Gerth Special Collections and University Archives, California State University, Sacramento.

34. Letter to Mr. J. M. Wedemeyer, Director Department of Social Welfare, from Richard A. Mcgee, Director of Corrections, July 7, 1961, Folder "Projects and Programs—Children of Women Prisoners, F3717:573," Projects and Programs Central Files, 1945-62, Department of Corrections Records, F3717, California State Archives.

35. Indeterminate sentencing also drove women's permanent loss of their children. Zietz noted that in at least one case a county welfare department representative expressed regret that the office had initiated an action for custody, but did so due to the belief that the woman would be incarcerated no less than fifty years. Zietz offered the correction that the "actual sentence was five years to life," but the county's estimation of fifty years was not unreasonable. The fact that parole boards were fully empowered to decide that a prisoner had not yet been

fully rehabilitated meant that actual time served could vary widely. This and all other quotes are contained in Dorothy Zietz, "Child Welfare Counseling Project, California Institution for Women, Corona, California," Summer 1960, pp. 2-4, Folder "Projects and Programs—Children of Women Prisoners, F3717:573," Projects and Programs Central Files, 1945-62, Department of Corrections Records, F3717, California State Archives (emphasis in original).

36. Of the 40 women included in Zietz's study, 19 had children in foster care and one did not know the whereabouts of her child. When the prison conducted its own survey a year after Zietz's study, 231 of the women indicated that their children were under some sort of state agency supervision, and 48 of these did not know which agency. While some of these children were under the supervision of friends and relatives who were working with the agencies, thereby potentially increasing women's chances of maintaining legal ties, Zietz's research makes clear, at least anecdotally, that agency involvement often led to the loss of custody. (Incarcerated mothers' fears that completing the survey would lead to unwanted state intervention with regards to their children's care arrangements, an observation noted in CIW's follow up study, further confirms this.) Moreover, 234 women indicated they had been unable to consult a social worker about their child's status. First reference to data taken from "Pertinent Data Relating to 40 Inmates and Expectant Mothers Included in the Family Counseling Project," California Institution for Women, Summer 1960, the data set included in Dorothy Zietz, "Child Welfare Counseling Project, California Institution for Women, Corona, California," Summer 1960. Second reference to data taken from "Study of Inmate-Child Relationships, California Institution for Women," Mar. 1961 [no author.] Both studies can be found in Folder "Projects and Programs—Children of Women Prisoners, F3717:573," Projects and Programs Central Files, 1945-62, Department of Corrections Records, F3717, California State Archives.

37. Dorothy Zietz, "Child Welfare Counseling Project California Institution for Women Corona, California," Summer 1960, pp. 4-5, Folder "Projects and Programs—Children of Women Prisoners, F3717:573," Projects and Programs Central Files, 1945-62, Department of Corrections Records, F3717, California State Archives.

38. Women also asserted their rights as single mothers when they argued that being required to name the father in exchange for the child to be eligible for state services was unfair. Dorothy Zietz, "Child Welfare Counseling Project California Institution for Women Corona, California," Summer 1960, p. 7, Folder "Projects and Programs—Children of Women Prisoners, F3717:573," Projects and Programs Central Files, 1945-62, Department of Corrections Records, F3717, California State Archives.

39. Serapio R. Zalba, *Women Prisoners and Their Families: A Monograph on a Study of the Relationships of a Correctional Institution and Social Agencies Working with Incarcerated Women and Their Children* (Los Angeles: Delmar, 1965), 8.

40. Ibid., 19–20.

41. Ibid., 2–3, 77, 119.

42. Ibid., 87, 60, 79.

43. For example, in her recommendations, Zietz reiterated CIW's "custodial treatment role" and its obligations to incarcerated women. She urged the Department of Corrections to improve its relationship with social service agencies so that it could make "known to these agencies what kinds of rehabilitative services the inmate has had, how she has responded to these and what the prognosis is for successful community adjustment. This kind of pre-emption would tend to identify the institution more clearly as a treatment resource, de-emphasize a preoccupation with the inmate's past criminal behavior and give the agency and community a more realistic and secure image of the 'treated' inmate." Dorothy Zietz, "Child Welfare Counseling Project California Institution for Women Corona, California," Summer 1960, p. 10, Folder "Projects and Programs—Children of Women Prisoners, F3717:573," Projects and Programs Central Files, 1945-62, Department of Corrections Records, F3717, California State Archives.

44. Zalba, *Women Prisoners and Their Families*, 41, 117–18.

45. See especially Khailil Muhammed, *The Condemnation of Blackness: Race, Crime, and the Making of Modern Urban America* (Cambridge, MA: Harvard University Press, 2011); Estelle Freedman, "'Uncontrolled Desires': The Response to the Sexual Psychopath, 1920–1960," *Journal of American History* 74, no. 1 (1987): 83–106. In Zietz's notes on her study participants, the vast majority of women are marked as "W" under the category titled "Race." See "Pertinent Data Relating to 40 Inmates and Expectant Mothers Included in the Family Counseling Project," California Institution for Women, Summer 1960, the data set included in Dorothy Zietz, "Child Welfare Counseling Project, California Institution for Women, Corona, California," Summer 1960, Folder "Projects and Programs—Children of Women Prisoners, F3717:573," Projects and Programs Central Files, 1945-62, Department of Corrections Records, F3717, California State Archives.

46. Zalba, *Women Prisoners and Their Families*, 78.

47. On the disparate responses to white and Black female "criminality" historically, see Hayley, *No Mercy Here*. On the historical link between blackness and criminality more generally, see Muhammed, *The Condemnation of Blackness*.

48. David A. Ward and Gene G. Kassebaum, *Women's Prison: Sex and Social Structure* (New Brunswick, NJ: Aldine Transaction, 1965), 2. The invocation of "pains of imprisonment" by Ward and Kassebaum references the influential works of Gresham M. Sykes, who coined the term, and Erving Goffman, who popularized the idea of the "total institution." Both works prompted sociologists to consider the psychological and social effects of confinement on prisoners and others held in institutions. Gresham M. Sykes, *The Society of Captives: A Study of a Maximum Security Prison* (Princeton, NJ: Princeton University Press,

1958); Erving Goffman, *Asylums: Essays on the Social Situation of Mental Patients and Other Inmates* (New York: Doubleday, 1961).

49. Ward and Kassebaum write, "Sykes has delineated the painful conditions of confinement which male prisoners must bear. . . . All these deprivations apply to female prisoners." Ward and Kassebaum, *Women's Prison*, 28.

50. Ibid., 14–15.

51. For a more detailed analysis of this interpretation of Ward and Kassebaum's study, see Regina Kunzel, *Criminal Intimacy: Prison and the Uneven History of Modern American Sexuality* (Chicago: University of Chicago Press, 2008), 126–29.

52. Letter to Ken Carpenter from Marilyn G. Haft, Barbara Swartz, Polly Feingold, Jan. 7, 1974, p. 1, ACLU Prison Project Papers, Folder "Women in Prison," Box 2999, Mudd Library, Princeton University.

53. American Friends Service Committee Newsletter MidWest Branch, 1976, Folder "Women in Prison," Box 2, FCL Series Prisons, Friends Committee on Legislation of California Records, Donald and Beverly Gerth Special Collections and University Archives, California State University, Sacramento.

54. Quote from "Mothers in Prison and Their Children: Breaking Down the Walls," *No More Cages: A Bi-monthly Women's Prison Newsletter* 2, no. 3 (Dec. 1980): 21, Folder "No More Cages," Carton 14 of 27, Inventory of the Nancy Stoller Papers Concerning Prison Inmate Health, 1970s–2000s, Archives and Special Collections, University of California, San Francisco; Young, "Sometimes I Feel Like a Motherless Child," *The Clarion*, July and Aug. 1974, Folder "Prisoner Writings," Carton 1 of 27, Inventory of the Nancy Stoller Papers Concerning Prison Inmate Health, 1970s-2000s, Archives and Special Collections, University of California, San Francisco.

55. Helen Gibson, "Women's Prisons: Laboratories for Penal Reform," *Wisconsin Law Review* 210 (1973): 224–25.

56. Annette M. Brodsky, "Planning for the Female Offender: Directions for the Future," *Criminal Justice and Behavior* 1, no. 4 (Dec. 1974): 395.

57. Kathleen Haley, "Mothers behind Bars: A Look at the Parental Rights of Incarcerated Women," *New England Journal on Prison Law* 4 (1977): 142.

58. Avery Eli Okin, "Inmates Rights to Motherhood," *Brooklyn Barrister*, n.d., Folder "Prison Nursery," Box 2, FCL Series Prisons, Friends Committee on Legislation of California Records, Donald and Beverly Gerth Special Collections and University Archives, California State University, Sacramento.

59. Sharon L. Fabian, "Toward the Best Interests of Woman Prisoners: Is the System Working?" *New England Journal on Prison Law* 6, no. 1 (Fall 1979): 24.

60. See, for example, Richard Palmer, "The Prisoner Mother and Her Child," *Capital University Law Review* 1 (1972); Haley, "Mothers behind Bars"; S. L. Hoffman, "On Prisoners and Parenting: Preserving the Tie That Binds," *Yale Law Journal* 87, no. 7 (June 1978): 1423–24; Fabian, "Toward the Best Interests

of Woman Prisoners," 58; Lynn Sametz, "Children of Incarcerated Women," *Social Work* 25, no. 4 (July 1980): 301.

61. Haley, "Mothers behind Bars," 154.

62. Palmer, "The Prisoner Mother and Her Child," 141–42. Palmer develops in depth the idea of "mother-release," but Haley also suggests that work-release could be extended to "provide a means for the mother to be released in order to perform her parental duties." Haley, "Mothers behind Bars," 154.

63. Palmer also argued for increased visitation that allowed privacy and physical contact for mother and child on the grounds that it had a rehabilitative promise. "It is submitted that extending the visitation privileges of the prisoner-mother to this extent would be a valuable aid to her rehabilitation, in that it would provide a type of family association which would otherwise be absent during her confinement. It is the duty of the legislatures to provide means for the prisoner-mother's rehabilitation. This program is such a means and should be implemented into the present programs that have been established by the legislatures." Palmer, "The Prisoner Mother and Her Child," 143.

64. Kay Nollenberger, "Jail Babies: Punishment of the Innocent," n.d., Folder "Women in Prison," Box 2, FCL Series Prisons, Friends Committee on Legislation of California Records, Donald and Beverly Gerth Special Collections and University Archives, California State University, Sacramento. In a similar vein, the director of The Program for Female Offenders, Inc., in Pittsburgh, PA, rejected placing women in a "large institution" and instead argued that women should be in "a community treatment center . . . close to their children or where their children can live with their mothers . . . where they can live in a family like setting." Charlotte Ginsburg, "Who Are the Women in Prison?" in *Women in Corrections,* ed. Barbara Hadley Olsson (American Correctional Association, 1981), 55.

65. "Keeping Mother and Child Together," *An Overview* 2, no. 9, Department of Health and Human Services Olympia, Washington, Sept. 1974, Folder "Assembly Bill 512: Retention of Children by Mother in Prison," Box 2, FCL Series Prisons, Friends Committee on Legislation of California Records, Library, California State University, Sacramento.

66. Kohler-Hausmann, *Getting Tough,* 250. While Julilly Kohler-Hausmann focuses on the consolidation of this logic throughout the 1970s, this chapter suggests a slightly slower timeline for rehabilitative initiatives that aimed to serve incarcerated women. That is, advocates' and prisoners' use of gender held open rehabilitation's imperfect potential and rhetoric slightly longer before being closed shut by the get-tough mandate.

67. Cardell v. Enomoto, No. 701-094 (Sup. Ct. San Francisco, 1976), Ellen Barry Personal Papers.

68. Terri L. Schupak, "Women and Children First: An Examination of the Unique Needs of Women in Prison," *Golden Gate University Law Review* 16, no. 3 (1986): 471.

69. "Testimony before the Assembly Select Committee on Corrections," presented by Claudia Bernard and Laurie Hauer of the Women's Litigation Unit of San Francisco Neighborhood Legal Assistance Foundation, Sept. 28, 1977, Ellen Barry Personal Papers.

70. "Unconstitutional to Take Infants from Incarcerated Mothers," *The Sun Reporter*, Nov. 11, 1976; "Prisoners' Rights to Personal Presence at Divorce and Family Court Hearings," n.d., p. 4, submitted by the Women's Litigation Unit of San Francisco Neighborhood Legal Assistance Foundation, Ellen Barry Personal Papers.

71. "Testimony before the Assembly Select Committee on Corrections," presented by Claudia Bernard and Laurie Hauer of the Women's Litigation Unit of San Francisco Neighborhood Legal Assistance Foundation, Sept. 28, 1977, Ellen Barry Personal Papers.

72. "Unconstitutional to Take Infants from Incarcerated Mothers," *The Sun Reporter*, Nov. 11, 1976; "Prisoners' Rights to Personal Presence at Divorce and Family Court Hearings," n.d., p. 4, submitted by the Women's Litigation Unit of San Francisco Neighborhood Legal Assistance Foundation, Ellen Barry Personal Papers.

73. Assembly Bill 512, Feb. 14, 1977, California State Legislature, Folder "Assembly Bill 512: Retention of Children by Mother in Prison," Box 2, FCL Series Prisons, Friends Committee on Legislation of California Records, Donald and Beverly Gerth Special Collections and University Archives, California State University, Sacramento.

74. "News from the Office of Assemblyman Terry Goggin," Feb. 14, 1977, Folder "Women in Prison," Box 2, FCL Series Prisons, Friends Committee on Legislation of California Records, Donald and Beverly Gerth Special Collections and University Archives, California State University, Sacramento.

75. "New Fixed Sentencing Takes Effect Today Statewide," *Recorder*, July 1, 1977, Folder "Senate Bill Implementation 1976–1977," Box 5, FCL Series Criminal Justice, Friends Committee on Legislation of California Records, Donald and Beverly Gerth Special Collections and University Archives, California State University, Sacramento.

76. Quoted in Candace Kruttschnitt and Rosemary Gartner, *Marking Time in the Golden State: Women's Imprisonment in California* (New York: Cambridge University Press, 2005), 13.

77. "Both Sides Now," Brent A. Barnhart, Legislative Representative ACLU of Northern California, Oct. 18, 1976, Folder "Senate Bill 42: Proposed Sentencing Law 1975–1976," Box 5, FCL Series Criminal Justice, Friends Committee on Legislation of California Records, Donald and Beverly Gerth Special Collections and University Archives, California State University, Sacramento.

78. For example, the Coordinating Council of Prisoner Organizations worked on amendments to the legislation in 1975. See "Proposed Amendments to SB 42,

draft," May 22, 1975, Folder "Senate Bill 42: Proposed Sentencing Law 1975–1976," Box 5, FCL Series Criminal Justice, Friends Committee on Legislation of California Records, Donald and Beverly Gerth Special Collections and University Archives, California State University, Sacramento.

79. For example, one amendment extended confinement for dangerous prisoners despite the fact that provisions excluding certain classes of criminals from benefitting from the new sentencing guidelines had been included in the original text. See "Struggling with SB 42," FCL Newsletter 26, no. 1 (Jan. 1977), Folder "Senate Bill 42 Implementation 1977," Box 5, FCL Series Criminal Justice, Friends Committee on Legislation of California Records, Donald and Beverly Gerth Special Collections and University Archives, California State University, Sacramento.

80. The nine groups included ACLU of Southern and Northern CA, Friends Committee on Legislation, AFSC, Committee for Prisoner Humanity and Justice, Community Alternatives to Prison, Prisoner's Health Project, Project Forum West, National Council on Crime and Delinquency, and the Unitarian Universalist Service Committee. The juvenile bills aimed to classify sixteen- and seventeen-year-olds as adult offenders. "Press Conference—Brown Criticized for Criminal Justice Stance," May 25, 1976, Folder "Senate Bill 42 Implementation 1977," Box 5, FCL Series Criminal Justice, Friends Committee on Legislation of California Records, Donald and Beverly Gerth Special Collections and University Archives, California State University, Sacramento.

81. J. J. Enomoto, "California's Need for New Prisons," *Los Angeles Times*, May 26, 1979.

82. As evidenced by the prison riot and the research conducted at CIW in the mid-1960s, this was business as usual for the CDC. Even during the supposed golden era of rehabilitation, incarcerated women in California were not beneficiaries. For example, a 1970 report examining the effects of vocational training on women's parole performance found that nearly all of the training options replicated the unskilled and semi-skilled labor capacities that inmates brought with them to CIW. The one program that did have a hundred percent success rate was cancelled after only a year of operation due to "administrative problems." The report stated, "It is obvious that the selection of the courses in the vocational training program at CIW was based on their practical contribution to the ongoing operation of the institution rather than an assessment of needs of either the labor market or the potential employee." Carol Spencer and John E. Berecochea, "Vocational Training at the California Institution for Women: An Evaluation," Research Report no. 41, Research Division, California Department of Corrections, pp. 30–33, Folder "Vocational Training in Women's Prisons," Box 2, FCL Series Prisons, Friends Committee on Legislation of California Records, Donald and Beverly Gerth Special Collections and University Archives, California State University, Sacramento. Five years later, minutes from an early Women's Prison

Coalition meeting indicated that if there had ever been any institutional support for women at CIW, it was on the decline. Budget cuts that year had forced the director of vocational training to suspend all work programs for women. The situation at county jails was even worse, and much of the efforts of the Women's Prison Coalition went towards forcing San Francisco County to create a work furlough program for women sentenced to San Bruno Jail, efforts that were largely unsuccessful. Women's Prison Coalition Meeting Minutes, Oct. 21, 1975, Ellen Barry Personal Papers.

83. Letter to Department of Corrections from Committee for Women and Children, "Program Development for Community Child Care Alternative," Oct. 1, 1979, Folder "Women in Prison: Articles and Newsletters," Box 2, FCL Series Prisons, Friends Committee on Legislation of California Records, Donald and Beverly Gerth Special Collections and University Archives, California State University, Sacramento.

84. Letter to Tony Antonuccio, CDC from A.B. 512 Task Force, "Implementation of Assembly Bill 512," Apr. 7, 1980, p. 5, Folder "Women in Prison: Articles and Newsletters," Box 2, FCL Series Prisons, Friends Committee on Legislation of California Records, Donald and Beverly Gerth Special Collections and University Archives, California State University, Sacramento.

85. Memorandum to Carole Shauffer, Rebecca Jurado, and Mark Rosenbaum from Ellen Barry, Feb. 12, 1985, p. 2, Ellen Barry Personal Papers.

86. From its original home base in the Bay Area, the organization continues to advocate on behalf of incarcerated people with children.

87. "Memorandum re: Mother-Infant Care Litigation" to Carole Shauffer, Rebecca Jurado, and Mark Rosenbaum from Ellen Barry, Feb. 21, 1985, Ellen Barry Personal Papers (emphasis in original).

88. "Declaration of Annette Harris," Aug. 21, 1985, Ellen Barry Personal Papers.

89. "Complaint for Declaratory and Injunctive Relief," Sept. 1, 1985, p. 10, Ellen Barry Personal Papers.

90. Ellen Barry, "Pregnant Prisoners," *Harvard Women's Law Journal* 12 (1989): 201-4, reference to Pregnancy-Related Health Care Team on p. 203.

91. Among a number of other changes, the settlement required the Parole and Community Services Division to issue monthly reports to the LSPC on the number of participants. "Rios v. Rowland, Settlement Agreement," May 22, 1990, Ellen Barry Personal Papers. A 2010 report issued by LSPC found that the program was still operating below capacity, even as California's three women's prisons continued to bulge at the seams. Karen Shain, Carol Strickman, and Robin Rederford, *California's Mother-Infant Prison Programs: An Investigation* (Oakland: Legal Services for Prisoners with Children, Nov. 2010).

92. Barry, "Pregnant Prisoners," 195.

93. Yvette Lehman was a professor of child development at Chabot Community College. Carolyn McCall was a recent PhD who had ties to the National

Council on Crime Delinquency (NCCD). It was Lehman who wondered what happened to the children of incarcerated mothers, and McCall who had the project management background. They also chose FCI, Pleasanton, rather than the state prison because they had heard FCI might be more amenable to such a program. Author interview. In one of the many grant proposals submitted by McCall on behalf of the program, she provided a brief history of the start of Prison MATCH. Given Warden Turnbo's counteroffer, the fact that they managed to agree upon full weekend visitation is noteworthy. See "Prison MATCH, a Research Proposal," submitted by the National Council on Crime Delinquency (NCCD), Feb. 22, 1980, p. 7, Denise Johnston Personal Papers.

94. Ibid., 1–3.

95. "The Pleasanton Children's Center Program Second-Year Report and Evaluation, 1979–1980," prepared by Carolyn McCall, NCCD, Feb. 14, 1980, pp. 1–3, Denise Johnston Personal Papers.

96. "Prison MATCH a Research Proposal," submitted by the NCCD, Feb. 22, 1980, p. 4, Denise Johnston Personal Papers.

97. Ibid., 15.

98. Child Development Associate Proposal submitted to HEW (Department of Health, Education, and Welfare) by Yvette Lehman, Nov. 17, 1978, p. 14, Denise Johnston Personal Papers. Commitment to this belief was further evidenced by the fact that the director of the children's center was hired in large part because she grew up with an incarcerated parent. Author interview.

99. Ibid., 11.

100. Ibid., 11–12.

101. Further still, foster parents had to be invested in the goal of reunification between mother and child, and the center encountered less than enthusiastic guardians who believed incarcerated mothers did not deserve to see their children. Ibid., 31.

102. "Prison MATCH: A Model Program for Imprisoned Mothers and Their Children," n.d., p. 6, Denise Johnston Personal Papers.

103. "Prison MATCH: The Pleasanton Children's Center, Mid-year Report, June–Dec., 1980," by Yvette K. Lehman for NCCD, Jan. 8, 1981, pp. 19–20, Denise Johnston Personal Papers.

104. Staff arranged for incarcerated women to have access to a birth center at a nearby hospital where they could use the services of a midwife. They also set up counseling program for pregnant women adjacent to the children's center. This effort would eventually prompt a study of perinatal services in three Bay Area correctional facilities, funded by the State Department of Health Services and undertaken largely by Carolyn McCall. The negative findings of the report no doubt contributed to strained relations between the program and prison officials. See Carolyn McCall, Jan Casteel, and Nancy S. Shaw, "Pregnancy in Prison: A Needs Assessment of Perinatal Outcome in Three California Penal Institutions,"

State of California Department of Health Services Maternal and Child Health Branch, Contract No. 84-84085 A-1, June 1985, Criminal Justice/NCCD Collection, John Cotton Dana Library, Rutgers University, Newark, New Jersey.

105. "The Pleasanton Children's Center Program, Quarterly Progress Report, July–September, 1979," NCCD, Oct. 11, 1979, p. 2, Denise Johnston Personal Papers.

106. "A Small Victim Is Doing Time . . . Information about Maternal Incarceration," n.d., p. 8, Denise Johnston Personal Papers.

107. "The Pleasanton Children's Center Program Second-Year Report and Evaluation, 1979–1980," prepared by Carolyn McCall, NCCD, Feb. 14, 1980, p. 38, Denise Johnston Personal Papers

108. "Objectives and Needs for This Assistance," Day Care Council of New York, Inc., n.d.; "Children's Center/Parenting Program at the Bronx House of Detention for Men," Osborne Association, Inc., Oct. 1984; "Helping Incarcerated Parents," Maine Department of Corrections, Dec. 30, 1987; "Technical Assistance by Prison MATCH to the Michigan Department of Corrections," National Institute of Corrections Technical Assistance, Oct. 1987. All files in Denise Johnston Personal Papers.

109. "Prison MATCH: Programs Needed in Federal Prisons for Women. A Proposal to Congress and the Bureau of Prisons," n.d., pp. 9–10, Denise Johnston Personal Papers.

110. In addition to participating in organized presentations at community agencies, conferences, and open houses hosted by the prison, women also developed a video of the program for distribution and wrote to media outlets requesting coverage. "The Pleasanton Children's Center Program, Quarterly Progress Report, July-September, 1979," Oct. 11, 1979, pp. 2–3; letter to Bob Lange from Barbara Mouzin, Feb. 28, 1985. Both files in Denise Johnston Personal Papers.

111. "Brief History of Prison MATCH—1978-1987," n.d., Denise Johnston Personal Papers.

112. Through some last-minute appeals, the organization was able to secure the annual 13,000-dollar grant from the BOP for that year. "Prison MATCH: Programs Needed in Federal Prisons for Women, a Proposal to Congress and the Bureau of Prisons," n.d., Denise Johnston Personal Papers.

113. At this point—1985—there was also a program at the federal prison in Fort Worth, TX, which was being run as a co-correctional facility. It was called Prison PACT. Prison MATCH staff was committed to making sure programs were also implemented at the federal facilities in Lexington, KY and Alderson, WV, so that all four federal prisons housing women would have the program. "Prison MATCH: Programs Needed in Federal Prisons for Women, a Proposal to Congress and the Bureau of Prisons," n.d., p. 13, Denise Johnston Personal Papers; "Brief History of Prison MATCH—1978-1987," n.d. Both files in Denise Johnston Personal Papers.

114. The line item was not mandatory and the BOP was in no way required to contract specifically with Prison MATCH. The amendment would resolve these concerns. Prison MATCH received 50,000 dollars from the BOP during these years. It made up the rest of the funds from foundation grants and community fundraising. "Prison MATCH History, Prepared for Pleasanton Children's Center Orientation Program: First Draft," n.d., Denise Johnston Personal Papers.

115. See Letter to Carolyn McCall and Janine Bertram from Robin, Nov. 14, 1986, Denise Johnston Personal Papers. In 1986, the BOP nearly cut funding to the program for a second time. See "Prison MATCH Amendment: Statement in Support of Amendment to H.R. 1400 Department of Justice Appropriation Authorization Act, Fiscal Year 1988," Representative Patricia Schroeder, n.d., Denise Johnston Personal Papers.

116. For example, the Comprehensive Crime Control Act eliminated parole for the federal prison system. For an overview of the political uses of the "war on drugs" from Richard Nixon to George H. W. Bush as well as Bill Clinton's own version of "tough on crime" politics, see Michelle Alexander, *The New Jim Crow: Mass Incarceration in the Age of Colorblindness* (New York: The New Press, 2010), 48–58. For a history that traces the roots of mass incarceration not to Reagan but to Lyndon Johnson and the distinct emergence of a federal program to criminalize "urban social programs" in the post–civil rights era, see Hinton, *From the War on Poverty to the War on Crime*, quote from p. 26.

117. Peter Kerr, "War on Drugs Straining Jails, U.S. Prison Officials See Overcrowding Getting Worse," *Chicago Tribune*, Sept. 25, 1987. Overcrowding at various levels of government taxed the federal system. For example, the District of Columbia's early problems with overcrowding meant that numerous incarcerated people were sent to federal institutions. For women, this meant going to Alderson, WV, as it was the closest federal facility for women. See Sari Horwitz, "D.C. Leans on U.S. Prisons; More Than 2,000 Local Inmates Housed in Federal Facilities," *Washington Post*, Aug. 25, 1988.

118. Notes by legal advocate, Dec. 11, 1987, and Letter to Congressman Thomas S. Foley from Lewis M. Schrawyer, Dec. 23, 1987, Denise Johnston Personal Papers.

119. Letter to Carolyn McCall from Dolores, Jan. 4, 1988, Denise Johnston Personal Papers.

120. Letter to Ellen Barry and Carolyn McCall from Katherine, Dec. 27, 1987, Denise Johnston Personal Papers.

121. Letter to Carolyn McCall from Lydia, Dec. 1, 1987, Denise Johnston Personal Papers.

122. Letter to Michael Quinlin from Janine, Dec. 11, 1987, Denise Johnston Personal Papers.

123. "Fall/Winter 1988 Effects on Inmate Mothers and Children of BOP Policies and Practices to Reduce Prison Overcrowding," submitted by Prison MATCH, Feb. 11, 1988, pp. 4–5, Denise Johnston Personal Papers.

124. "Notes on Congressional Visit, Early March, 1989, Prison MATCH," n.d., Denise Johnston Personal Papers.

125. Ruth M. Glick and Virginia V. Neto, "National Study of Women's Correctional Programs," National Institute of Law Enforcement and Criminal Justice Law Enforcement Assistance Administration, U.S. Department of Justice, Washington, DC, June 1977, p. 208.

126. Natalie J. Sokoloff, Barbara Raffel Price, and Jeanne Flavin, "The Criminal Law and Women," in *The Criminal Justice System and Women: Offenders, Prisoners, Victims, and Workers*, ed. Barbara Raffel Price and Natalie J. Sokoloff (Boston: McGraw Hill, 2004), 11; Aleks Kajstura, *Women's Mass Incarceration: The Whole Pie, 2019* (Easthampton, MA: Prison Policy Initiative, Oct. 29, 2019).

127. Lynne Haney, "Motherhood as Punishment: The Case of Parenting in Prison," *Signs* 39, no. 1 (2013): 108.

128. Gilmore, *Golden Gulag*, 7.

129. Barbara and David Steinhart, *Why Punish the Children? A Reappraisal of the Children of Incarcerated Mothers in America* (Oakland: National Council on Crime and Delinquency, 1992), 26; Christopher J. Mumola, "Bureau of Justice Statistics Special Report: Incarcerated Parents and Their Children," U.S. Department of Justice, Aug. 2000, p. 5.

130. For example, many facilities require that children be accompanied by a legal guardian, a status that may not extend to grandparents, extended family, or family friends. And foster parents, while legal guardians, must believe that it is in the best interest of the child to see their mother. See Lindsey Cramer, Margaret Goff, Bryce Peterson, and Heather Sandstrom, *Parent-Child Visiting Practices in Prisons and Jails: A Synthesis of Research and Practice* (Washington, DC: Urban Institute, Apr. 2017), 20.

131. By and large, these programs are built around the programmatic elements of the MATCH model. Bloom and Steinhart, *Why Punish the Children?*, appendix.

132. A 1992 NCCD study showed that mother-child prison visitation declined from 92 percent in 1978 to less than 50 percent in 1992. Katherine Gabel and Denise Johnston, eds., *Children of Incarcerated Parents* (New York: Lexington Books, 1995), 16. Additionally, the proportion of mothers who reported monthly visits with children fell from 17.9 percent in 1991 to 14.3 percent in 1997. Elizabeth I. Johnson and Jane Waldfogel, "Parental Incarceration: Recent Trends and Implications for Child Welfare," *Social Service Review* 76, no. 3 (Sept. 2002): 471. This is at least in part due to the fact that by 2019, nearly half of incarcerated women were held in jails, which have the highest barriers to family visitation or contact.

133. Eli Hager and Anna Flagg, *How Incarcerated Parents Are Losing Their Children Forever* (New York: The Marshall Project, Dec. 2, 2018), https://www .themarshallproject.org/2018/12/03/how-incarcerated-parents-are-losing-their -children-forever (accessed Jan. 2020).

134. Haney, "Motherhood as Punishment," 127.

135. More succinctly, "imprisoning parents increases the total amount of state supervision of Black children." Dorothy Roberts, *Shattered Bonds: The Color of Child Welfare* (New York: Basic Books, 2002), 203, 213.

136. As Lynne Haney has argued, this scholarship has largely focused on what happens when fathers and male partners are incarcerated, particularly how women are then required to absorb caretaking and breadwinning responsibilities as well as the maintenance of family ties. For this discussion, see Haney, "Motherhood as Punishment," 108. For a model that examines the diverse effects of criminalization and imprisonment across different members of the familial unit, see Roberts, *Shattered Bonds,* 200–220. For work that examines other aspects of care work produced by mass incarceration, such as mothers advocating on behalf of their incarcerated children, see Ruth Wilson Gilmore, "Pierce the Future for Hope: Mothers and Prisoners in the Post-Keynesian California Landscape," in *Global Lockdown: Race, Gender, and the Prison-Industrial Complex,* ed. Julia Sudbury and Julia Chinyere Oparah (New York: Routledge, 2004).

137. A recent study from the Prison Policy Initiative found that among women who could not make bail, their median income was 11,071 dollars. Within this group, Black women had a median annual income of 9,083 dollars. It is especially this inability to afford bail that contributes to family separation. The same study found that Black women, Native American women, and queer women are disproportionately subject to incarceration. See Kajstura, *Women's Mass Incarceration.*

138. For example, a special report on incarcerated parents and their children published by the Bureau of Justice in 2000 found that nearly 20 percent of mothers in state prison had been homeless in the year prior to their incarceration. Mumola, "Bureau of Justice Special Report," 9. A 2016 report published by the Vera Institute for Justice on the rising numbers of women held in jails since 1970 stated, "women often become involved with the justice system as a result of efforts to cope with life challenges such as poverty, unemployment, and significant physical or behavioral health struggles, including those related to past histories of trauma, mental illness, or substance abuse . . . 60 percent of women in jail did not have full-time employment prior to their arrest . . . and nearly 30 percent of incarcerated women receive public assistance." Elizabeth Swavola, Kristine Riley, and Ram Subramanian, *Overlooked: Women and Jails in an Era of Reform* (New York: Vera Institute of Justice, 2016), 9–10.

CHAPTER 3. THE LABOR OF SURVIVAL

Epigraph: Coalition to Fight Infant Mortality (newsletter), vol. 1, no. 2, July 1980, p. 3, Folder "CFIM Brochures 79–80," Series I. Administration, Box 1 of 7, Third World Women's Alliance Records, Sophia Smith Collection, Smith College, Northampton, MA.

1. Ibid.

2. Coalition to Fight Infant Mortality (newsletter), vol. 1, no. 1, Apr. 1980, p. 1, Folder "CFIM-Brochures 79–80," Series I. Administration, Box 1 of 7, Third World Women's Alliance Records, Sophia Smith Collection, Smith College.

3. Ibid., 3.

4. Ronald Reagan, Inaugural Address, Jan. 20, 1981.

5. On the argument that "the neoliberal critique of social insurance had acquired something akin to commonsense status by the end of the decade," see Cooper, *Family Values*, 185–88, quote on p. 186. The quote from Joseph Bort that follows is from p. 2 of the Apr. 1980 Coalition to Fight Infant Mortality (newsletter) cited in note 2 above.

6. For a detailed overview of changes to social programs instituted by the Reagan administration, see John L. Palmer and Isabel V. Sawhill, eds., *The Reagan Record: An Assessment of America's Changing Domestic Priorities* (Cambridge, MA: Ballinger, 1984). Of course, scholarship on the rightward shift in American politics traces the retreat of state government, popularly associated with Reagan, as a process well under way before his presidential victory. See David Harvey, *A Brief History of Neoliberalism* (New York: Oxford University Press, 2005); Stein, *Pivotal Decade*. Recent scholarship has shown that, in contrast to the dominant narrative of austerity so central to the free-market ideology that marked this period, there were in fact moments where social insurance was made to expand, though always through complicated logics and with contradictory results. See Gabriel Winant, "A Place to Die: Nursing Home Abuse and the Political Economy of the 1970s," *Journal of American History* 105, no. 1 (2018); Jonathan Bell, "Rethinking the 'Straight State': Welfare Politics, Health Care, and Public Policy in the Shadow of AIDS," *Journal of American History* 104, no. 4 (2018); Benjamin Holtzman, "'Shelter Is Only a First Step': Housing the Homeless in 1980s New York City," *Journal of Social History* 52, no. 3 (2019).

7. Sandra J. Tanenbaum, "Medicaid Eligibility Policy in the 1980s: Medical Utilitarianism and the Deserving Poor," *Journal of Health Politics, Policy and Law* 20, no. 4 (Winter 1995): 933. By the early 2000s, Medicaid expansion meant that the government was covering nearly half of all deliveries in the United States. Kosali I. Simon and Arden Handler, "Welfare Reform and Insurance Coverage during the Pregnancy Period: Implications for Preconception and Interconception Care," *Women's Health Issues* 78, no. 6 (2008).

8. For histories of such models, see Alondra Nelson, *Body and Soul: The Black Panther Party and the Fight against Medical Discrimination* (Minneapolis: University of Minnesota Press, 2013); Jenna Lloyd, *Health Rights Are Civil Rights: Peace and Justice Activism in Los Angeles, 1963-1978* (Minneapolis: University of Minnesota Press, 2014); and Jennifer Nelson, *More Than Medicine: A History of the Feminist Women's Health Movement* (New York: NYU Press, 2015).

9. "Special Report: Regionalized Perinatal Services," Robert Wood Johnson Foundation, no. 2/1978, Folder 580, "The Expert Panel on Infant Mortality, City of Philadelphia: Meeting Materials, Reports, Supporting Research: 1981–1985," Box 46, Maternity Care Coalition Records, Kislak Center for Special Collections, University of Pennsylvania, Philadelphia, PA.

10. Nelson, *More Than Medicine* (quoting the Economic Opportunity Act of 1966), 26.

11. Christopher J. L. Murray, "Rethinking DALYs [disability-adjusted life years]," in *The Global Burden of a Disease: A Comprehensive Assessment of Mortality and Disability from Diseases, Injuries, and Risk Factors in 1990 and Projected to 2020*, ed. Christopher J. L. Murray and Alan D. Lopez (Cambridge, MA: Harvard School of Public Health, 1996).

12. "Healthier Mothers and Babies—1900-1999," *Morbidity and Mortality Weekly Report*, published in the *Journal of American Medical Association* 282, no. 19 (Nov. 17, 1999): 1808. Whereas advances in neonatal medicine and regionalized perinatal services accounted for the decrease that defined the mid-1960s through the 1970s, it is generally agreed that the decrease that began at the start of the twentieth century occurred mostly in post-neonatal infant mortality, a category that is understood as resulting more from socioeconomic factors than congenital factors or incidents related to the birth. For more on the regionalization of perinatal care implemented throughout the 1960s, see "Special Report: Regionalized Perinatal Services," Robert Wood Johnson Foundation, no. 2/1978, Folder 580, "The Expert Panel on Infant Mortality, City of Philadelphia: Meeting Materials, Reports, Supporting Research: 1981–1985," Box 46, Maternity Care Coalition Records, University of Pennsylvania.

13. Between 1965 and 1969 the rate of "other than white" infant deaths declined at a faster speed than the rate of white infant deaths, momentarily bringing groups closer together than they had been or would be again until the twenty-first century. I use "other than white" here in reference to the language of the source, which did not further specify racial categories beyond "white" and "all other." See Joseph Garfinkel et al., *Infant, Maternal, and Childhood Mortality in the United States, 1968-1973*, U.S. Department of Health, Education and Welfare Publication no. 75-5013 (1975), p. 3; Douglas Almond, Kenneth Y. Chay, and Michael Greenstone, "Civil Rights, the War on Poverty, and Black-White Convergence in Infant Mortality in the Rural South and Mississippi," MIT Department of Economics Working Paper 07-04 (Dec. 31, 2006), p. 1.

The 2006 MIT study concludes that the narrowing of the racial disparity that took place between 1965 and the 1970s represents the "sole period of large reductions in the black-white infant mortality gap since World War II." However, the respective rates did not decline at the same pace, with the rate of white infant death decreasing at a faster pace than the Black infant death rate. The ratio of infant mortality rates for Blacks compared with whites increased 20 percent between 1980 and 1991, by which point Black infants had a 2.2 greater likelihood of dying before their first birthday than white infants. This divergence would ultimately carry over into the twenty-first century. Garfinkel et al., *Infant, Maternal, and Childhood Mortality in the United States, 1968–1973*, 3; Gopal Singh and Stella Yu, "Infant Mortality in the United States: Trends, Differentials and Projections, 1950–2010," *American Journal of Public Health* 85, no. 7 (July 1995): 957; "Differences in Infant Mortality Between Blacks and Whites—United States, 1980–1991," *Mortality and Morbidity Weekly Report,* published in the *Journal of American Medical Association* 271, no. 20 (May 25, 1994): 43; Myron Wegman, "Infant Mortality in the 20th Century, Dramatic but Uneven Progress," *Journal of Nutrition* 131, no. 2 (Feb. 1, 2001): 403s.

14. Infant mortality was considered a crisis by the mid-1980s in part because the immense progress made over the course of the twentieth century in reducing rates of infant death slowed significantly during the 1970s. While infant mortality did not decline at a consistent pace across the decades, the United States nevertheless experienced a decline in the rate of infant deaths from the start of the century on. The period immediately preceding the slowdown that began in the late 1970s was not only one of more rapid decline, but also initiated a reduction in the Black-white disparity that has long been a defining feature of infant mortality in the United States. This speedup was followed by an abrupt slowing in rates that greatly reduced U.S. standing in relation to other industrialized countries. While in 1960 the United States ranked 10th in comparison to other industrialized nations, by 1988 it stood at 23rd. "Healthier Mothers and Babies—1900–1999," 1808; *Infant, Maternal, and Childhood Mortality in the United States, 1968–1973*, 3; Singh and Yu, "Infant Mortality in the United States," 957.

15. "East Oakland's Shocking Rate of Infant Deaths," *San Francisco Chronicle,* May 9, 1978.

16. Ibid.

17. Coalition to Fight Infant Mortality (newsletter), vol. 1, no. 1, Apr. 1980, p. 1, Folder "CFIM-Brochures 79–80," Series I. Administration, Box 1 of 7, Third World Women's Alliance Records, Sophia Smith Archives, Smith College.

18. "Coalition to Fight Infant Mortality Newsletter," vol. 1, no. 2, July 1980, pp. 3, 8, Folder "CFIM-Brochures 79–80," Series I. Administration, Box 1 of 7, Third World Women's Alliance Records, Sophia Smith Archives, Smith College.

19. Ibid., 8.

20. Susan Stern, "Infant Mortality Rate Cited, Highland Investigation Ordered," *Synapse* 24, no. 3, n.d., Folder "CFIM Clippings, 78–79," Series I. Administration, Box 1 of 7, Third World Women's Alliance Records, Sophia Smith Archives, Smith College.

21. "County Hospitals Project," vol. 1, 1978, Folder "CFIM Statistics 77–79," Series I. Administration Box 1 of 7, and "Looking at Pediatric and Ob-Gyn Services at Highland Hospital: A Report from Supervisor John George's Health Advisory Task Force," Jan. 1978, pp. 2–5, Folder "CFIM Statistics 77–79," Series I. Administration, Box 1 of 7, both in Third World Women's Alliance Records, Sophia Smith Archives, Smith College. That same year Highland's application for Title V support was denied because, according to the chief of maternal and child health, its well-documented problems with maternity services made it uncompetitive for state funding. See Letter to Stewart Gross from Siegerie A. Centerwell, May 5, 1978, Folder "CFIM Third Party Correspondence," Series I. Administration, Box 2 of 7, Third World Women's Alliance Records, Sophia Smith Archives, Smith College.

22. "Excerpts from Statements of Support Submitted to the Coalition to Fight Infant Mortality from Community Groups and Agencies," Sept. 11, 1979, Folder "CFIM Press Releases, 79–80," Series I. Administration, Box 1 of 7, Third World Women's Alliance Records, Sophia Smith Archives, Smith College.

23. "Comparison of Perinatal Mortality Rates, 1977," Department of Health, Maternal, and Child Health Branch, Office of Statewide Health Planning and Development, State of California, n.d., Folder "CFIM Press Releases, 79–80," Series I. Administration, Box 1 of 7, Third World Women's Alliance Records, Sophia Smith Archives, Smith College.

24. Susan Stern, "Infant Mortality Rate Cited, Highland Investigation Ordered," *Synapse* 24, no. 3, n.d., Folder "CFIM Clippings, 78–79," Series I. Administration, Box 1 of 7, Third World Women's Alliance Records, Sophia Smith Archives, Smith College.

25. "For Immediate Release," Sept. 27, 1979, CFIM Press release, "CFIM Press Releases, 79–80," Series I. Administration, Box 1 of 7, Third World Women's Alliance Records, Sophia Smith Archives, Smith College.

26. Susan Stern, "Infant Mortality Rate Cited, Highland Investigation Ordered," *Synapse* 24, no. 3, n.d., Folder "CFIM Clippings, 78–79," Series I. Administration, Box 1 of 7, Third World Women's Alliance Records, Sophia Smith Archives, Smith College.

27. "Report to the Alameda County Grand Jury, California Medical Associates," Apr. 1980, pp. 30–33, Folder "CFIM Grand Jury: Correspondence; Report, 1979–1980," Series I. Administration, Box 1 of 12, Alliance Against Women's Oppression Papers, Sophia Smith Archives, Smith College.

28. Ronald L. Williams, "Vital Record Data for Use in the Planning of Obstetric and Newborn Care with Special Reference to: HSA-5 (East Bay) in California,"

First Rough Draft, Nov. 5, 1979, Folder "CFIM Grand Jury: Correspondence; Report, 1979–1980," Series I. Administration, Box 1 of 12, Alliance Against Women's Oppression Papers, Sophia Smith Archives, Smith College.

29. Williams compared the "expected perinatal mortality rate" to the "observed perinatal mortality rate" by dividing the latter by the former and multiplying the result by one hundred to produce the "indirectly standardized perinatal mortality ratio," which served as the index of effectiveness capable of assessing three areas of variation in the observed "perinatal mortality rate": that resulting from newborn risk differentials (risk), that attributable to differences in perinatal care (care), and that attributable to chance (sampling error). Ibid.

30. Similar findings held true for key cities in Alameda County, including Richmond, Berkeley and Oakland, with Oakland exhibiting the highest indexes of Black infants born out of wedlock to teen mothers with no reported prenatal care. Ibid.

31. Ibid.

32. Grand Jury Report Submitted to the Board of Supervisors for Alameda County, June 18, 1980, pp. 5–7, 10, Folder "CFIM Grand Jury: Correspondence; Report, 1979–1980," Series I. Administration, Box 1 of 12, Alliance Against Women's Oppression Papers, Sophia Smith Archives, Smith College.

33. The report defined community members as "women, primarily ethnic minorities, who were either pregnant, or had used obstetric/gynecologic services in the past, or who knew women who had used OB/GYN services." "The Report of the Community Investigation of Alameda County's High Infant Mortality Rate," Investigating Team, Aug. 1980, p. 4, Folder "Coalition to Fight Infant Mortality, Community Investigation, I-Team, Original 1980," Series I. Administration, Box 1 of 12, Alliance Against Women's Oppression Papers, Sophia Smith Archives, Smith College.

34. Ibid., 10, 16.

35. Ibid., 84; Coalition to Fight Infant Mortality, "The Investigating Team vs. The Grand Jury," Oct. 14, 1980, Folder "Coalition to Fight Infant Mortality, Community Investigation, I-Team, Letters of Introduction; Questionnaires; Statements; 1979–n.d.," Series I. Administration, Box 1 of 12, Alliance Against Women's Oppression Papers, Sophia Smith Archives, Smith College, Smith College.

36. Coalition to Fight Infant Mortality, "The Investigating Team vs. The Grand Jury," Oct. 14, 1980, Folder "Coalition to Fight Infant Mortality, Community Investigation, I-Team, Letters of Introduction; Questionnaires; Statements; 1979–n.d.," Series I. Administration, Box 1 of 12, Alliance Against Women's Oppression Papers, Sophia Smith Archives, Smith College.

37. Coalition to Fight Infant Mortality Newsletter, "WIC Food Program Slashed," vol. 2, no. 2, July 1981, p. 2; Coalition to Fight Infant Mortality Newsletter, "Alta Bates Cuts Back Community Obstetrical Services," vol. 3, no. 2, May 1982, p. 7;

Coalition to Fight Infant Mortality Newsletter, "New Coalition Responds to Deuk's Cutbacks," vol. 4, no. 3, Dec. 1983, p. 4; Art Goldberg, "The Medi-Cal Crisis," *East Bay Express* 4, no. 17 (Feb. 12, 1982)—all in Folder "CFIM newsletters, clippings, press releases, 1979–84, n.d.," Series I. Administration, Box 1 of 12, Alliance Against Women's Oppression Papers, Sophia Smith Archives. Smith College.

38. CFIM Newsletter, "County Stalls on CFIM Proposals," vol. 4, no. 3, Dec. 1983, Folder "CFIM Newsletters, Clippings, Press Releases, 1979–84, n.d.," Series I. Administration, Box 1 of 12, Alliance Against Women's Oppression Papers, Sophia Smith Archives, Smith College.

39. The Maternity Care Coalition (MCC) was a collaboration between the city's Welfare Rights Organization, faculty running the Health Law Project at the University of Pennsylvania, practitioners with the Association for Nurse-Midwives, and activists from a reproductive rights group called CHOICE. Ed Sparer, MCC co-founder and leading architect of the field of legal aid for the poor, wrote to the nascent coalition in 1980: "We do have an extraordinary opportunity to build an unusual and effective maternity care coalition. The very nature of our cross-class group, coupled with the active interest and efforts of the nurse-midwives, testifies to that." Letter from Ed Sparer to Annette Lynch, Mar. 4, 1980, Folder 608 "MCC Programs, Meetings, Correspondence: 3/4/1980–9/24/1981," Box 49, Maternity Care Coalition Records, University of Pennsylvania. For more on Sparer, see his obituary: Sylvia A. Law, "Edward V. Sparer," *University of Pennsylvania Law Review* 132 (1984).

40. "The Maternity Care Coalition of Greater Philadelphia by Walter J. Lear, draft 7/5/83," pp. 3, 5, Folder 578 "The Expert Panel on Infant Mortality, City of Philadelphia: Meetings, Minutes and Correspondence, 1981–9/7/1983," Box 45, Maternity Care Coalition Records, University of Pennsylvania.

41. A representative example of how the MCC understood the relationship between individual and societal transformation was described in the MCC Plan of Action. "True, grassroots outreach and consumer education including: block-by-block, direct contact; poster/flyer campaigns; educational seminars sponsored by community groups; and tours of maternity facilities. MCC outreach teams are trained by the Philadelphia Welfare Rights Organization, known for its extraordinary effectiveness in reaching poor people with consumer education." "General Problem Analysis Statement," by Sr. Teresita Hinnegan, Apr. 1982, p. 3, Folder 609 "MCC Programs, Meetings, and Correspondence 1982, 2/20/1982-12/30/1982," Box 49, Maternity Care Coalition Records, University of Pennsylvania.

Many members drew on past experiences of improving medical services for the indigent through consumer choice, which ensured the MCC prioritized community participation in all of its organizational initiatives. A flyer that illustrates this ethic reads, "Your community needs you to help tell presbyterian what kind of maternity services we need. What is a maternity center? It is a special service planned by the people living in the community. It can stop unnecessary deaths and reach out to young mothers. Women from the neighborhood, young and old, can get quality maternity and gynecology services." Flyer, Folder 611, "MCC Program Mtgs and Correspondence 10/1983-12/1983," Box 49, Maternity Care Coalition Records, University of Pennsylvania.

42. "The Maternity Care Coalition of Greater Philadelphia by Walter J. Lear, draft 7/5/83," pp. 3–4, Folder 578 "The Expert Panel on Infant Mortality, City of Philadelphia: Meetings, Minutes and Correspondence, 1981–9/7/1983," Box 45, Maternity Care Coalition Records, University of Pennsylvania.

43. "Minutes of Board Meeting of May 16, 1984," p. 3, Folder 602 "MCC Board Mtg Mins 9/14/1983–6/13/1985," Box 48, Maternity Care Coalition Records, University of Pennsylvania.

44. The demand for intervention increased as rising unemployment left more Americans uninsured, creating a population that was both ineligible for Medicaid and unable to obtain coverage privately. "Minutes from 3/15/83"; "A Pledge to the Women of Philadelphia"; "A Petition to the Hospitals of Philadelphia," Folder 600 "MCC Board of Directors, Meetings, Agendas, Minutes, 1/7/1981–11/29/1983," Box 47, Maternity Care Coalition Records, University of Pennsylvania.

45. "Minutes of Special Board Meeting, December 30, 1982," p. 2; "Board Meeting Minutes 2/83." Both files in Folder 600 "MCC Board of Directors, Meetings, Agendas, Minutes, 1/7/1981–11/29/1983," Box 47, Maternity Care Coalition Records, University of Pennsylvania.

46. "A Summary of Six Months' Work: March–September 1981"; "Memorandum to Board Members, Active Friends, and Community Workers of the Maternity Care Coalition from Ed Sparer, August 20, 1981," p. 5, Folder 608 "MCC Programs, Meetings, Correspondence: 3/4/1980–9/24/1981," Box 49, Maternity Care Coalition Records, University of Pennsylvania.

47. "General Problem Analysis Statement," Sr. Teresita Hinnegan, Apr. 1982, Folder 609 "MCC Programs, Meetings, and Correspondence 1982, 2/20/1982–12/30/1982," Box 49, Maternity Care Coalition Records, University of Pennsylvania.

48. The state also allocated less funding to the city for MIC, shrinking the grant from 1.5 million dollars in 1981 to 1.1 million dollars in 1982. "Prenatal Plan Is Altered," *Philadelphia Inquirer,* June 5, 1983, Folder 600 "MCC Board of Directors, Meetings, Agendas, Minutes, 1/7/1981–11/29/1983," Box 47, Maternity Care Coalition Records, University of Pennsylvania.

49. Ibid.

50. I acknowledge the critique that this statement sets up a false dichotomy. But when MCC members filling the role of WIC program administrators (who were absent due to administrative cuts) made sure that their own education and outreach programs focused on enrolling women, it is fair to say that MCC was taking on service provision at the expense of its broader aim of establishing community maternity centers. "Maternal and Infant Care Fact Sheet," n.d.; "Minutes

of Meeting of Board of Directors, January 10, 1983," p. 2. Both files in Folder 600 "MCC Board of Directors, Meetings, Agendas, Minutes, 1/7/1981–11/29/1983," Box 47, Maternity Care Coalition Records, University of Pennsylvania.

51. "A Report on Client Advocacy, July 1984–November 1984," Folder 568 "MCC Program Advocacy in the Community, Report of the Community Organization Project 7/7/1982–4/10/1985, ND," Box 45, Maternity Care Coalition Records, University of Pennsylvania. The need for client advocacy was so great that it prompted an expansion of the client advocacy program. Based on a year of experiences like that of Thorton's, MCC members proposed a "unified program of advocacy for individuals and empowerment of neighborhood people for self-advocacy to help people in the target area get the maternity and infant care services they need." "Future Plans—Advocacy in the Community," Folder 568 "MCC Program Advocacy in the Community, Report of the Community Organization Project 7/7/1982–4/10/1985 ND," Box 45, Maternity Care Coalition Records, University of Pennsylvania.

52. Barbara Clinton, Maternal and Infant Health Outreach Worker Project, Interim Report, Nov. 7, 1983, Folder 579 "The Expert Panel on Infant Mortality City of Philadelphia Meetings, Mins, and Correspondence 6/13/1984–8/6/1985," Box 46, Maternity Care Coalition Records, University of Pennsylvania.

53. Letter to "MCC Board Member" from Walter J. Lear, July 9, 1984, Folder 590 "MCC Position Paper on the Mayor's Commission on Health in the Eighties, Correspondence, 1983–4/1/1985, ND," Box 46, Maternity Care Coalition Records, University of Pennsylvania.

54. "Position Paper on the Recommendations of the Mayor's Commission on Health in the Eighties by MCC of Greater Philadelphia, Final Draft, 12/84," p. 16, Folder 588 "MCC Position Paper on Records of the Mayor's Commission on Health in the Eighties (4 copies of final draft)," 12/1984, Box 46, Maternity Care Coalition Records, University of Pennsylvania.

55. Walter Lear, "What Is the Mission of the Maternity Care Coalition?" Jan. 26, 1990, Folder 620 "MCC Programs, Meetings, Correspondence 1/1990–12/1990," Box 51, Maternity Care Coalition Records, University of Pennsylvania.

56. *Health Mothers and Babies: Pay Now or Pay Later,* Kentucky Coalition for Maternal and Child Health, Apr. 1983, Fol. 610 "MCC Programs, Mtgs, Correspondence 1/1983–9/1983," Box 49; "Public Interest Health Consortium Maternal and Child Health Task Force," 1983, Fol. 611, "MCC Programs, Mtgs, Correspondence 10/1983–12/1983, ND," Box 49; "Letter to Healthy Mothers/Healthy Babies Coalition Member" from Kathleen Stoll, Oct. 18, 1985, Fol. 614 "MCC Programs, Mtgs, Correspondence, 1/4/1985–2/31/1985," Box 50, all in Maternity Care Coalition Records, Univ. of Penn.; CFIM newsletter, Mar. 1983, "As Infant Mortality Rises," Fol. "CFIM newsletters, clippings, press releases, 1979–84, n.d.," Series I Administration, Box 1 of 12, Alliance Against Women's Oppression Papers, Sophia Smith Archives, Smith College.

57. Quoted on p. 10 of Oversight on Efforts to Reduce Infant Mortality and to Improve Pregnancy Outcome, June 30, 1980, Subcommittee on Child and Human Development, Committee on Labor and Human Resources, Senate.

58. It was initially projected that Medicaid would add 250 million dollars to the federal government's healthcare expenditures. Charles N. Oberg and Cynthia Longseth Polich, "Medicaid: The Third Decade," Health Affairs, 7, no. 4 (Fall 1988): 84. Instead, by 1976, governmental expenditures were expected to be 14 billion dollars. When unemployment began to rise in 1974, states scrambled to make cuts so as to avoid the rising costs of their Medicaid programs. See Karen Davis, "Medicaid Payments and Utilization of Medical Services by the Poor," Inquiry 13, no. 2 (June 2, 1976): 122.

59. This was partially due to wide variation between states' eligibility mechanisms (making some states far more generous Medicaid providers than others) and partially due to the growing number of Americans who were uninsured but who did not qualify for Medicaid because they did not meet eligibility requirements (through either AFDC or SSI). For example, in 1976 only 17 percent of Medicaid payments were made in the Southern region of the country despite nearly half of the nation's poor living there. Ibid., 132.

60. Better Health for Our Children: A National Strategy. The Report of the Select Panel for the Promotion of Child Health to the United States Congress and the Secretary of Health and Human Services, Vol. 1, U.S. Department of Health and Human Services, Publication No. 79-55071, 1981, p. 1.

61. Martin Tolchin, "More Health Funds for Children Urged," New York Times, Nov. 30, 1980. See also Better Health for Our Children: A National Strategy.

62. The GAO report echoed concerns raised by community organizations about services at the local level, evidencing the magnitude of disorganization that advocates were up against: "For the most part, these services have been administered independently and frequently without coordination with the MCH program at the Federal, State, and local levels." Quoted on p. 17 of Oversight on Efforts to Reduce Infant Mortality and to Improve Pregnancy Outcome, June 30, 1980, Subcommittee on Child and Human Development, Committee on Labor and Human Resources, Senate.

63. The widespread practice of physicians refusing Medicaid patients due to low reimbursement rates as compared to private insurance also hindered access, and was rampant in every state GAO researchers visited. Ibid., 23–24.

64. Or, as Karen Davis put it, "that [it] is built upon the Federal-State welfare system." Davis, "Medicaid Payments and Utilization of Medical Services by the Poor," 122.

65. Federal law required states to provide Medicaid to those receiving benefits through AFDC and Supplemental Security Income (SSI). See Karl Kronebusch, "Children's Medicaid Enrollment: The Impacts of Mandates, Welfare

Reform, and Policy Delinking," *Journal of Health Politics, Policy, and Law* 26, no. 6 (Dec. 2001). Also see Robert Stevens and Rosemary Stevens, *Welfare Medicine in America: A Case Study of Medicaid* (New York: The Free Press, 1974). The creation of Supplemental Security Income in 1972 was one such distancing attempt. SSI put the aged, blind, and disabled into a single federal program, which meant a single federal eligibility standard. Poor mothers and their children remained dependent on states for assessing eligibility. See Colleen Grogan and Eric M. Patashnik, "Between Welfare Medicine and Mainstream Entitlement: Medicaid at the Political Crossroads," *Journal of Health Politics, Policy and Law* 28, no. 5 (Oct. 2003): 829.

66. On the various practices used to restrict families' access to welfare since its inception and through the 1960s, see Nadasen, *Welfare Warriors*, 4–13. On the argument that leaving such restriction criteria up to the states was a demand made by and granted to Southern congressman in order to ensure ADC's passage, see Jill Quadagno, *The Transformation of Old Age Security: Class Politics in the American Welfare State* (Chicago: University of Chicago Press, 1988), 115.

67. In 1981, Diana Pearce wrote, "The real value of the average welfare payment, accounting for inflation and the declining size of recipient households, has decreased by approximately 20 percent in the last decade." Diana Pearce and Harriette McAdoo, *Women and Children: Alone and In Poverty* (National Advisory Council on Economic Opportunity, 1981), 10.

68. Grogan and Patashnik, "Between Welfare Medicine and Mainstream Entitlement," 830.

69. Stakeholders included: Public Advocates, Inc., a public interest law firm located in San Francisco; the Children's Defense Fund (CDF); the Congressional Black Caucus; the Food and Action Research Center (FARC); and other key allies in Congress. Key players of this coalition, notably congressional representative and chairman of the subcommittee on Health and the Environment of the House Committee on Energy and Commerce Henry Waxman and the Children's Defense Fund, had attempted to circumvent the AFDC–state problem by pushing for passage of the Child Health Assurance Act under Carter's administration, which would have operated through a national income eligibility standard distinct from state AFDC income eligibility levels. It was aimed at improving the poorly administered Early and Periodic Screening, Diagnostic and Treatment (EPSDT) program. What would become the Child Health Assurance Program would not get through Congress until 1984. For more on the Child Health Assurance Act, see Child Health Assurance Act, Hearings before the Subcommittee on Health and the Environment of the Committee on Interstate and Foreign Commerce House of Representatives, June 7 and 11, 1979. For further discussion of delinking Medicaid from AFDC, see Kronebusch, "Children's Medicaid Enrollment." The Children's Defense Fund (CDF), founded by civil rights and feminist activist Marian Wright Edelman in 1973, also became a leading voice in the

campaign for Medicaid expansion. The organization accused the administration of declaring "a war on children" and started a Child Watch program that enlisted church groups to assess the impact of cuts on social programs. "Impact of the Administration's Proposed Budget Cuts on Children," Joint Hearing Before the Subcommittee on Oversight, Committee on Ways and Means, and the Subcommittee on Health and the Environment, Committee on Energy and Commerce, Mar. 3, 1982, p. 112.

70. Congresswoman Mikulski quote can be found ibid., 66. Other examples taken from testimony submitted to Congress by the National Health Law Program, the CDF, the Food and Action Research Center (FARC), Child Welfare League of America, and representatives from community health centers. Ibid. The coalition was not unique in its approach. Take a medical study about prenatal care in New York City for example. Contrasting the issue of accessible healthcare to the rapid advancements in neonatal technologies that had done so much to reduce infant death over the course of the 1960s, expert testimony pointed out that these infants "were not the victims of a profession's intellectual or scientific inadequacies. They were not boys and girls born too soon—because certain fatal diseases have yet to be understood and made responsive to medical treatment. They were boys and girls who, *with their mothers of course*, needed only what millions of others received: adequate medical attention. Their deaths were, by and large, utterly avoidable" (emphasis mine). Infant Mortality, Subcommittee on Fiscal Affairs and Health, Committee on the District of Columbia. House; Committee on the District of Columbia Serial No. 96–15, May 7–8, 1980, p. 172. It is important to note that other frameworks were available. For example, the National Women's Health Network was not content to simply discuss access to care but emphasized *quality* of care, and framed infant mortality and poor infant outcomes as a product of aggressive and unnecessary obstetric interventions during delivery typical of the medical establishment's patriarchal approach to women's health. Oversight on Efforts to Reduce Infant Mortality and to Improve Pregnancy Outcome, June 30, 1980, Subcommittee on Child and Human Development, Committee on Labor and Human Resources. Senate; Committee on Labor and Human Resources, p. 350.

71. The CDF's written testimony also made sure to highlight the insufficiencies in the delivery of maternal and child healthcare prior to the Reagan administration's cuts. "Impact of Federal Spending on Maternal and Child Health Care," Subcommittee on Economic Goals and Intergovernmental Policy of the Joint Economic Committee, Nov. 17, 1983, pp. 5, 25.

72. Letter to John D. Dingell from the Congressional Black Caucus, Jan. 30, 1984; "The Infant Mortality Gap in the U.S.A—Excerpts from Public Advocates' Administrative Petition," Folder 571, MCC Press Conference on High Mortality Rates of Black Infants in Philadelphia, 1/30/1984–4/2/1984, Box 45, Maternity Care Coalition Records, University of Pennsylvania.

73. Ibid.; see also "News Advisory—Public Health Organizations to Outline Black/White Infant Mortality Gap," Folder 571, Box 45, MCC Records.

74. Carl T. Rowan, "Do Only the Unborn Matter?" *Washington Post*, Feb. 7, 1984; "Equal Rights for Infants," *New York Times*, Jan. 17, 1984.

75. "Community Activists Charge Federal Inaction on Preventable Deaths of Black Infants," Mar. 16, 1984, Folder 571, "MCC Press Conference on High Mortality Rates of Black Infants in Philadelphia, 1/30/1984–4/2/1984," Box 45, Maternity Care Coalition Records, University of Pennsylvania.

76. As mentioned earlier, the 1980 GAO report painted a depressing picture of dysfunctional public programs. "Medicaid, Community Health Centers, National Health Services Corps, Family Planning, Health Planning, and WIC"— just to name a few—not only often replicated the services originally set forth in Title V, but were carried out with little to no oversight by state maternal and child health personnel. There was also little to no outreach, which resulted in low participation of services.

77. Infant Mortality Rates: Failure to Close the Black-White Gap, Hearing before the Subcommittee on Oversight and Investigations and the Subcommittee on Health and the Environment of the Committee on Energy and Commerce House of Representatives, Mar. 16, 1984, p. 9.

78. Ibid., 15, 18.

79. Ibid., 102. Brandt based his comments on special analysis he requested from the National Center for Health Statistics (NCHS) after receiving the petition from Public Advocates. Once again the debate over statistical data took center stage, as NCHS analysts squared off with FARC and the CDF. The director of NCHS's Division of Analysis prepared a special analysis of race-specific trends in response to the claims made by the two advocacy groups. While both reports linked IMR statistics to state and city cutbacks, federal researchers pointed out that analyzing variation within a one- to two-year period was unreliable, as infant mortality was an unsteady phenomenon. Best practice was to compare longer periods of time. They also showed that for seven of the states for which FARC reported increases in Black IMR in 1981, those rates decreased the following year: "The major social, economic, and health system changes during the 1970s produced a complex web of interacting forces upon infant mortality. It is therefore possible to create a number of equally plausible scenarios to account for the decrease and subsequent increase in the black/white IMR ratio. Counterarguments to any such scenario can also be developed. Although the decline in the black/white ratio coincided with increasing activity in Maternal and Infant Care programs and Neighborhood Health centers the sharp increase in 1976 did not coincide with a sharp cutback in these programs. In fact, the proportion of black women who began prenatal care in the first trimester of pregnancy continued to increase through the late 1970s." The report also cited numerous discrepancies between the data offered by the CDF and FARC and the data obtained by

the NCHS. For example, the CDF reported that 21.1 percent of nonwhite women in the District of Columbia received late or no prenatal care in 1982. But when the NCHS obtained data from the district, it showed that the number was much lower, only 8.2 percent. Furthermore, over the period 1978–1981, the CDF showed an increase in women with no prenatal care whereas the District's and NCHS's data showed slight decreases. Ibid., 198, 206.

80. Ibid., 222.

81. Ibid., 228.

82. Ibid., 230–32 (emphasis mine).

83. CDF Newsletter, July 2, 1984, Folder 593, "MCC's Involvement in Children's Coalition of Greater Philly, 2/1984–2/26/1986," Box 46, Maternity Care Coalition Records, University of Pennsylvania.

84. Letter to H. Arnold Muller, Secretary of Health for Pennsylvania from Edward Brandt, Secretary of Health, 1/8/1985, Folder 614, "MCC Programs, Meetings, Correspondence, 1/4/1985–2/31/1985," Box 50, Maternity Care Coalition Records, University of Pennsylvania. For an overview of directions made to Brandt by the co-chairman of the PHS working group on low birth weight, see "Note to Dr. Brandt" from Vince L. Hutchins, Oct. 30, 1984, Folder 614, ibid.

85. "Appendix G, Effective Pregnancy and Infant Care," p. 4, n.d., Folder 614, Box 50, Maternity Care Coalition Records.

86. Southern Regional Task Force on Infant Mortality, *Final Report: For the Children of Tomorrow*, Southern Governors' Association (Nov. 1985), 24.

87. Margaret Heckler, *Report of the Secretary's Task Force on Black and Minority Health, Volume 1: Executive Summary* (Washington, DC: U.S. Government Printing Office, 1985).

88. Committee to Study the Prevention of Low Birthweight, Division of Health Promotion and Disease Prevention, *Preventing Low Birthweight*, Institute of Medicine (Washington, DC: National Academies Press, 1985).

89. C. Arden Miller, "Infant Mortality in the U.S.," *Scientific American* 253, no. 1 (July 1985).

90. "Preventing Infant Mortality: Intergovernmental Dimensions of a National Problem," Joint Hearings before the Subcommittee on Intergovernmental Relations of the Committee on Governmental Affairs and the Committee on the Budget, on S. 1209 to establish the national commission to prevent infant mortality and report, Sept. 11, 1985.

91. Committee to Study the Prevention of Low Birthweight, *Preventing Low Birth Weight*, 17.

92. "Preventing Infant Mortality: Intergovernmental Dimensions of a National Problem," Joint Hearings before the Subcommittee on Intergovernmental Relations of the Committee on Governmental Affairs and the Committee on the Budget, on S. 1209 to establish the national commission to prevent infant mortality and report, Sept. 11, 1985, p. 3.

93. Committee to Study the Prevention of Low Birth Weight, *Preventing Low Birth Weight*, 56.

94. Sandra R. Gregg, "The Black-White Health Gap: Disparity Widening, Congressional Caucus Is Told," *Washington Post*, Oct. 10, 1984.

95. "Preventing Infant Mortality: Intergovernmental Dimensions of a National Problem," Joint Hearings before the Subcommittee on Intergovernmental Relations of the Committee on Governmental Affairs and the Committee on the Budget, on S. 1209 to establish the national commission to prevent infant mortality and report, Sept. 11, 1985, p. 30.

96. For example, Philadelphia mayor Wilson Goode established a coalition to prevent adolescent pregnancy in 1985. During this period MCC board members noted the shift in focus on the part of foundations; being turned down encouraged them to move in this direction. See MCC Board Meeting Minutes, Sept. 12, 1985, and Nov. 14, 1985, Folder 603, "MCC Board and Directors Meeting Minutes 3/20/1985–1/14/1985," Maternity Care Coalition Records, University of Pennsylvania.

97. For example, this recommendation appears first in the 1985 "Expert Panel on Infant Mortality" report convened by Mayor Goode for Philadelphia. Folder 585, "The Expert Panel on Infant Mortality Report, Recommendations for the Reduction of Infant Mortality in Philadelphia, 8/1985–10/30/1985," Box 46, Maternity Care Coalition Records, University of Pennsylvania.

98. MCC Board Meeting Minutes, Apr. 16, 1987, Folder 615 "MCC Programs, Meetings, Correspondence: 1/3/1986–12/12/1986," Box 50, Maternity Care Coalition Records, University of Pennsylvania. CDF also created campaign materials to distribute to communities that wanted to start local initiatives. See materials in Folder 596 "Public Awareness Materials for Children's Defense Fund and Women's Agenda, 1986–1989," Box 46, ibid.

99. Andrew H. Malcom, "New Generation of Poor Youths Emerges in U.S.," *New York Times*, Oct. 20, 1985.

100. For more on Moynihan's contributions to debates over welfare during this period, see Kornbluh and Mink, *Ensuring Poverty*, 38–41

101. See Ian T. Hill, "Improving State Medicaid Programs for Pregnant Women and Children," *HealthCare Financing Review*, Annual Supplement (1990): 76.

102. Waxman quoted in Tanenbaum, "Medicaid Eligibility in the 1980s," 945. I am grateful to both Tanenbaum's article and a personal exchange with her for the point about the parsing of populations.

103. To be considered an active participant in the Medicaid program a provider had to bill for at least 300 claims per year. See "SOBRA Monitoring Project: Summary of Findings," Women's Agenda, Oct. 2, 1989, Folder 619 "MCC Programs, Meetings, Correspondence 7/1/1989–12/1989," Box 50, Maternity Care Coalition Records, University of Pennsylvania.

104. MCC grant application to the Allen Hilles Fund, 1988 Proposal Summary, Folder 617 "MCC Programs, Meetings, Correspondence 1/1988–12/1988," Box 46, Maternity Care Coalition Records, University of Pennsylvania.

105. "Advocacy in the Community," n.d., Folder 614 "MCC Programs, Meetings, Correspondence, 1/4/1985–2/31/1985," Box 50, Maternity Care Coalition Records, University of Pennsylvania.

106. Susan Fitzgerald, "A Bleak Record on Infant Death," *Philadelphia Inquirer,* Apr. 26, 1987.

107. Arline T. Geronimus, "The Effects of Race, Residence, and Prenatal Care on the Relationship of Maternal Age to Neonatal Mortality," *American Journal of Public Health* 76, no. 12 (Dec. 1986): 1416.

108. For example, whereas social science research was concerned with socioeconomic determinants of mortality that offered correlates but not causes, biomedical research was concerned with biological processes of disease that too often ignored socioeconomic determinants. Arline T. Geronimus, "On Teenage Childbearing and Neonatal Mortality in the United States," *Population and Development Review* 13, no. 2 (June 1987): 247.

109. Such a framework offered a way to capture how social conditions, such as poverty and racism, operated through other biological factors, such as nutrient deficiency, to determine morbidity and mortality. W. Henry Mosley and Lincoln C. Chen, "An Analytical Framework for the Study of Child Survival in Developing Countries," *Population and Development Review* 10 (1984): 29.

110. Geronimus, "On Teenage Childbearing and Neonatal Mortality in the United States," 253.

111. Geronimus, "The Effects of Race, Residence, and Prenatal Care on the Relationship of Maternal Age to Neonatal Mortality," 1416–21.

112. When Geronimus linked birth and infant death certificate registers for three states, she attempted to isolate the effects of maternal age at first birth from the maternal characteristics of racial identification, adequacy of prenatal care, and residency. Despite the fact that, across the board, teenage mothers faced a number of environmentally induced risk factors resulting from socioeconomic disadvantage, Geronimus's study showed that Black women exhibited higher rates of low birth weight and neonatal mortality than their white counterparts. One of the problems with research investigating the causes of infant mortality was the presumption that risk indicators were uniformly distributed; for all women of childbearing age (itself a large span of time that was rarely controlled for), poverty's effects would be considered to be the same for pregnancy at any age, for example. Geronimus hypothesized that the presumption of universality did not reflect reality and was skewing researchers' findings as a result. Specifically, she questioned the idea that the "prime" childbearing years (twenties

through early thirties) should be applied as a universal standard predicting optimal birth outcomes across different populations.

113. Arline T. Geronimus and John Bound, "Black/White Differences in Women's Reproductive-Related Health Status: Evidence from Vital Statistics," *Demography* 27, no. 3 (Aug. 1990).

114. Ibid., 464. See also Arline T. Geronimus, H. F. Andersen, and J. Bound, "Differences in Hypertension Prevalence among U.S. Black and White Women of Childbearing Age," paper presented at the Annual Meeting of the American Public Health Association, Chicago, 1989.

115. For example, in addition to suggestions like Geronimus's countering the presumed negative outcomes of teen pregnancy, researchers were also challenging the routinely invoked argument that the U.S. was experiencing an "epidemic" of pregnant teenagers. See Maris Vinovskis, *An "Epidemic" of Adolescent Pregnancy? Some Historical and Policy Considerations* (New York: Oxford University Press, 1988). The "forcefully" quote is taken from sociologist Frank Furstenberg's discussion of the unfolding debate, where he also relayed Geronimus's presentation at the American Association for the Advancement of Science. See Frank F. Furstenberg, "As the Pendulum Swings: Teenage Childbearing and Social Concern," *Family Relations* 40, no. 2 (1991): 128. Among the researchers suggesting that teen pregnancy might actually pose advantages, sociologist Kristen Luker began publishing work in 1990 on what would become *Dubious Conceptions: The Politics of Teenage Pregnancy* (Cambridge, MA: Harvard University Press, 1996). For a contemporary overview of the literature that has continued in these two veins (teenage pregnancy does not cause poverty and because of inequality it offers some advantages), see Briggs, *How All Politics Became Reproductive Politics,* 55–56.

116. Tamar Lewin, "Studies Cause Confusion on Impact of Teen-Age Pregnancy," *New York Times,* Mar. 7, 1990.

117. Chris Raymond, "Researchers Say Teenage Pregnancy Is a Symptom of Societal Ills with No Simple Solution," *Chronicle of Higher Education,* Feb. 28, 1990.

118. Rosann Wisman, "A Wise Decision?" *Washington Post,* Mar. 12, 1990.

119. Colbert I. King, "Buying into White Supremacy," *Washington Post,* May 31, 1991.

120. For example, Geronimus succinctly righted the distortion offered by Hulbert in a letter to the editor that concluded, "I am deeply troubled that lack of access to healthcare, child care, education, and employment opportunities makes teen childbearing a tolerable choice in some poor communities. This is true not because poor teens face ideal circumstances for childbearing now, but because unless there are radical changes in social policy, their circumstances will never be ideal." Arline T. Geronimus, "Baby Talk," *New Republic,* Dec. 24, 1990.

Geronimus also exposed a CDF report authored by Pittman that distorted research on infant mortality. In her report, Pittman argued that Geronimus's findings were based on neonatal mortality, which should not be generalized to all infant mortality. But Pittman counted on lay readers not knowing that neonatal mortality accounted for two thirds of the overall infant mortality rate. When Geronimus analyzed the figures in Pittman's report, she argued that Pittman's distinction—that rates of infant death within the first year would "tell a different story" than the one told by Geronimus—in fact did not. In this same article, Geronimus also took on Frank Furstenberg and Ann Hulbert. See Arline T. Geronimus, "Teenage Childbearing and Social and Reproductive Disadvantage: The Evolution of Complex Questions and the Demise of Simple Answers," *Family Relations* 40, no. 4 (Oct. 1991): 467.

121. Ibid., 466. As Laura Briggs discusses, citing researchers who demonstrated there are sometimes social benefits to teen pregnancy by examining sibling pairs who have children at different ages, support such as help from family allows teen mothers still living with their parents to spend more years accruing education and work without associated costs of things like child care. See Briggs, *How All Politics Became Reproductive Politics*, 56.

122. Arline T. Geronimus, "The Weathering Hypothesis and the Health of African-American Women and Infants: Evidence and Speculation," *Ethnicity and Disease* 2, no. 3 (Summer 1992): 26.

123. General Accounting Office, *Prenatal Care: Early Success in Enrolling Women Made Eligible by Medicaid Expansions* (Washington, DC: GAO, Feb. 1991).

124. Greg R. Alexander and Milton Kotelchuck, "Assessing the Role and Effectiveness of Prenatal Care: History, Challenges and Directions for Future Research," *Public Health Reports* 116 (July/Aug. 2001): 309.

125. Southern Governors' Association, *Coming of Age: Ten Years in the Campaign against Infant Mortality*, Southern Regional Project on Infant Mortality, 1984-1994, Report No. C100-9400 (1994).

126. On the politics of "preconception care," see Miranda R. Waggoner, *The Zero Trimester: Pre-pregnancy Care and the Politics of Reproductive Risk* (Berkeley: University of California Press, 2017).

127. Indeed, at least 104 lawmakers told Speaker of the House Newt Gingrich in June of 1996 that "you've got to decouple the Medicaid and the welfare because we've got to send him a bill that he can sign." Quoted in Kornbluh and Mink, *Ensuring Poverty*, 76. Thanks to Medicaid expansion, this decoupling was already underway. See Teresa A. Coughlin, *Medicaid since 1980: Costs, Coverage, and the Shifting Alliance Between the Federal Government and the States* (Washington, DC: The Urban Institute Press, 1994), 2.

128. Simon and Handler, "Welfare Reform and Insurance Coverage During the Pregnancy Period."

129. Walter Lear, "What Is the Mission of the Maternity Care Coalition?" Jan. 26, 1990, Folder 620, MCC Programs, Mtgs, Correspondence 1/1990–12/1990, Box 51, Maternity Care Coalition Records, University of Pennsylvania.

130. Dána-Ain Davis, *Reproductive Injustice: Racism, Pregnancy, and Premature Birth* (New York: NYU Press, 2019).

CHAPTER 4. THE LABOR OF RISK

Epigraph: Women's AIDS Network (WAN) Meeting Minutes, Feb. 5, 1990, Folder "Minutes: Jan-Dec, 1991," Carton 1 of 1, WAN Records, UCSF Library, Archives and Special Collections, University of California, San Francisco.

1. "Women's Health: Report of the Public Health Service Task Force on Women's Health Issues," *Public Health Reports* 100, no. 1 (1985): 84, 74. Chapter title references Paula A. Treichler, *How to Have Theory in an Epidemic: Cultural Chronicles of AIDS* (Durham, NC: Duke University Press, 1999).

2. Bureau of Labor Statistics, *Perspectives on Working Women: A Databook,* Bulletin 2080 (Washington, DC, 1980), 10.

3. Solinger, *Beggars and Choosers,* 196 (for quote and statistic).

4. Janice Peterson, "The Feminization of Poverty," *Journal of Economic Issues* 21, no. 1 (Mar. 1987): 329, 331, 333.

5. Solinger, *Beggars and Choosers,* 194, 196.

6. Cooper, *Family Values,* 189.

7. "Women's Health: Report," 74, 79.

8. Treichler, *How to Have Theory in an Epidemic,* 69.

9. Jennifer Brier, *Infectious Ideas: U.S. Political Responses to the AIDS Crisis* (Chapel Hill: University of North Carolina Press, 2009), 80. Reagan's first public address specifically dedicated to the epidemic would not happen until April 1, 1987. See Paula Treichler, *How to Have Theory in An Epidemic,* 57.

10. In the CDC's first-year update on the disease, 4 percent of the 355 reported cases were women, and the report acknowledged that "this proportion of heterosexuals (16%) is higher than previously described." See Treichler, *How to Have Theory in an Epidemic,* 49. On the myopic association between AIDS and gay men, Melinda Cooper has recently written that "as late as 1982, in fact, scientists were still debating whether the strange new immune condition afflicting young gay men could be attributed to the repeated lifestyle stresses of dancing, poppers, and sodomy." See Cooper, *Family Values,* 202.

11. Cindy Patton, *Last Served? Gendering the HIV Pandemic* (London: Taylor and Francis, 1994), 11.

12. The CDC changed its definition in 1991 due to immense and prolonged activist pressure. For an overview of women's activism on this and related issues, see Brier, *Infectious Ideas,* 171–77.

13. See Evelyn Hammonds, "Missing Persons: African American Women, AIDS, and the History of the Disease," *Radical America* 24, no. 2 (1992), and "Toward a Genealogy of Black Female Sexuality: The Problematic of Silence," in *Feminist Genealogies, Colonial Legacies, Democratic Futures,* ed. M. Jacqui Alexander and Chandra Talpade Mohanty (New York: Routledge, 1997); Patton, *Last Served?;* Catherine Waldby, *AIDS and the Body Politic: Biomedicine and Sexual Difference* (New York: Routledge, 1996); Nancy Goldstein and Jennifer L. Manlowe, eds., *The Gender Politics of HIV/AIDS in Women: Perspectives on the Pandemic in the United States* (New York: NYU Press, 1997); Treichler, *How to Have Theory in an Epidemic;* Cathy Cohen, *The Boundaries of Blackness: AIDS and the Breakdown of Black Politics* (Chicago: University of Chicago Press, 1999), 324–32. Gena Corea's *The Invisible Epidemic: The Story of Women and AIDS* (New York: Perennial Press, 1993) is a quintessential example of the invisibility framework.

14. Patton outlined the ways that "women-who-do-not-count-as-women," such as sex workers, intravenous drug users, and irresponsible mothers carelessly infecting their babies, were made hypervisible in order to preserve the idea that white, heterosexual, middle-class women were immune to infection. Patton, *Last Served?*, 5, 109. Oftentimes, advocacy groups appealed to both formulations. For example, the AIDS Coalition to Unleash Power (ACT UP) popularized the slogans "Women Don't Get AIDS, They Just Die from It" and "Women Cannot Wait 'til Later, We Are Not Your Incubators," which communicate the two different positions outlined here.

15. Solinger, *Beggars and Choosers*, 193–200.

16. Risa Denenberg, "What the Numbers Mean," in *Women, AIDS, and Activism*, ed. ACT UP/NY Women and AIDS Book Group (Boston: South End Press, 1990), 1.

17. By 1994, women comprised 18 percent of new AIDS cases, which represented a threefold increase since 1985. See *HIV Surveillance, Reporting and Testing Policies: Controversial Issues for Women* (Washington, DC: Center for Women Policy Studies, Oct. 1995).

18. Chris Norwood, "Alarming Rise in Deaths: Are Women Showing New 'AIDS' Symptoms?" *Ms.*, July 1988, pp. 65–67.

19. Sheldon H. Landesman, Howard L. Minkoff, and Anne Willoughby, "HIV Disease in Reproductive Age Women: A Problem of the Present," *Journal of the American Medical Association* 261, no. 9 (Mar. 3, 1989): 1327.

20. Judy Gerber, "Black Women and AIDS: The Second Epidemic," *Breakthrough* 16, no. 1 (Summer 1992), Marion Banzhaf Personal Papers.

21. Vito Russo, "Why We Fight," speech, https://actupny.org/documents/whfight.html (accessed Aug. 5, 2020).

22. On AIDS service organizations (ASOs) see Deborah B. Gould, *Moving Politics: Emotion and ACT UP's Fight against AIDS* (Chicago: University of Chi-

cago Press, 2009), ch. 1. On the limits and exclusions that characterized many early ASOs, see Brier, *Infectious Ideas,* ch. 2. On the early efforts of Black gay activists to respond to AIDS in their community followed by broader responses on the part of "more traditional black leaders," see Cathy Cohen, *The Boundaries of Blackness: AIDS and the Breakdown of Black Politics* (Chicago: University of Chicago Press, 1999), ch. 3.

23. Risa Denenberg, "What the Numbers Mean," 2. Two studies that do high-light the precarity and inequality that characterized the early 1980s and set the context for the epidemic's early years are Melinda Cooper's *Family Values* and Cathy Cohen's *Boundaries of Blackness.* Cooper is interested in how gay sex and queer kinship were forced into the social insurance afforded by marital monog-amy, and her study highlights the immense insecurity, particularly with regard to public health and any kind of care infrastructure, that made such private insur-ance a necessary option (see especially ch. 5). Cohen explores "the political and economic context of black communities in which AIDS emerged," which for Cohen meant that in the first years of the epidemic "black activists turned their attention, instead, to the new and old crisis plaguing black communities." Cohen traces the numerous anti-Black, anti-poor initiatives enacted by the Reagan administration (see especially ch. 3). My contribution is an examination of the gender inequality and reproductive labor that such conditions produced and necessitated.

24. Indeed, it was white, gay men's access to private health insurance that "shaped the very profile of the epidemic" in the first place because "for AIDS to be recognized as an identifiable illness . . . it was necessary for a sufficient number of people of a certain demographic to have access to premium medical practitioners in direct contact with the highest levels of public health surveil-lance." This "certain demographic" also needed to be "healthy" in order for the immune deficiency to seem out of the ordinary (rather than easily attributable to other illnesses more commonly seen in poor people, homeless people, and intra-venous drug users). See Cooper, *Family Values,* 204–5.

25. As Cooper puts it, "In the early 1980s, municipal governments had endured more than a decade of inflating social service costs and were in the full throes of a fiscal crisis induced by the Volcker shock." Ibid., 188.

26. Laurie Hauer, "Women's AIDS Network Acceptance Speech," Mar. 29, 1987, Folder "Minutes: April, 1987," Carton 1 of 1, Women's Aids Network (WAN) Records, UCSF Library, Archives and Special Collections, University of California, San Francisco.

27. "Memo to WAN members from Nancy Shaw," Dec. 26, 1984, Folder "Min-utes: Sept, Oct, Dec," Carton 1 of 1, WAN Records, UCSF Library, Archives and Special Collections, University of California, San Francisco.

28. Judy Clark and Kathy Boudin, "Community of Women Organize Them-selves to Cope with the AIDS Crisis: A Case Study from Bedford Hills Correc-tional Facility," *Social Justice* 17, no. 2 (1990), Marion Banzhaf Personal Papers.

29. ACE Statement of Purpose, Sept. 10, 1988, Marion Banzhaf Personal Papers.

30. "History," WARN Pamphlet, n.d., Folder, "Women and AIDS Resource Network," Box "W," Barnard Archives and Special Collections, Barnard College, New York.

31. Nelson, *More Than Medicine*, 158–59.

32. Untitled newsletter, Women and AIDS Project, Feb. 1, 1987, p. 2, Linda Loffredo Personal Papers.

33. Cohen, *Boundaries of Blackness*, 84. Jennifer Brier has cautioned against painting with too broad a brush the Reagan administration's response to the epidemic. She charts the internal disagreements among Reagan's officials and argues that moral conservatism did not necessarily win the day, as evidenced by Surgeon General Everett Koop's success in releasing to the public his report on AIDS in 1986. Koop was guided by "scientific reasoning and Christian compassion" rather than the moralizing about the so-called evils of homosexuality characteristic of other officials, such as Gary Bauer. My concern is less about the power of New Right ideology (though Brier's point that it was not all-powerful is well taken) and more about how these internal debates delayed necessary action in the early, critical years, which Brier acknowledges. See Brier, *Infectious Ideas*, ch. 3.

34. Nelson, *More Than Medicine*, 160.

35. For example, as late as 1989, WAN received a request for materials from an assistant AIDS program coordinator in the Health Program Office in Tampa, FL. "Minutes, WAN Meeting November 7, 1989," Folder "Minutes: November 1988," Carton 1 of 1, WAN Records, UCSF Library, Archives and Special Collections, University of California, San Francisco.

36. On how cuts to HUD were especially damaging to poor Americans, see Mauro F. Guillen and Charles Perrow, *The AIDS Disaster: The Failure of Organizations in New York and the Nation* (New Haven, CT: Yale University Press, 1990). On the rise of family homelessness, see Peter Rossi, "The Old Homeless and the New Homelessness in Historical Perspective," *American Psychologist* 45, no. 8 (1990).

37. D. Lee Bawden and John L. Palmer, "Social Policy," in *The Reagan Record: An Assessment of America's Changing Domestic Priorities*, ed. John L. Palmer and Isabel V. Sawhill (Cambridge, MA: Ballinger, 1984), 204.

38. Cooper, *Family Values*, 194.

39. "Women with AIDS and ARC in San Francisco," Sept. 17, 1987, "Testimony of WAN Members, 1986–1987," Carton 1 of 1, WAN Records, UCSF Library, Archives and Special Collections, University of California, San Francisco.

40. WARN Pamphlet, n.d., Folder "Women and AIDS Resource Network," Box "W," Folder, "Women and AIDS Resource Network," Box "W," Barnard Archives and Special Collections, Barnard College, New York.

41. Ibid.

42. "Executive Summary," n.d., Folder "Women and AIDS Resource Network," Box "W," Barnard Archives and Special Collections, Barnard College, New York.

43. Letter to SF Human Rights Commission from Nancy Stoller Shaw, Feb. 4 and 5, 1986, Folder "Testimony of WAN members 1986–1987," Carton 1 of 1, WAN Records, UCSF Library, Archives and Special Collections, University of California, San Francisco.

44. WAN Meeting Minutes, June 3, 1986, Folder "Minutes: Feb–March; May–Sept, 1986," Carton 1 of 1, WAN Records, UCSF Library, Archives and Special Collections, University of California, San Francisco.

45. WARN Pamphlet, n.d., Folder "Women and AIDS Resource Network," Box "W," Barnard Archives and Special Collections, Barnard College, New York.

46. WAN Meeting Minutes, June 3, 1986, Folder "Minutes: Feb–March; May–Sept, 1986," Carton 1 of 1, WAN Records, UCSF Library, Archives and Special Collections, University of California, San Francisco.

47. WAN Meeting Minutes, Jan. 6, 1987, Folder "Minutes: January, 1987," Carton 1 of 1, WAN Records, UCSF Library, Archives and Special Collections, University of California, San Francisco.

48. Letter to Caroline Mufford from Ruth Mota, Dec 1, 1986, Folder "Minutes: December 1986," Carton 1 of 1, WAN Records, UCSF Library, Archives and Special Collections, University of California, San Francisco.

49. Cooper, *Family Values*, 189.

50. Mary G. Boland and Ruth Maring Klug, "AIDS: The Implications for Home Care," *The American Journal of Maternal Child Nursing*, vol. 11 (Nov.–Dec. 1986), Folder "Minutes, February, 1987," Carton 1 of 1, WAN Records, UCSF Library, Archives and Special Collections, University of California, San Francisco.

51. Letter to David Werdegar from Nancy Shaw, Dec. 9, 1986, Folder "Minutes: December, 1986," Carton 1 of 1, WAN Records, UCSF Library, Archives and Special Collections, San Francisco.

52. "Women with AIDS and ARC in San Francisco," Sept. 17, 1987, "Testimony of WAN Members, 1986–1987," Carton 1 of 1, WAN Records, UCSF Library, Archives and Special Collections, San Francisco.

53. "Open Letter to the Health Commission," Folder "Minutes: March 1987," Carton 1 of 1, WAN Records UCSF Library, Archives and Special Collections, San Francisco. As with many ASOs, WAN combined public funds with private resources. The same year that WAN and others petitioned the city for more funding, they received 10 percent of the proceeds from the International Ms. Leather contest, which added 800 dollars to the organization's budget. Women's AIDS Network, Apr. 7, 1987, Folder "Minutes: April, 1987," Carton 1 of 1, WAN Records, UCSF Library, Archives and Special Collections, San Francisco.

54. "CAAA Reports," vol. 1, no. 4, June–July 1987, Folder "Minutes: July, 1987," Carton 1 of 1, WAN Records, UCSF Library, Archives and Special Collections, San Francisco.

55. "Minutes, Women's AIDS Network, August 4, 1987," Folder "Minutes: August, 1987," Carton 1 of 1, WAN Records, UCSF Library, Archives and Special Collections, San Francisco.

56. This entailed urging the San Francisco Department of Public Health to charge a special group with issuing recommendations on the needs of women with AIDS. "Board of Directors Resolution Shanti Project," n.d., Folder "Agenda and Minutes: November, 1987," Carton 1 of 1, WAN Records, UCSF Library, Archives and Special Collections, San Francisco.

57. Interview with Ruth Schwartz by Rebecca Issacs, "Women and AIDS," *The Exchange (Publication of the National Lawyers Guild AIDS Network)*, no. 7, Mar. 1988, p. 2, Folder "Minutes: April 1988," Carton 1 of 1, WAN Records, UCSF Library, Archives and Special Collections, San Francisco.

58. "Executive Summary," n.d., Folder "Women and AIDS Resource Network," Box "W," Barnard Archives and Special Collections, Barnard College, New York.

59. Ruth Schwartz, "Testimony to Democratic Party Platform Hearings, December 12, 1987," Folder "Minutes December, 1987," Carton 1 of 1, WAN Records, UCSF Library, San Francisco.; "Women and AIDS," *The Exchange*, no. 7, Mar. 1988, p. 2, Folder "Minutes: April 1988," Carton 1 of 1, WAN Records, UCSF Library, Archives and Special Collections, San Francisco.

60. Brier, *Infectious Ideas*, 97–96.

61. "Alliance Initiates Project on Women's Centers and AIDS in New York State and New Jersey, Press Release," Feb. 4, 1988, Folder "Minutes: March, 1988," Carton 1 of 1, WAN Records, UCSF Library, Archives and Special Collections, San Francisco.

62. See, for example, Vickie M. Mays and Susan D. Cochran, "Issues in the Perception of AIDS Risk and Risk Reduction Activities by Black and Hispanic/Latina Women," *American Psychologist* 43, no. 11 (Nov. 1988); Interview with Ruth Schwartz by Rebecca Issacs, "Women and AIDS," *The Exchange (Publication of the National Lawyers Guild AIDS Network)*, no. 7, Mar. 1988, p. 2, Folder "Minutes: April 1988," Carton 1 of 1, WAN Records, UCSF Library, Archives and Special Collections, San Francisco; Chris Norwood, "Alarming Rise in Deaths: Are Women Showing New 'AIDS' Symptoms?" *Ms.*, July 1988.

63. Letter to Ruth Schwartz from Patrick Mulcahey, May 18, 1988, Folder "Minutes: May 1988," Carton 1 of 1, WAN Records, UCSF Library, Archives and Special Collections, San Francisco.

64. "WAN Meeting Minutes, 5/3/88," Folder "May: 1988," Carton 1 of 1, WAN Records, UCSF Library, Archives and Special Collections, San Francisco.

65. "Women, Children and AIDS: A Statement to the 1988 4th International AIDS Conference," International Working Group on Women and AIDS, Folder

"Minutes: August, 1988," Carton 1 of 1, WAN Records, UCSF Library, Archives and Special Collections, San Francisco.

66. Nancy Stoller Shaw, "Preventing AIDS among Women: The Role of Community Organizing," *Socialist Review* 18, no. 4 (Fall 1988): 80.

67. Quoted in Cooper, *Family Values*, 190. As Cooper makes clear, "The early AIDS service organizations were well aware of the catch 22 in which they found themselves."

68. "WAN Minutes: Jan 3, 1989," Folder "Minutes: January, 1989," Carton 1 of 1; and "WAN Minutes, Mar. 7, 1989," Folder "Minutes: March, 1989," Carton 1 of 1, both in WAN Records, UCSF Library, Archives and Special Collections, San Francisco. Of course, volunteer and donation-based efforts were also increasingly strapped. The volunteer therapist program run by UCSF's AIDS Health Project was faced with a growing waiting list of clients who could not afford private therapy while Catholic Charities, which had extended over 300,000 dollars to cover medical-related needs for people with AIDS and ARC the two years prior, announced that it would need to close its Emergency Health Fund to new applicants. WAN also felt the squeeze as the San Francisco AIDS Foundation faced the budget crunch and pulled back on sharing its office resources (such as photocopying) with the organization. Letter from James W. Dilley, n.d., Folder "Minutes: April, 1989," Carton 1 of 1; Letter to "AIDS Service Provider" from Bob Nelson, Mar. 17, 1989, Folder "Minutes: May, 1989," Carton 1 of 1; "Minutes WAN Meeting June 6 1989," Folder "Minutes: June, 1989," Carton 1 of 1, all in WAN Records, UCSF Library, Archives and Special Collections, San Francisco.

69. "WAN Minutes, March 7, 1989," Folder "Minutes: March 1989," Carton 1 of 1, WAN Records, UCSF Library, Archives and Special Collections, San Francisco.

70. Letter to Honorable George Deukmejian from Rand Martin, Executive Director of LIFE AIDS Lobby, Mar. 9, 1989, Folder "Minutes: April, 1989," Carton 1 of 1, WAN Records, UCSF Library, Archives and Special Collections, San Francisco.

71. "WAN Minutes: January 3, 1989," Folder "Minutes: January, 1989," Carton 1 of 1, WAN Records, UCSF Library, Archives and Special Collections, San Francisco.

72. "Minutes of WAN Meeting July 2, 1991," Folder "Minutes: Jan–Dec, 1991," Carton 1 of 1, WAN Records, UCSF Library, Archives and Special Collections, San Francisco.

73. WAN Meeting Minutes, Feb. 5, 1990, Folder "Minutes: Jan–Dec, 1991," Carton 1 of 1, WAN Records, UCSF Library, Archives and Special Collections, San Francisco.

74. "Minutes of WAN Meeting March 5, 1990," Folder "Minutes: Jan–Dec, 1991," Carton 1 of 1, WAN Records, UCSF Library, Archives and Special Collections, San Francisco.

75. Author interview.

76. In 1990, the Women and AIDS Project (WAP) urged its members to support WARN with donations. "WARN remains, to our knowledge, the only women's specific AIDS service agency in New York State, perhaps in the country. That it must struggle continually for money is something that is not surprising to us, but is surely infuriating." "Women and AIDS Project," Spring 1990, p. 3, Linda Loffredo Personal Papers. WAP's main strategy for getting prominent New York City women's organizations and philanthropists to invest resources in the AIDS epidemic was by hosting invitation-only "leadership breakfasts" in which women well known in the fields of AIDS research and advocacy would speak on different issues pertaining to women and the epidemic. This tactic was quite successful. In 1990, *Vogue* magazine hosted the leadership breakfast with Diane Sawyer acting as master of ceremonies. This breakfast in particular would help to secure the necessary funding for Iris House's opening. Author interviews.

77. "Neighborhood Report: Harlem; A Center to Help Women with AIDS," *New York Times*, Sept. 19, 1993; Author interview.

78. WARN's philosophy of establishing trust in order to facilitate empowerment was applied at the smallest level of detail, such as sending nonresidential clients their information in envelopes without return addresses in the event the women had not shared their status with their families. Author interview.

79. Dázon Dixon Diallo, interview by Loretta Ross, Apr. 4, 2009, transcript of video recording, p. 27, Voices of Feminism Oral History Project, Sophia Smith Collection, Smith College; Nelson, *More Than Medicine*, 162.

80. Nelson, *More Than Medicine*, 160–63.

81. Dázon Dixon Diallo interview, 27.

82. Nelson, *More Than Medicine*, 163.

83. Lisa M. Koonin, Tedd V. Ellerbrock, and Hani K. Atrash, "Pregnancy Associated Deaths due to AIDS in the United States," *Journal of the American Medical Association* 261, no. 9 (1989): 1308.

84. AIDS activists had long criticized regulatory drug policies that made approval of new drugs a nearly decade-long process. But by the late 1980s, the movement had begun to successfully intervene in drug testing procedures, offering their own thoroughly researched suggestions of how the FDA and National Institute of Allergy and Infectious Diseases (NIAID) could expand access to experimental HIV and AIDS drugs, speed up approval, and make clinical testing more humane. For example, by 1989 NIAID director Anthony Fauci had expressed public support for activists' "parallel track" model for expanding access to AIDS drugs. For a thorough discussion of this and other changes that resulted from AIDS activism, see Mary M. Dunbar, "Shaking Up the Status Quo: How AIDS Activists Have Challenged Drug Development and Approval Procedures," *Food, Drug, Cosmetic Law Journal* 46, no. 5 (1991); and Steven Epstein, *Impure Science: AIDS, Activism, and the Politics of Knowledge* (Berkeley:

University of California Press, 1996), 208–94. For a discussion of how activists' greater involvement with AIDS officials caused tensions within the direct-action AIDS movement, particularly between members of ACT UP, see Gould, *Moving Politics*, 267–438; Epstein, *Impure Science*, 265–329.

85. For detailed overviews of this political process, see Carol Sachs Weisman, *Women's Health Care: Activist Traditions and Institutional Change* (Baltimore: Johns Hopkins University Press, 1998), 77–93; Steven Epstein, *Inclusion: The Politics of Difference in Medical Research* (Chicago: University of Chicago Press, 2007), 74, 83.

86. The Alcohol, Drug Abuse and Mental Health Administration (ADAMHA) also sponsored the policy, but this too had little impact. Furthermore, any sort of guideline for implementing the new policy was not published until three years after NIH's announcement that researchers needed to include women in clinical trials. See U.S. General Accounting Office (GAO), *National Institutes of Health: Problems in Implementing Women in Study Populations*, 1990, "Statement of Mark V. Nadel before the Subcommittee on Health and the Environment, Committee on Energy and Commerce, House of Representatives," GAO/T-HRD-90-50. For a more detailed account of how Representatives Snowe and Schroeder decided to go after the NIH's policies in order to leverage their broader goals for women's health such as passage of the Women's Health Equity Act, see Epstein, *Inclusion*, 76–78.

87. U.S. General Accounting Office (GAO), *National Institutes of Health: Problems in Implementing Women in Study Populations*, 1990, "Statement of Mark V. Nadel before the Subcommittee on Health and the Environment, Committee on Energy and Commerce, House of Representatives," GAO/T-HRD-90-50, p. 1.

88. Epstein, Steven, *Inclusion*, 78.

89. As Sally J. Kenney has argued, the thalidomide tragedy significantly shaped the way the United States thought about reproductive hazards. See Sally J. Kenney, *For Whose Protection? Reproductive Hazards and Exclusionary Policies in the United States and Britain* (Ann Arbor: University of Michigan Press, 1992), 16–17.

90. Pharmaceutical companies' more conservative approach to participants was targeted primarily at women. Tracey Johnson and Elizabeth Fee, "Women's Participation in Clinical Research: From Protectionism to Access," in *Women and Health Research: Ethical and Legal Issues of Including Women in Clinical Trials*, vol. 2, ed. Anna C. Mastroianni, Ruth Faden, and Daniel Federman (Washington, DC: National Academies Press, 1994), 1–10. For an analysis of the evolving contours of "the research subject" in U.S. history, see Epstein, *Inclusion*, 30–52.

91. Department of Health, Education, and Welfare, "Protection of Human Subjects: Fetuses, Pregnant Women, and In Vitro Fertilization," *Federal Register* 40, no. 154 (1975).

92. "Women of childbearing age" was defined as "a premenopausal female capable of becoming pregnant. This includes women on oral, injectable, or mechanical contraception; women who are single; women whose husbands have been vasectomized or whose husbands have received or are utilizing mechanical contraceptive devices." The animal reproduction studies did not happen until a drug had been found safe and somewhat effective in phase 1 and 2 trials, leaving women ineligible until these studies were completed and phase 3 trials were underway. Food and Drug Administration, "General Considerations for the Clinical Evaluations of Drugs," HEW Publication no. (FDA) 77-3040 (1977). For a discussion of how protective legislation has often meant discrimination and restriction, see Kenney, *For Whose Protection?*, ch. 1.

93. Mark V. Nadel, "Women's Health: FDA Needs to Ensure More Study of Gender Differences in Prescription Drug Testing" (Washington, DC: General Accounting Office, Oct. 1992).

94. Epstein, *Inclusion*, 63.

95. See, for example, Maxine Wolfe and Iris Long, "Through the Eye of a Needle: Women's Access to Drug Treatments through Clinical Trials," Women and AIDS, Section 3.C, Reel 54, Box 73, Folder 12; and Iris Long, "Women's AIDS Treatment Issues: 1991 Update," Reel 137, Box 166, Folder 9, both in ACT UP New York Records, New York Public Library, New York City.

96. This left Lucey with no other treatment options, as the negative side effects she experienced from AZT were the original reason her doctor suggested enrolling in the trial. See Theresa M. McGovern, Martha S. Jones, and Martha Davis, "Memorandum on the FDA's Proposed Guideline for the Study and Evaluation of Gender Differences in the Clinical Evaluation of Drugs," Oct. 18, 1993, pp. 1–2, Folder "National Organization for Women," Box "N," Barnard Archives and Special Collections, Barnard College (hereafter HLP Memorandum, 1993).

97. These organizations included NOW Legal Defense and Education Fund, AIDS Project of the ACLU, AIDS Service Center Lower Manhattan, ACT UP Women's FDA Working Group, AIDS Counseling and Education for Women in Transition from Correctional Facilities, New Jersey Women and AIDS Network, Housing Works, as well as Mary Lucey, who brought the original case to HIV Law Project (HLP). "Citizen Petition," Dec. 15, 1992, signed by AIDS Service Center, HIV Law Project, Records of the NOW Legal Defense and Education Fund, and ACLU AIDS Project, in HIV Law Project Private Papers, New York City (hereafter HLP Citizen Petition, 1992).

98. HLP Citizen Petition, 1992, p. 9.

99. See Hazel Sandomire, "Women in Clinical Trials: Are Sponsors Liable for Fetal Injury?" *Journal of Law, Medicine, and Ethics* 21, no. 2 (1993); L. Elizabeth Bowles, "The Disfranchisement of Fertile Women in Clinical Trials: The Legal Ramifications of and Solutions for Rectifying the Knowledge Gap," *Vanderbilt Law Review* 45, no. 4 (1992).

100. See Janice K. Bush, "The Industry Perspective on the Inclusion of Women in Clinical Trials," *Academic Medicine* 69, no. 9 (1994): 713.

101. Howard Minkoff, Jonathan D. Moreno, and Kathleen R. Powderly, "Fetal Protection and Women's Access to Clinical Trials," *Journal of Women's Health* 1, no. 2 (1992): 138.

102. See Ruth B. Merkatz and Suzanne White Junod, "Historical Background of Changes in FDA Policy on the Study and Evaluation of Drugs in Women," *Academic Medicine* 69, no. 9 (1994): 703.

103. Department of Health and Human Services, "Guideline for the Study and Evaluation of Gender Differences in the Clinical Evaluation of Drugs: Notice," *Federal Register* 58, no. 139 (1993): 39406.

104. Quoted in Ruth B. Merkatz and Suzanne White Junod, "Historical Background of Changes in FDA Policy on the Study and Evaluation of Drugs in Women," p. 706.

105. In addition to article cited in the text, see Ruth B. Merkatz et al., "Women in Clinical Trials of New Drugs—A Change in Food and Drug Administration Policy," *New England Journal of Medicine* 329 (1993); Ruth B. Merkatz, "FDA: Making a Difference in Women's Health," *Journal of the American Medical Women's Association* 49, no. 4 (1994); Linda Ann Sherman, Robert Temple, and Ruth B. Merkatz, "Women in Clinical Trials: An FDA Perspective," *Science* 269, no. 5225 (Aug. 1995): 793–95; Ruth B. Merkatz and Elyse I. Summers, "Including Women in Clinical Trials: Policy Changes at the Food and Drug Administration," in *Women's Health Research: A Medical and Policy Primer*, ed. Florence P. Haseltine and Beverly Greenberg Jacobson (Washington, DC: Health Press International, 1997).

106. Merkatz et al., "Women in Clinical Trials of New Drugs," 295.

107. For scholarship that attributes the victory to AIDS activists, see Theresa M. McGovern, Martha Davis, and Mary Beth Caschetta, "FDA Policy on Women in Drug Trials," *New England Journal of Medicine* 329, no. 4 (1993): 1815; Oonagh P. Corrigan, "'First in Man': The Politics and Ethics of Women in Clinical Drug Trials," *Feminist Review* 72, no. 1 (2002): 40–52; Epstein, *Inclusion*, 55. For scholarship that acknowledges the negative impact the policy had on both women with AIDS and AIDS research during this period, see Leslie Laurence and Beth Weinhouse, *Outrageous Practices: The Alarming Truth about How Medicine Mistreats Women* (New York: Fawcett Columbine, 1994), 149–52; Treichler, *How to Have Theory in an Epidemic*, 247–51; Epstein, *Impure Science*, 260–61.

108. In contrast, the women's health lobby that celebrated the reversal were not as concerned with getting women into early phases of trials as they were with including women in large enough numbers so that results could eventually be analyzed for gender-based differences. The distinction between phases of trials was of little concern to this group. The 1992 GAO report evaluating the FDA's practices explicitly tabled whether or not the 1977 guideline was applied to

phase 1 and 2 trials—advocates for women's health were largely concerned with including women in representative numbers before trials were completed. U.S. General Accounting Office (GAO), "Women's Health: FDA Needs to Ensure More Study of Gender Differences in Prescription Drug Testing," 1992, Report to congressional requesters, GAO/HRD-93-17, p. 2. This distinction is also evidenced in women's health advocates' subsequent engagement with FDA officials. Following the reversal, these advocates continued pressing the FDA to apply stricter requirements for analyzing study results for gender-based differences. Accounting for the gendered effects of treatment rather than gaining women access to the early phases of trials remained the goal of the women's health lobby into the early 2000s. See Epstein, *Inclusion*, 167–68.

109. HLP Citizen Petition, 1992, pp. 23, 75.

110. Sherman, Temple, and Merkatz, "Women in Clinical Trials," 794.

111. See Iris Long, "What Happened at the Aug 9th 1993 Meeting with the FDA? Summary," 1993, Folder 9, Reel 137, Box 166, ACT UP New York Papers, New York Public Library.

112. HLP Memorandum, 1993, p. 4. This fear was valid, especially when it came to individual institutional review boards approving or not approving women's entry. See Epstein, *Inclusion*, 65.

113. Letter to HLP from the Department of Health and Human Services, Oct. 27, 1994, p. 12, HIV Law Project Private Papers, New York City.

114. Iris Long and Juan "Alex" Leger, "Women's Access to Government Sponsored AIDS/HIV Clinical Trials: Status Report, Critique and Recommendations," Sept. 14, 1994, pp. 1–2, 6, 14, Folder 9, Reel 137, Box 166, ACT UP NY Papers, New York Public Library.

115. Machelle Allen, "The Dilemma for Women of Color in Clinical Trials," *Journal of the American Medical Women's Association* 49, no. 4 (1994); Vanessa Northington Gamble and Bonnie Ellen Blustein, "Racial Differentials in Medical Care: Implications for Research on Women," in *Women and Health Research: Ethical and Legal Issues of Including Women in Clinical Studies*, vol. 2 (Washington, DC: National Academies Press, 1994).

116. HLP Citizen Petition, 1992, p. 12.

117. W. El-Sadr and L. Capps, "The Challenge of Minority Recruitment in Clinical Trials for AIDS," *Journal of American Medical Association* 267, no. 7 (1992).

118. Diane B. Stoy, "Recruitment and Retention of Women in Clinical Studies: Theoretical Perspectives and Methodological Considerations" and Janet L. Mitchell, "Recruitment and Retention of Women of Color in Clinical Studies," both in *Women and Health Research: Ethical and Legal Issues of Including Women in Clinical Studies,* vol. 2 (Washington, DC: National Academies Press, 1994). There is evidence that at least some FDA representatives were interested in how to make AIDS trial sites more accommodating to women, such as at Bel-

levue Hospital in New York City, which offered child care and whole family treatment when a woman came in for her own primary care. This setup seems to have been one of few, however. See David Fiegel's comments in Iris Long, "What Happened at the Aug 9th 1993 Meeting with the FDA? Summary," Aug. 22, 1993, Reel 137, Box 166, Folder 9, ACT UP New York Papers, New York Public Library.

119. Letter to Commissioner Kessler from Theresa M. McGovern, Dec. 6, 1995, pp. 11, 13, HIV Law Project Private Papers, New York City. McGovern was assigned to the National Task Force on AIDS Drugs Development by the Clinton administration, where she continued to push for further reforms to the FDA guidelines.

120. Department of Health and Human Services, "Investigational New Drug Applications: Proposed Amendments to Clinical Hold Regulations for Products Intended for Life-Threatening Diseases," *Federal Register* 62, no. 185 (1997): 49946–54; Department of Health and Human Services, "Clinical Hold for Products Intended for Life-Threatening Conditions," *Federal Register* 65, no. 106 (2000): 34963–71.

121. Theresa McGovern first introduced the clinical hold rule in the report she wrote while serving on the Presidential Advisory Council on HIV/AIDS. According to the *Federal Register*, the clinical hold rule was by and large a response to these recommendations. Theresa McGovern, "Proposal to Eliminate Obstacles Facing Women in the Drug Development Process: A Recommendation to the National Task Force on AIDS Drug Development," June 30, 1994, p. 31, HIV Law Project Private Papers, New York City; *Federal Register* 65, no. 106 (2000): 34970.

122. Letter to HLP from Department of Health and Human Services, Oct. 27, 1994, p. 6, HIV Law Project Private Papers, New York City.

123. In November of 2000, HLP held a community forum titled "HIV, Women, and Clinical Trials" to publicize passage of the clinical hold rule in order to "help HIV positive women and their advocates learn more about a new rule that can potentially increase the number of women who access clinical drug trials." Letter to Roma Baran from Andrea B. Williams of the HIV Law Project, Oct. 26, 2000, HIV Law Project Private Papers, New York City.

124. *Federal Register* 65, no. 106 (2000): 34966–67.

125. *Federal Register* 62, no. 185 (1997): 49953.

126. Ibid.

127. Judith Walker, "Mothers and Children," in *Women, AIDS, and Activism*, ed. ACT UP/NY Women and AIDS Book Group (Boston: South End Press, 1990), 165.

128. John Henkel, "Attacking AIDS with a 'Cocktail' Therapy: Drug Combo Sends Deaths Plummeting," *Food and Drug Administration Consumer*, July 1, 1999; Suzanne K. Whitmore, "Epidemiology of HIV/AIDS among Non-Hispanic Black Women in the United States," *Journal of the National Medical Association* 97, no. 7 (July 2005).

129. Kathryn Whetten and Susan Reif, "Overview: HIV/AIDS in the Deep South Region of the United States," *AIDS Care* 18 (2006).

130. Paula M. Frew et al., "Socioecological Factors Influencing Women's HIV Risk in the United States: Qualitative Findings from the Women's HIV Seroincidence Study (HPTN 064)," *BMC Public Health* 16, no. 803 (2016): 14.

131. Ellen Pinnow et al., "Increasing Participation of Women in Early Phase Clinical Trials Approved by the FDA," *Women's Health Issues* 19 (2009); Yang et al., "Participation of Women in Clinical Trials for New Drugs Approved by the Food and Drug Administration in 2000–2002," *Journal of Women's Health* 2009 18, no. 3 (2013).

132. Rita Poon et al., "Participation of Women and Sex Analyses in Late-Phase Clinical Trials of New Molecular Entity Drugs and Biologics Approved by the FDA in 2007–2009," *Journal of Women's Health* 22, no. 7 (2013).

133. Marcy C. Blehar, Catherine Song, and Janine A. Clayton, "Enrolling Pregnant Women: Issues in Clinical Research," *Women's Health Issues* 23, no. 1 (2013); Kristine Shields and Anne Drapkin Lyerly, "Exclusion of Pregnant Women from Industry-Sponsored Clinical Trials," *Obstetrics and Gynecology* 122, no. 5 (2013).

134. Self, *All in the Family*, 394. For a discussion on "invisible" AIDS deaths, see Cooper, *Family Values*, 205.

135. Centers for Disease Control, *Fact Sheet: HIV among Women*, Mar. 2014.

CHAPTER 5. THE LABOR OF "CHOICE"

Epigraph: Elizabeth Gleick, "Where Can Pregnant Teens Turn?" *Time*, Feb. 20, 1995, Folder "24:13 CAC," Box 024, Institute for First Amendment Studies Records, Tisch Library, Tufts University, Medford, MA.

1. Lisa McIntire, *Crisis Pregnancy Centers Lie: The Insidious Threat to Reproductive Freedom* (Washington, DC: NARAL Pro-Choice America, 2015), 1.

2. Eleanor Zehala, "Lifeline Volunteer Poses as Client at Pittsburgh Abortion Clinic," *Heartbeat Magazine* 1, no. 1 (1978), bMS 404/9, George Huntston Williams Papers, Harvard Divinity School Repository, Harvard University, Cambridge, MA.

3. For work that specifically addresses the potential costs and rewards of publicly acknowledging such complex realities, see Lisa H. Harris, "Second Trimester Abortion Provision: Breaking the Silence and Changing the Discourse," *Reproductive Health Matters* 16, no. 31 (2008); Jeannie Ludlow, "The Things We Cannot Say: Witnessing the Trauma-tization of Abortion in the United States," *Women's Studies Quarterly* 36, no. 1/2 (2008). For recent histories that have also contributed to a more diverse range of abortion narratives immediately

following *Roe*, see Johanna Schoen, *Abortion after Roe* (Chapel Hill: University of North Carolina Press, 2017); Nelson, *More Than Medicine*.

4. The public seems most familiar with the term "crisis pregnancy centers" (CPCs), but current movement participants prefer "pregnancy resource centers" (PRCs) or "pregnancy care centers." The movement originally referred to itself as "emergency pregnancy services" (EPS). For the most part, I use EPS when discussing the movement in its historical context, and otherwise rely on the commonly used term CPCs.

5. By the end of the 1970s, less than one-third of young mothers who became pregnant out of wedlock had married by the time their infants were born. See Thistle, *From Marriage to the Market*, 50.

6. Ibid.

7. For a brief discussion of crisis pregnancy center practices and the opposition they engendered, including lawsuits brought by clients in the 1980s and early 1990s, see Kimberly Kelly, "In the Name of the Mother: Renegotiating Conservative Women's Authority in the Crisis Pregnancy Center Movement," *Signs* 38, no. 1 (2012): 211; Karissa Haugeberg, *Women against Abortion: Inside the Largest Moral Reform Movement of the Twentieth Century* (Champaign: University of Illinois Press, 2017), 23.

8. See Faye Ginsburg, *Contested Lives: The Abortion Debate in an American Community* (Berkeley: University of California Press, 1998) 119–21; Dallas A. Blanchard, *The Anti-Abortion Movement and the Rise of the Religious Right: From Polite to Fiery Protest* (New York: Twayne, 1994), ch. 7; Suzanne Staggenborg, *The Pro-Choice Movement: Organization and Activism in the Abortion Conflict* (New York: Oxford University Press, 1991), 129–30.

9. See, for example, Dawn Stacey, "The Pregnancy Center Movement: History of Crisis Pregnancy Centers," Crisis Pregnancy Center Watch, n.d., available at https://motherjones.com/wp-content/uploads/cpchistory2.pdf; Meagan McElroy, "Protecting Pregnant Pennsylvanians: Public Funding of Crisis Pregnancy Centers," *University of Pittsburgh Law Review* 76 (2015); Brittany A. Campbell, "The Crisis Inside Crisis Pregnancy Centers: How to Stop These Facilities from Depriving Women of Their Reproductive Freedom," *Boston College Journal of Law and Social Justice* 37, no. 1 (2017). Rob Pearson, who founded Pearson Foundation in 1970 to oversee the development of other CPCs, believed that "abortion-seeking women" needed to be "educated in what abortion really is," the murder of an innocent life. "The Pearson Foundation: Saving Babies and Their Mothers," n.d., MC 496, Carton 78, Folder "CPCs 'Fake Clinics,' 1985," NOW Records, 1959–2002 (Inclusive), Schlesinger Library, Radcliffe Institute, Harvard University, Cambridge, MA.

10. An important corrective has recently been written by Karissa Haugeberg. See Haugeberg, *Women against Abortion*, ch. 1.

11. For example, see Campbell, "The Crisis Inside Crisis Pregnancy Centers," 15.

12. Kimberly Kelly puts the number much lower, around 4 percent. For both the official 20 percent espoused by movement leaders and Kelly's adjusted percentage, see Kimberly Kelly, "Evangelical Underdogs: Intrinsic Success, Organizational Solidarity, and Marginalized Identities as Religious Movement Resources," *Journal of Contemporary Ethnography* 43, no. 4 (2014): 423.

13. As with most standard talking points on the abortion debate, abortion care immediately following *Roe* was more complicated than EPS volunteers' assessment. As Johanna Schoen has shown, "What kind of abortion services women were to receive and how they experienced legal abortion depended not only on the kind of abortion provider a woman visited but also on the philosophical orientation and organizational structures which shaped abortion services inside the clinic walls." Schoen explores the differences between medical and feminist models of abortion care, and shows that individual patients sought out each model for different reasons—not all women cared to politicize their reproductive healthcare, they just wanted quality care. However, she reminds us that the feminist critique of medicine honed by women's health activists remained necessary after abortion care became more accessible. "In more traditional clinic settings, it was most frequently physicians and insensitive staff that drew patient criticism." It is possible to find actual evidence of the uncaring abortion provider that anti-abortion narratives depict as representative of *all* abortion providers. The fact that legalization "did not guarantee that patients received respectful treatment" was partially what drove women's health activists to demand control over the procedure in the first place. See Schoen, *Abortion after Roe*, 45–55.

14. Sara Dubow argues that beginning in the 1980s, pro-life organizations developed a "new rhetorical strategy that emphasized the ways that abortion hurt women and fetuses." Dubow traces how the claim that abortion is psychologically damaging to women worked its way into medical literature and legal decisions. For volunteers providing emergency pregnancy services in the early 1970s, however, abortion did not represent a psychological threat but an abandonment of pregnant women on the part of the state, a law that "helped" women by providing them with only one avenue for addressing an unplanned pregnancy. EPS volunteers set out to provide women with the "meaningful alternatives" the state would not. See Dubow, *Ourselves Unborn*, 153.

15. For discussion of the distinct ways white and Black nonmarital pregnancy and single motherhood was theorized and addressed in the decades preceding *Roe*, see Solinger, *Wake Up Little Susie*.

16. Sue Kincaid, *The Cleveland Press*, Dec. 14, 1970.

17. For a discussion of how pro-life activist Marjory Mecklenburg helped popularize this view in her Minnesota-based organization American Citizens Con-

cerned for Life, which also directed pro-life women to EPS work following *Roe,* see Haugeberg, *Women against Abortion,* ch. 1.

18. Such abortion referral services predated changes at the state level, of course, and underground networks were vital for women seeking quality, though typically illicit, abortion care. The Jane Collective is perhaps the most well-known abortion collective that helped women access the procedure in Chicago, with some members even learning how to perform abortions themselves. The Consultation Clergy Services (CCS) was another prominent referral service that assisted women across the United States and Canada. See Laura Kaplan, *The Story of Jane: The Legendary Underground Feminist Abortion Service* (Chicago: University of Chicago Press, 1995).

19. Nelson, *More Than Medicine,* 58.

20. Pregnancy Counseling Service report, Mar. 1971, bMS 404/2, George Huntston Williams Papers, Harvard Divinity School Repository, Harvard University.

21. "Proposal to Establish a Medical Facility at the Crittenton Hastings House in Conjunction with the Pregnancy Counseling Service, Inc.," Mar. 1971, bMS 404/2, and "Volcom Speaks . . ." newsletter, Oct. 1972, bMS 404/2, both in George Huntston Williams Papers, Harvard Divinity School Repository, Harvard University.

22. "Statement before the Massachusetts Conference of Bishops," Sept. 25, 1971, bMS 404/2, George Huntston Williams Papers, Harvard Divinity School Repository, Harvard University.

23. For example, in the Value of Life Committee's statement to the Massachusetts Conference of Bishops, they cited the Pregnancy Counseling Services' number of clients as evidence of the fact that despite their attempts with the Pregnancy Guidance hotline, they were not reaching "the majority of these pregnant and troubled girls." "Statement before the Massachusetts Conference of Bishops," Sept. 25, 1971, bMS 404/1, George Huntston Williams Papers, Harvard Divinity School Repository, Harvard University.

24. Minnesota Citizens Concerned For Life, Inc. newsletter, Jan. 1972, bMS 404/3, George Huntston Williams Papers, Harvard Divinity School Repository, Harvard University.

25. Undated Right to Life training materials, International Life Services Papers, Los Angeles.

26. Author interview.

27. *Heartbeat Magazine* 5, no. 1 (Spring 1982): 5, bMS 479/1, George Huntston Williams Papers, Harvard Divinity School Repository, Harvard University.

28. Undated Right to Life training materials, International Life Services Papers, Los Angeles.

29. For example, the Right to Life League helped women in Fond du Lac, WI, start a similar service, "Pregnancy Health Line, Inc.," in 1978. See "LifeLine

Training Program," "Pregnancy Health Line, Inc. 1978–1979 Annual Report, November 15, 1979," International Life Services Papers, Los Angeles.

30. Peggy Hartshorn, *Foot Soldiers Armed with Love: Heartbeat International's First Forty Years* (Virginia Beach, VA: The Donning Company Publishers, 2011), 17–34.

31. Letter to Bishop from Maier, Folder Bishop Correspondence, Heartbeat International Papers, Columbus, OH.

32. *Heartbeat Bulletin* 5, no. 1 (July 1973), bMS 404/8, and *Heartbeat Bulletin* 7, no. 6 (Dec. 1974), bMS 404/9, both in George Huntston Williams Papers, Harvard Divinity School Repository, Harvard University.

33. *Heartbeat Bulletin* 5, no. 4 (Oct. 1973), bMS 404/8, George Huntston Williams Papers, Harvard Divinity School Repository, Harvard University (emphasis in original).

34. *Heartbeat Bulletin* 7, no. 5 (1974), bMS 404/9, George Huntston Williams Papers, Harvard Divinity School Repository, Harvard University.

35. AAI went from having 181 affiliates in 1972 to 467 affiliates in 1973. AAI's Worldwide Directory of Emergency Pregnancy Services, Aug. 1972 and Dec. 1973 editions, George Huntston Williams Papers, Harvard Divinity School Repository, Harvard University.

36. Letter to Senator Birch Bayh from Lore Maier, Dec. 4, 1975, Heartbeat International Papers, Columbus, OH.

37. *Heartbeat Bulletin* 8, no. 1 (Jan. 1975), bMS 404/9, George Huntston Williams Papers, Harvard Divinity School, Harvard University.

38. Ibid.

39. "Counseling Tips," AAI Education Committee-Sister Paula Vandegaer, June 1972, bMS 404/8, George Huntston Williams Papers, Harvard Divinity School Repository, Harvard University.

40. Paula Vandegaer, "Reflections on Professional and Para-professional Pro-Life Services," *Heartbeat Magazine* 4, no. 2 (1981), bMS 438/3, George Huntston Williams Papers, Harvard Divinity School Repository, Harvard University (emphasis mine).

41. Letter to David Matthews, Secretary for the Department of Health, Education and Welfare, from Lore Maier, Dec. 4, 1975, Heartbeat International Papers, Columbus, OH.

42. Letter to AAI from Ritaellen B., Sept. 16, 1979, Letter to Friends of Life from Sister Paula, Folder "EPS Correspondence," International Life Services Papers, Los Angeles, CA.

43. *Heartbeat Bulletin* 5, no. 5 (Nov. 1973), bMS 404/8, George Huntston Williams Papers, Harvard Divinity School Repository, Harvard University.

44. *Heartbeat Bulletin* 7, no. 6 (Dec. 1974), bMS 404/9, George Huntston Williams Papers, Harvard Divinity School Repository, Harvard University.

45. *Heartbeat Bulletin* 2, no. 1 (Jan. 1972), bMS 404/9, George Huntston Williams Papers, Harvard Divinity School Repository, Harvard University.

46. "Increasing Your Client Outreach through a Good Public Relations Strategy," *Heartbeat Magazine*, bMS 479/2, George Huntston Williams Papers, Harvard Divinity School Repository, Harvard University.

47. Ibid.

48. *Heartbeat Magazine* 7, no. 4 (Winter 1984): 7, bMS 438/3, George Huntston Williams Papers, Harvard Divinity School Repository, Harvard University.

49. For a discussion of how federal budget cuts imperiled community health clinics, especially women's health clinics, see Sandra Morgen, *Into Our Own Hands: The Women's Health Movement in the United States, 1969–1990* (New Brunswick, NJ: Rutgers University Press, 2002), ch. 8.

50. Author interview.

51. "News from Affiliates," *Heartbeat Quarterly Newsletter*, Fall 1995, p. 3, Heartbeat International Papers, Columbus, OH.

52. Judy Thorton for MCC, "A report on client advocacy July 1984–Nov 1984," p. 2, Folder "MCC Program Advocacy in the Community, Report of the Community Organization Project: 7/7/1982–4/10/1985, N.D.," Maternity Care Coalition Records, Kislak Center for Special Collections, University of Pennsylvania.

53. Author interview.

54. "News from Affiliates," *Heartbeat Newsletter*, Spring 1995, p. 4, Heartbeat International Papers, Columbus, OH.

55. "Meet an Affiliate," *Heartbeat Newsletter*, Summer 1995, p. 4, Heartbeat International Papers, Columbus, OH.

56. Author interview.

57. "Meet an Affiliate," *Heartbeat Newsletter*, Summer 1994, p. 3, Heartbeat International Papers, Columbus, OH.

58. *Heartbeat Newsletter*, Winter 1996, p. 3, and *Heartbeat Newsletter*, Spring 1995, pp. 4–5, both in Heartbeat International Papers, Columbus, OH.

59. Leaders describe this shift as the second wave of the EPS movement. See Hartshorn, *Foot Soldiers Armed with Love*, 58–59.

60. Focus on the Family and Jerry Falwell also began funding CPCs in the 1980s. Gary Bergel, "A Release of Virtue: Alternatives to Abortion," n.d., MC 496, Box 74, Folder "Fake Clinics, 1984," NOW Records, 1959–2000 (Inclusive), Schlesinger Library, Radcliffe Institute, Harvard University; "Abortion, It's a Lonely Word," Christian Action Council Newsletter, Dec. 1, 1984, bMS 438/3, George Huntston Williams Papers, Harvard Divinity School Repository, Harvard University.

61. While the following description captures a more recent version of the relationship between Care Net and Heartbeat, it is still helpful in illuminating the shift that was set in motion with the influx of evangelical leadership: "Thus,

while Heartbeat is officially interdenominational and Care Net is stricter about enforcing evangelical goals, these differences represent more a question of degree than kind." See Kelly, "In the Name of the Mother," 206–7.

62. Through debate with the heads of major affiliate organizations, and at the urging of Care Net's general counsel Kurt Entsminger, movement leaders eventually agreed to draft a Commitment of Care document meant to guide all volunteers on their interactions with clients. While an original draft stated that clients would be treated in a "non-judgmental caring manner," the national director of Christian Life Resources reminded the coalition that "faith-based judgment is always to be void of *self-righteous* judgment," but "it is not non-judgmental.'" Such "faith-based judgment involves witnessing with God's Word which is oftentimes very judgmental." As a result, the number two principle was changed to promise that center staff and volunteers would treat clients "with kindness, compassion, and in a caring manner." Letter to International Life Services from Care Net's General Counsel Kurt Entsminger, Feb. 12, 2001; Letter to Kurt Entsminger from Pastor Robert Fleishmann, National Director of Christian Life Resources, May 16, 2000; Letter to Sister Paula from Kurt Entsminger, Dec. 13, 1999, all in International Life Services Papers, Los Angeles.

63. "Focus on an Affiliate," Heartbeat International, Quarterly Newsletter, Fall 1995, p. 4, Heartbeat International Papers, Columbus, OH.

64. Care Net president Curt Young explained that his decision to assess the impact of EPS centers was motivated by increasing numbers of anecdotal reports that centers were seeing "services only" clients far more than clients "at risk" for abortion. "Assessing Center Impact—Increasing Center Effectiveness," Marketing Research Analysis presented to the Crisis Pregnancy Center Movement at Focus on the Family, Feb. 5, 1998, Folder "Center-Marketing," International Life Services Papers, Los Angeles.

65. Solinger, *Beggars and Choosers*, 209. On welfare myths, see Roberts, *Killing the Black Body*, 217–25.

66. For a discussion of the development of family cap legislation, see Roberts, *Killing the Black Body*, 205–13.

67. Frederica Mathewes-Green, "Pro-Life Dilemma: Pregnancy Centers and the Welfare Trap," *Policy Review* 78 (Jul.–Aug. 1996): 40–41. Mathewes-Green has been an outspoken critic of this aspect of crisis pregnancy centers. See also Frederica Mathewes-Green, "Seeking Abortion's Middle Ground," *Washington Post*, July 28, 1996; Frederica Mathewes-Green, "Unplanned Parenthood: Easing the Pain of Crisis Pregnancy," *Policy Review* 57 (Summer 1991).

68. Elizabeth Gleick, "Where Can Pregnant Teens Turn?" *Time*, Feb. 20, 1995, Folder "24:13 CAC," Box 024, Institute for First Amendment Studies Records, Tisch Library, Tufts University, Medford, MA.

69. Curt Young, "Assessing Center Impact—Increasing Center Effectiveness," Marketing Research Analysis presented to the Crisis Pregnancy Center Move-

ment at Focus on the Family, Feb. 5, 1998, Folder "Center-Marketing," International Life Services Papers, Los Angeles.

70. Ibid.

71. Hartshorn, *Foot Soldiers Armed with Love*, 66–70.

72. Pulse Newsletter, First Quarter, 2001, p. 1, Heartbeat International Papers, Columbus, OH.

73. "Claim That Most Abortion Clinics Are Located in Black or Hispanic Neighborhoods Is False," *Guttmacher Advisory*, 2014, available at https://www.guttmacher.org/claim-most-abortion-clinics-are-located-black-or-hispanic-neighborhoods-false.

74. Author interview; "Abortion Hub Research," Aug. 10, 2004, Heartbeat International Papers, Columbus, OH; Hartshorn, *Foot Soldiers Armed with Love*, 71. For a sociological discussion that takes a contemporary snapshot of these campaigns and situates them within larger racial reconciliation efforts by white evangelicals, see Kimberly Kelly and Amanda Gochanour, "Racial Reconciliation or Spiritual Smokescreens? Blackwashing the Crisis Pregnancy Center Movement," *Qualitative Sociology* 41 (2018).

75. Hartshorn, *Foot Soldiers Armed with Love*, 72.

76. "Heartbeat of Miami," www.heartbeatofmiami.org/about/#2.

77. Hartshorn, *Foot Soldiers Armed with Love*, 72.

78. Care Net Report, May–June 2007, available at https://cdn2.hubspot.net/hub/367552/file-2208992161-pdf/Newsletter_Archive/cnrMayJun07.pdf; Care Net Report, Sept.–Oct. 2007 (no longer accessible online, PDF on file with author); Kimberly Kelly and Amanda Gochanour, "Racial Reconciliation or Spiritual Smokescreens?" 434. While it is clear that this initiative marks the first time Heartbeat and Care Net, predominantly white organizations, invoked an explicitly racialized narrative in their work, there is evidence that it was not the first time EPS centers were started by advocates of color. See, for example, Greg Keath, "Abortion Is Not a Civil Right," *Wall Street Journal*, Sept. 27, 1989.

79. Quoted in Haugeberg, *Women against Abortion*, 14–15.

80. Loretta J. Ross, "Trust Black Women: Reproductive Justice and Eugenics," in *Radical Reproductive Justice: Foundations, Theory, Practice, Critique*, ed. Loretta J. Ross et al. (New York: Feminist Press, 2017). For a thorough discussion of historical debates among African Americans over the uses of birth control, see Roberts, *Killing the Black Body*, 98–103.

81. For an analysis that weaves together these historical claims with more contemporary versions of this argument while keeping Black women's reproductive autonomy in view, see Ross, "Trust Black Women Reproductive Justice and Eugenics."

82. NARAL, "The Truth about Crisis Pregnancy Centers," Jan. 1, 2014.

83. According to the movement's own estimates based on participating centers, women who visited a clinic in 2015 considering abortion made up less than

10 percent of clients. Available at https://www.ekyros.com/Pub/Default.aspx? tabindex=3&tabid=16 (data also on file with author).

84. Laura A. Hussey, "Crisis Pregnancy Centers, Poverty, and the Expanding Frontiers of American Abortion Politics," *Politics and Policy* 41, no. 6 (2013): 999.

85. "A Report on Client Advocacy, July 1984–November 1984," Folder 568, MCC Program Advocacy in the Community, Report of the Community Organization Project 7/71982–4/10/1985 ND, Box 45, Maternity Care Coalition Records, University of Pennsylvania.

86. CPCs and other pro-life services such as maternity homes, Catholic Social Services, and Catholic Charities in Pennsylvania grew from 92 operations in 1983 to 150 operations in 1989. AAI Worldwide Directories, 1983, 1989, Heartbeat International Papers, Columbus, OH.

87. Hussey, "Crisis Pregnancy Centers, Poverty, and the Expanding Frontiers of American Abortion Politics," 1001.

88. My conversation with an employee at Maternity Care Coalition (an organization that identifies as pro-choice and provides both abortion and contraception counseling and referrals) about the relationship between MCC and crisis pregnancy centers and other pro-life social services confirmed for Philadelphia and the surrounding counties of Delaware and Montgomery what other researchers have found. Centers do not shy away from partnerships with other organizations or from helping women obtain publicly available aid and support.

89. Kelly, "In the Name of the Mother," 214.

90. Vitoria Lin and Cynthia Dailard, "Crisis Pregnancy Centers Seek to Increase Political Clout, Secure Government Subsidy," *Guttmacher Report on Public Policy* 5, no. 2 (2002): 5.

91. Kimberly Kelly, "In the Name of the Mother," 218.

92. For a representative example, see Sheila Bapat, "Ohio Diverts TANF Dollars to CPCs, Revealing Connection between Reproductive, Economic Justice," *Rewire*, July 22, 2013.

93. Kimberly Kelly's ethnographic work in CPCs has shown that "CPC counselors . . . eschew a dogmatic focus on traditional solutions and consider each client's situation individually." Kelly, "In the Name of the Mother," 218-19.

94. CPCs fall under what Melinda Cooper and others call "faith-based welfare," which grew considerably following Clinton's welfare reform bill due to the opening of social service contracts to faith-based organizations. See Cooper, *Family Values*, 266–310; quotes from pp. 309 and 301, respectively.

95. Melinda Delahoyde and Kristen Hansen, "Pregnancy Centers: A Practical Response to the Abortion Dilemma," *Religion and Society Report* 23, no. 3 (2006).

96. Ross, "Trust Black Women: Reproductive Justice and Eugenics."

97. Pam Belluck (quoting Jeanneane Maxon), "Pregnancy Centers Gain Influence in Anti-Abortion Arena," *New York Times*, Jan. 4, 2013.

98. Katrina Kimport, "Pregnant Women's Reasons for and Experiences of Visiting Antiabortion Pregnancy Resource Centers," *Perspectives on Sexual and Reproductive Health* 52, no. 1 (2020): 54.

EPILOGUE

1. Diana Greene Foster, *Ten Years, a Thousand Women, and the Consequences of Having—or Being Denied—an Abortion* (New York: Simon and Schuster, 2020).

2. *The Harms of Denying a Woman a Wanted Abortion: Findings from the Turnaway Study,* fact sheet (Oakland: Advancing New Standards in Reproductive Health), available at https://www.ansirh.org/sites/default/files/publications/files/the_harms_of_denying_a_woman_a_wanted_abortion_4-16-2020.pdf.

3. Michael Madowitz and Diana Boesch, *The Shambolic Response to the Public Health and Economic Crisis Has Women on the Brink as the Job Recovery Stalls* (Washington, DC: Center for American Progress, Oct. 2020); Amanda Barroso and Rakesh Kochhar, *In the Pandemic, the Share of Unpartnered Moms at Work Fell More Sharply Than among Other Parents* (Washington, DC: Pew Research Center, Nov. 2020); Jocelyn Frye, *On the Frontlines at Work and at Home: The Disproportionate Economic Effects of the Coronavirus Pandemic on Women of Color* (Washington, DC: Center for American Progress, April 2020).

4. Ai-jen Poo, *The Age of Dignity: Preparing for the Elder Boom in a Changing America* (New York: The New Press, 2016).

5. Mignon Duffy and Kim Price-Glynn, "A 'Care' Agenda Is Essential Policy," NPR, Apr. 8, 2021.

6. "Fact Sheet: The American Families Plan" (Washington, DC: White House, Apr. 2021), available at https://www.whitehouse.gov/briefing-room/statements-releases/2021/04/28/fact-sheet-the-american-families-plan/.

7. Rakeen Mabud and Lenore Palladino, "The Nation's Moment of Truth: The Economic and Moral Case for Investing in Caregivers," *Ms.*, Apr. 30, 2021.

8. Emily Peck, "Policymakers Used to Ignore Child Care. Then Came the Pandemic," *New York Times*, May 9, 2021.

9. Aja Beckham, "D.C. Mothers Facing Housing Insecurity Worry about What Happens When the Eviction Moratorium Ends," *DCist*, Apr. 29, 2021.

Selected Bibliography

MANUSCRIPT COLLECTIONS

Andover-Harvard Theological Library, Harvard Divinity School Repository, Cambridge, MA

George Huntston Williams Papers

Bancroft Library, University of California, Berkeley, Berkeley, CA

Cathy Cade Photograph Archive

Barnard Archives and Special Collections, Barnard College, New York, NY

Women and AIDS Resource Network (WARN)
National Organization for Women (NOW)

Sallie Bingham Center, David M. Rubenstein Rare Book and Manuscript Library, Duke University, Durham, NC

Atlanta Lesbian Feminist Alliance Archives Collection
Atlanta Lesbian Feminist Alliance Periodicals Collection
Feminist Women's Health Center Records
Lesbian Health Resource Center Records

Women's and Lesbian, Gay, Bisexual, and Transgender Movements (LGBT)
 Periodicals Collection

California State Archives, Sacramento, CA

Institutions—California Institution for Women, Tehachapi (CIW), Department
 of Correctional Records

*Gay, Lesbian, Bisexual, and Transgender Historical Society, San
Francisco, CA*

Cheri Pies Papers
Donna Hitchens Papers
Phyllis Lyon and Del Martin Papers

*Donald and Beverly Gerth Special Collections and University
Archives, California State University, Sacramento, CA*

Friends Committee on Legislation of California Records

*James C. Hormel LGBTQIA Center, San Francisco Public Library,
San Francisco, CA*

Patti Roberts Papers

*Kislak Center for Special Collections, University of Pennsylvania,
Philadelphia, PA*

Maternity Care Coalition Records

Mudd Library, Princeton University, Princeton, NJ

ACLU Prison Project Papers

*New York Public Library, Manuscripts and Archives Division,
New York City, NY*

ACT UP New York Records

*Schlesinger Library, Radcliffe Institute, Harvard
University, Cambridge, MA*

National Organization for Women (NOW) Records
National Organization for Women (NOW) Additional Records
Records of the NOW Legal Defense and Education Fund

Records of Sojourner Truth

Sophia Smith Collection, Smith College, Northampton, MA

Alliance Against Women's Oppression Records
Crimes, Prisons, and Reform Schools Collection
Gena Corea Papers
Third World Women's Alliance, Bay Area Chapter Records
Voices of Feminism Oral History Project

Snell Library, Northeastern University, Boston, MA

Fenway Community Health Center Historical Records

Tamiment Library, New York University, New York, NY

WHAM! (Women's Health Action and Mobilization) Records

Tisch Library, Tufts University, Medford, MA

Institute for First Amendment Studies Records

UCSF Library, Archives and Special Collections, University of California, San Francisco, San Francisco, CA

Nancy Stoller Papers Concerning Prison Inmate Health
Women's AIDS Network (WAN) Records

Wilson Library, University of North Carolina-Chapel Hill, Chapel Hill, NC

Office of the Dean of the School of Medicine of the University of North Carolina
    at Chapel Hill Records
William W. Dow Papers

PRIVATE COLLECTIONS

Marion Banzhaf Personal Papers
Ellen Barry Personal Papers
Heartbeat International Papers, Columbus, OH
HIV Law Project Papers, New York, NY
International Life Services Papers Los Angeles, CA
Denise Johnston Personal Papers

Linda Loffredo Personal Papers
Louise Rosenkrantz Personal Papers
Marie St. Cyr Personal Papers
The Sperm Bank of California Berkeley, CA

PUBLISHED SOURCES

ACT UP/NY Women and AIDS Book Group, ed. *Women, AIDS, and Activism.* Boston: South End Press, 1990.

Agigian, Amy. *Baby Steps: How Lesbian Alternative Insemination Is Changing the World.* Middletown, CN: Wesleyan University Press, 2004.

Aizley, Harlyn. *Buying Dad: One Woman's Search for the Perfect Sperm Donor.* New York: Alyson Books, 2003.

Allen, Machelle. "The Dilemma for Women of Color in Clinical Trials." *Journal of the American Medical Women's Association* 49, no. 4 (1994).

Almeling, Rene. *Sex Cells: The Medical Market for Eggs and Sperm.* Berkeley: University of California Press, 2011.

Almond, Douglas, Kenneth Y. Chay, and Michael Greenstone. "Civil Rights, the War on Poverty, and Black-White Convergence in Infant Mortality in the Rural South and Mississippi." MIT Department of Economics Working Paper 07-04, Dec. 31, 2006.

American Friends Service Committee. *Struggle for Justice: A Report on Crime and Punishment in America.* New York: Hill and Wang, 1971.

Arditti, Rita, Renate Klein, and Shelley Minden. *Test Tube Women: What Future for Motherhood?* London: Pandora Press, 1984.

Barry, Ellen. "Pregnant Prisoners." *Harvard Women's Law Journal* 12 (1989).

Bassichis, D. Morgan. *It's War in Here: A Report on the Treatment of Transgender and Intersex People in New York State Men's Prisons.* New York: Sylvia Rivera Law Project, 2007.

Batza, Katie. "From Sperm Runners to Sperm Banks: Lesbians, Assisted Conception, and Challenging the Fertility Industry, 1971–1983." *Journal of Women's History* 28, no. 2 (2016).

Bawden, D. Lee, and John L. Palmer. "Social Policy." In *The Reagan Record: An Assessment of America's Changing Domestic Priorities,* ed. John L. Palmer and Isabel V. Sawhill. Cambridge, MA: Ballinger, 1984.

Beal, Frances. "Double Jeopardy: To Be Black and Female." In *Words of Fire: An Anthology of African American Feminist Thought,* ed. Beverly Guy-Sheftall. New York: The New Press, 1995.

Bell, Jonathan. "Rethinking the 'Straight State': Welfare Politics, Health Care, and Public Policy in the Shadow of AIDS." *Journal of American History* 104, no. 4 (2018).

Ben-Moshe, Liat. *Decarcerating Disability: Deinstitutionalization and Prison Abolition.* Minneapolis: University of Minnesota Press, 2020.

Berger, Dan, and Toussaint Losier. *Rethinking the American Prison Movement.* New York: Routledge, 2018.

Berlant, Lauren. *The Queen of America Goes to Washington City: Essays on Sex and Citizenship.* Durham, NC: Duke University Press, 1997.

Berry, Mary Frances. *The Politics of Parenting: Child Care, Women's Rights, and the Myth of the Good Mother.* New York: Viking, 1993.

Bhatia, Rajani, Jade S. Sasser, Diana Ojeda, Anne Hendrixson, Sarojini Nadimpally, and Ellen E. Foley. "A Feminist Exploration of 'Populationism': Engaging Contemporary Forms of Population Control." *Gender, Place, and Culture* 27, no. 3 (2019).

Blanchard, Dallas A. *The Anti-Abortion Movement and the Rise of the Religious Right: From Polite to Fiery Protest.* New York: Twayne, 1994.

Blehar, Marcy C., Catherine Song, and Janine A. Clayton. "Enrolling Pregnant Women: Issues in Clinical Research." *Women's Health Issues* 23, no. 1 (2013).

Bloom, Barbara, and David Steinhart. *Why Punish the Children? A Reappraisal of the Children of Incarcerated Mothers in America.* Oakland: National Council on Crime and Delinquency, 1992.

Boonstra, Heather, and Elizabeth Nash. "A Surge of State Abortion Restrictions Puts Providers and the Women They Serve—in the Crosshairs." *Guttmacher Policy Review* 17, no. 1 (Mar. 1, 2014).

Boris, Eileen, and Jennifer Klein. *Caring for America: Home Health Workers in the Shadow of the Welfare State.* New York: Oxford University Press, 2012.

Bowles, Elizabeth L. "The Disfranchisement of Fertile Women in Clinical Trials: The Legal Ramifications of and Solutions for Rectifying the Knowledge Gap." *Vanderbilt Law Review* 45, no. 4 (1992).

Boyd, Nan Alamilla. *Wide-Open Town: A History of Queer San Francisco to 1965.* Berkeley: University of California Press, 2005.

Brier, Jennifer. *Infectious Ideas: U.S. Political Responses to the AIDS Crisis.* Chapel Hill: University of North Carolina Press, 2011.

Briggs, Laura. *Reproducing Empire: Race, Sex, Science, and U.S. Imperialism in Puerto Rico.* Berkeley: University of California Press, 2002.

———. "Of Lesbians and Technosperm." *GLQ* 15, no. 2 (2009).

———. *Somebody's Children: The Politics of Transracial and Transnational Adoption.* Durham, NC: Duke University Press, 2012.

———. *How All Politics Became Reproductive Politics: From Welfare Reform to Foreclosure to Trump.* Berkeley: University of California Press, 2017.

———. *Taking Children: A History of American Terror.* Berkeley: University of California Press, 2020.

Brodsky, Annette M. "Planning for the Female Offender: Directions for the Future." *Criminal Justice and Behavior* 1, no. 4 (Dec. 1974).

Brown, Jenny. *Birth Strike: The Hidden Fight Over Women's Work.* Oakland: PM Press, 2019.

Brown, Wendy. "Neo-Liberalism and the End of Liberal Democracy." *Theory and Event* 7, no. 1 (2003).

Bush, Janice K. "The Industry Perspective on the Inclusion of Women in Clinical Trials." *Academic Medicine: Journal of the Association of American Medical Colleges* 69, no. 9 (1994).

Campbell, Brittany A. "The Crisis Inside Crisis Pregnancy Centers: How to Stop These Facilities from Depriving Women of Their Reproductive Freedom." *Boston College Journal of Law and Social Justice* 37, no. 1 (2017).

Canaday, Margot. *The Straight State: Sexuality and Citizenship in Twentieth-Century America.* Princeton, NJ: Princeton University Press, 2009.

Carroll, Tamar W. *Mobilizing New York: AIDS, Antipoverty, and Feminist Activism.* Chapel Hill: University of North Carolina Press, 2015.

Carter, Dan T. *The Politics of Rage: George Wallace, the Origins of the New Conservatism, and the Transformation of American Politics.* New York: Simon and Schuster, 1995.

Chang, Grace. *Disposable Domestics: Immigrant Women Workers in the Global Economy.* Chicago: Haymarket Books, 2016.

Chappell, Marisa. "Rethinking Women's Politics in the 1970s: The League of Women Voters and the National Organization for Women Confront Poverty." *Journal of Women's History* 13, no. 4 (2002).

———. *The War on Welfare: Family, Poverty, and Politics in Modern America.* Philadelphia: University of Pennsylvania Press, 2009.

Chesney-Lind, Meda. "Women and Crime: The Female Offender." *Signs* 2 (1986).

Chu, S. Y., J. W. Buehler, and R. L. Berkelman. "Impact of the Human Immuno-deficiency Virus Epidemic on Mortality in Women of Reproductive Age, United States." *Journal of the American Medical Association* 264 (1990).

Cisler, Lucinda. "Unfinished Business: Birth Control and Women's Liberation." In *Sisterhood Is Powerful,* ed. Robin Morgan. New York: Vintage, 1970.

Clark, Judy, and Kathy Boudin. "Community of Women Organize Themselves to Cope with the AIDS Crisis: A Case Study from Bedford Hills Correctional Facility." *Social Justice* 17, no. 2 (1990).

Cohen, Cathy, "Punks, Bulldaggers, and Welfare Queens: The Radical Potential of Queer Politics?" *GLQ* 3, no. 4 (1997).

———. *The Boundaries of Blackness: AIDS and the Breakdown of Black Politics.* Chicago: University of Chicago Press, 1999.

Coker, Donna. "The Story of Wanrow: The Reasonable Woman and the Law of Self Defense." In *Criminal Law Stories,* ed. Donna Coker and Robert Weisberg. New York: Foundation Press, 2013.

Collins, James W., Jr., Richard J. David, Arden Handler, Stephen Wall, and Steven Andes. "Very Low Birthweight in African American Infants: The Role of Maternal Exposure to Interpersonal Racial Discrimination." *American Journal of Public Health* 94, no. 12 (2004).

Combahee River Collective. *The Combahee River Collective Statement: Black Feminist Organizing in the Seventies and Eighties*. Albany, NY: Kitchen Table Women of Color Press, 1986.

Constable, Nicole. "The Commodification of Intimacy: Marriage, Sex and Reproductive Labor." *Annual Review of Anthropology* 38 (2009).

Cooper, Melinda. *Family Values: Between Neoliberalism and the New Social Conservatism*. New York: Zone Books, 2017.

Copelon, Rhonda. "From Privacy to Autonomy: The Conditions for Sexual and Reproductive Freedom." In *From Abortion to Reproductive Freedom: Transforming a Movement*, ed. Marlene Gerber Fried. Boston: South End Press, 1990.

Corea, Gena. *The Invisible Epidemic: The Story of Women and AIDS*. New York: Perennial Press, 1993.

Corrigan, Oonagh P. "'First in Man': The Politics and Ethics of Women in Clinical Drug Trials." *Feminist Review* 72, no. 1 (2002).

Cott, Nancy F. *Public Vows: A History of Marriage and the Nation*. Cambridge, MA: Harvard University Press, 2000.

Coughlin, Teresa A. *Medicaid Since 1980: Costs, Coverage, and the Shifting Alliance Between the Federal Government and the States*. Washington, DC: Urban Institute Press, 1994.

Cowie, Jefferson. *Capital Moves: RCA's Seventy-Year Quest for Cheap Labor*. New York: The New Press, 2001.

Cramer, Lindsey, Margaret Goff, Bryce Peterson, and Heather Sandstrom. *Parent-Child Visiting Practices in Prisons and Jails: A Synthesis of Research and Practice*. Washington, DC: Urban Institute, Apr. 2017.

Crittenden, Ann. *The Price of Motherhood: Why the Most Important Job in the World Is Still the Least Valued*. New York: Owl Books, 2001.

Cromer, Risa. "Racial Politics of Frozen Embryo Personhood in the US Anti-abortion Movement." *Transforming Anthropology* 27, no. 1 (2019).

Curie-Cohen, Martin, Lesleigh Luttrell, and Sander Shapiro. "Current Practice of Artificial Insemination by Donor in the United States." *New England Journal of Medicine* 300, no. 11 (1979).

Dalla Costa, Mariarosa. *Women and the Subversion of the Community: A Mariarosa Dalla Costa Reader*, ed. Camille Barbagallo. Oakland: PM Press, 2019.

Dalton, Susan E. "From Presumed Fathers to Lesbian Mothers: Sex Discrimination and the Legal Construction of Parenthood." *Michigan Journal of Gender and Law* 9, no. 2 (2003).

Davis, Angela Y. *Women, Race, and Class*. New York: Vintage Books, 1981.

Davis, Dána-Ain. *Reproductive Injustice: Racism, Pregnancy, and Premature Birth*. New York: NYU Press, 2019.

Davis, Karen. "Medicaid Payments and Utilization of Medical Services by the Poor." *Inquiry* 13, no. 2 (June 2, 1976).

Daniel, Clare. *Mediating Morality: The Politics of Teen Pregnancy in the Post-Welfare Era*. Amherst: University of Massachusetts Press, 2017.

Daniels, Cynthia R., and Erin Heidt-Forsythe. "Gendered Eugenics and the Problematic of Free Market Reproductive Technologies: Sperm and Egg Donation in the United States." *Signs* 37, no. 3 (2012).

Delahoyde, Melinda, and Kristen Hansen, "Pregnancy Centers: A Practical Response to the Abortion Dilemma." *Religion and Society Report* 23, no. 3 (2006).

Denenberg, Risa. "What the Numbers Mean." In *Women, AIDS, and Activism*, ed. ACT UP/NY Women and AIDS Book Group. Boston: South End Press, 1990.

Díaz-Cotto, Juanita. *Gender, Ethnicity, and the State: Latina and Latino Prison Politics*. Albany: State University of New York Press, 1996.

Dinner, Deborah. "The Costs of Reproduction: History and the Legal Construction of Sex Equality." *Harvard Civil Rights–Civil Liberties Law Review* 46 (2011).

———. "Strange Bedfellows at Work: Neomaternalism in the Making of Sex Discrimination Law." *Washington University Law Review* 91, no. 3 (2014).

Donovan, Carol A. "The Uniform Parentage Act and Nonmarital Motherhood-by-Choice." *NYU Review of Law and Social Change* 11 (1982).

Douglas, Susan, and Meredith Michaels. *The Mommy Myth: The Idealization of Motherhood and How It Has Undermined Women*. New York: The Free Press, 2004.

Dubow, Sara. *Ourselves Unborn: A History of the Fetus in Modern America*. New York: Oxford University Press, 2011.

Duggan, Lisa. *The Twilight of Equality: Neoliberalism, Cultural Politics, and the Attack on Democracy*. Boston: Beacon Press, 2004.

Duffy, Mignon. "Doing the Dirty Work: Gender, Race, and Reproductive Labor in Historical Perspective," *Gender and Society* 21, no. 3 (2007).

Dunbar, Mary M. "Shaking Up the Status Quo: How AIDS Activists Have Challenged Drug Development and Approval Procedures." *Food, Drug, Cosmetic Law Journal* 46, no. 5 (1991).

Eckman, Anne. "Beyond 'The Yentl Syndrome': Making Women Visible in Post-1990 Women's Health Discourse." In *Visible Woman: Imaging Technologies, Gender, and Science,* ed. Paula A. Treichler, Lisa Cartwright, and Constance Penley. New York: NYU Press, 1998.

Editors. "On Prisoners and Parenting: Preserving the Tie That Binds." *Yale Law Journal* 87 (1978).

Ehrenreich, Barbara, and Arlie Hochschild, eds. *Global Woman: Nannies, Maids, and Sex Workers in the New Economy.* New York: Henry Holt, 2002.

El-Sadr, W., and L. Capps. "The Challenge of Minority Recruitment in Clinical Trials for AIDS." *Journal of American Medical Association* 267, no. 7 (1992).

Engemann, Kristie M., and Michael T. Owyang. "Social Changes Lead Married Women into Labor Force." *The Regional Economist,* Apr. 2006.

Epstein, Steven. *Impure Science: AIDS, Activism, and the Politics of Knowledge.* Berkeley: University of California Press, 1996.

———. *Inclusion: The Politics of Difference in Medical Research.* Chicago: University of Chicago Press, 2007.

Fabian, Sharon L. "Toward the Best Interests of Women Prisoners: Is the System Working." *New England Journal on Prison Law* 6, no. 1 (Fall 1979).

Farmer, Ashley. *Remaking Black Power: How Black Women Transformed an Era.* Chapel Hill: University of North Carolina Press, 2017.

Federici, Silvia. *Wages against Housework.* Bristol and London: Power of Women Collective; Falling Wall Press, 1975.

———. *Caliban and the Witch: Women, the Body, and Primitive Accumulation.* Brooklyn, NY: Autonomedia, 2004.

———. *Revolution at Point Zero: Housework, Reproduction, and Feminist Struggle.* Oakland: PM Press, 2012.

Finegold, Wilfred. *Artificial Insemination.* 1st ed. Charles C. Thomas, 1964.

Fineman, Martha. *The Neutered Mother, the Sexual Family and Other Twentieth Century Tragedies.* New York: Routledge, 1995.

Flavin, Jeanne. *Our Bodies, Our Crimes: The Policing of Women's Reproduction in America.* New York: NYU Press, 2009.

Folbre, Nancy. "'Holding Hands at Midnight': The Paradox of Caring Labor." *Feminist Economics* 1, no. 1 (1995).

Fortunati, Leopoldina. *The Arcane of Reproduction: Housework, Prostitution, Labor and Capital.* Brooklyn: Autonomedia, 1995.

Foucault, Michel. *Society Must Be Defended: Lectures at the Collège de France, 1975–1976.* New York: St. Martin's Press, 1997.

Frank, Gil. "'The Civil Rights of Parents': Race and Conservative Politics in Anita Bryant's Campaign against Gay Rights in 1970s Florida. *Journal of the History of Sexuality* 22, no. 1 (Jan. 2013).

Franke, Katherine. *Wedlocked: The Perils of Marriage Equality: How African Americans and Gays Mistakenly Thought the Right to Marry Would Set Them Free.* New York: NYU Press, 2015.

Fraser, Nancy. *Fortunes of Feminism: From State-Managed Capitalism to Neoliberal Crisis.* New York: Verso Books, 2013.

———. "Crisis of Care? On the Social-Reproductive Contradictions of Contemporary Capitalism." In *Social Reproduction Theory: Remapping Class, Recentering Oppression,* ed. Tithi Bhattacharya. London: Pluto Press, 2017.

Fraser, Nancy, and Linda Gordon. "A Genealogy of 'Dependency': Tracing a Keyword of the American Welfare State." *Signs* 19 (Winter 1994).

Freedman, Estelle. "'Uncontrolled Desires': The Response to the Sexual Psychopath, 1920–1960." *Journal of American History* 74, no. 1 (1987).

Frew, Paula M., et al. "Socioecological Factors Influencing Women's HIV Risk in the United States: Qualitative Findings from the Women's HIV Seroincidence Study (HPTN 064)." *BMC Public Health* 16, no. 803 (2016).

Furstenberg, Frank F. "As the Pendulum Swings: Teenage Childbearing and Social Concern." *Family Relations* 40, no. 2 (1991).

———. *Destinies of the Disadvantaged: The Politics of Teen Childbearing.* New York: Russell Sage Foundation, 2007.

Gabel, Katherine, and Denise Johnston, eds. *Children of Incarcerated Parents.* New York: Lexington Books, 1995.

Gagne, Patricia. *Battered Women's Justice: The Movement for Clemency and the Politics of Self-Defense.* New York: Twayne, 1998.

Gamble, Vanessa Northington, and Bonnie Ellen Blustein. "Racial Differentials in Medical Care: Implications for Research on Women." In *Women and Health Research: Ethical and Legal Issues of Including Women in Clinical Studies.* Vol. 2. Washington, DC: National Academies Press, 1994.

Garfinkel, Joseph et al. *Infant, Maternal, and Childhood Mortality in the United States, 1968–1973.* U. S. Department of Health, Education and Welfare Publication no. 75-5013. 1975.

Garland, David. *The Culture of Control: Crime and Social Order in Contemporary Society.* Chicago: University of Chicago Press, 2001.

Gerber Fried, Marlene, ed. *From Abortion to Reproductive Freedom: Transforming a Movement.* Boston: South End Press, 1990.

Geronimus, Arline T. "The Effects of Race, Residence, and Prenatal Care on the Relationship of Maternal Age to Neonatal Mortality." *American Journal of Public Health* 76, no. 12 (Dec. 1986).

———. "On Teenage Childbearing and Neonatal Mortality in the United States." *Population and Development Review* 13, no. 2 (June 1987).

———. "Teenage Childbearing and Social and Reproductive Disadvantage: The Evolution of Complex Questions and the Demise of Simple Answers." *Family Relations* 40, no. 4 (Oct. 1991).

———. "The Weathering Hypothesis and the Health of African-American Women and Infants: Evidence and Speculation." *Ethnicity and Disease* 2, no. 3 (Summer 1992).

Geronimus, Arline T., and John Bound. "Black/White Differences in Women's Reproductive-Related Health Status: Evidence from Vital Statistics." *Demography* 27, no. 3 (Aug. 1990).

Geronimus, Arline T., and Sanders Korenman. "Maternal Youth or Family Background? On the Health Disadvantages of Infants with Teenage Mothers." *American Journal of Epidemiology* 137, no. 2 (1993).

Gibson, Helen. "Women's Prisons: Laboratories for Penal Reform." *Wisconsin Law Review* 210 (1973).

Gilbert, Dorie J., and Ednita M. Wright. *African American Women and HIV/ AIDS: Critical Responses*. Westport, CT: Praeger Publishers, 2003.

Gilmore, Ruth Wilson. "Pierce the Future for Hope: Mothers and Prisoners in the Post-Keynesian California Landscape." In *Global Lockdown: Race, Gender, and the Prison-Industrial Complex*, ed. Julia Sudbury and Julia Chinyere Oparah. New York: Routledge, 2004.

———. *Golden Gulag: Prisons, Surplus, Crisis, and Opposition in Globalizing California*. Berkeley: University of California Press, 2007.

Ginsburg, Faye. *Contested Lives: The Abortion Debate in an American Community*. Berkeley: University of California Press, 1989.

———. "Saving America's Souls: Operation Rescue's Crusade against Abortion." In *Fundamentalisms and the State: Remaking Polities, Economies, and Militance*, ed. Martin E. Marty and R. Scott Appleby. Chicago: University of Chicago Press, 1993.

Ginsburg, Faye, and Rayna Rapp. *Conceiving the New World Order: The Global Politics of Reproduction*. Berkeley: University of California Press, 1995.

Girshick, Lori. "Out of Compliance: Masculine-Identified People in Women's Prisons." In *Captive Genders: Trans Embodiment and the Prison Industrial Complex*, 2nd ed., ed. Eric A. Stanley and Nat Smith. Oakland: AK Press, 2015.

Glenn, Evelyn Nakano. "From Servitude to Service Work: Historical Continuities in the Racial Division of Paid Reproductive Labor." *Signs* 18, no. 1 (1992).

———. "Creating a Caring Society." *Contemporary Sociology* 29, no. 1 (Jan. 2000).

———. *Unequal Freedom: How Race and Gender Shaped American Citizenship and Labor*. Cambridge, MA: Harvard University Press, 2002.

———. *Forced to Care: Coercion and Caregiving in America*. Cambridge, MA: Harvard University Press, 2012.

Glick, Ruth M., and Virginia V. Neto. *National Study of Women's Correctional Programs*. Washington, DC: U. S. Department of Justice, National Institute of Law Enforcement and Criminal Justice Law Enforcement Assistance Administration, June 1977.

Goffman, Erving. *Asylums: Essays on the Social Situation of Mental Patients and Other Inmates*. New York: Doubleday, 1961.

Goldmann, Bonnie J. "A Drug Company Report: What Is the Same and What Is Changing with Respect to Inclusion/Exclusion of Women in Clinical Trials." *Food and Drug Law Journal* 48 (1993).

Goldstein, Nancy, and Jennifer L. Manlowe, eds. *The Gender Politics of HIV/ AIDS in Women: Perspectives on the Pandemic in the United States.* New York: NYU Press, 1997.

Goodwin, Michelle. *Baby Markets: Money and the New Politics of Creating Families.* Cambridge: Cambridge University Press, 2010.

Gordon, Linda. "Who Is Frightened of Reproductive Freedom for Women and Why? Some Historical Answers." *Frontiers: A Journal of Women Studies* 9, no. 1 (1986).

———. *Pitied but Not Entitled: Single Mothers and the History of Welfare, 1890–1935.* New York: The Free Press, 1994.

Gottschalk, Marie. *The Prison and the Gallows: The Politics of Mass Incarceration in America.* New York: Cambridge University Press, 2006.

Gould, Deborah B. *Moving Politics: Emotion and ACT UP's Fight against AIDS.* Chicago: University of Chicago Press, 2009.

Greene Foster, Diana. *Ten Years, a Thousand Women, and the Consequences of Having—or Being Denied—an Abortion.* New York, NY: Simon and Schuster, 2020.

Grimes, D. A., et al. "An Epidemic of Antiabortion Violence in the United States." *American Journal of Obstetrics and Gynecology* 165 (1991).

Grogan, Colleen, and Eric M. Patashnik. "Between Welfare Medicine and Mainstream Entitlement: Medicaid at the Political Crossroads." *Journal of Health Politics, Policy and Law* 28, no. 5 (Oct. 2003).

Guillen, Mauro F., and Charles Perrow. *The AIDS Disaster: The Failure of Organizations in New York and the Nation.* New Haven, CT: Yale University Press, 1990.

Gumbs, Alexis Pauline, China Martens, and Mai'a Williams. *Revolutionary Mothering: Love on the Front Lines.* Oakland: PM Press, 2016.

Gurr, Barbara. *Reproductive Justice: The Politics of Health Care for Native American Women.* New Brunswick, NJ: Rutgers University Press, 2014.

Gutiérrez, Elena R. *Fertile Matters: The Politics of Mexican-Origin Women's Reproduction.* Austin: University of Texas Press, 2008.

Hager, Eli, and Anna Flagg. *How Incarcerated Parents Are Losing Their Children Forever.* New York: The Marshall Project, Dec. 2, 2018.

Haley, Kathleen. "Mothers behind Bars: A Look at the Parental Rights of Incarcerated Women." *New England Journal on Prison Law* 4 (1977).

Hamilton, Dona C., and Charles V. Hamilton. *The Dual Agenda: Race and Social Welfare Policies of Civil Rights Organizations.* New York: Columbia University Press, 1997.

Hammonds, Evelynn. "Missing Persons: African American Women, AIDS, and the History of the Disease." *Radical America* 24, no. 2 (1992).

———. "Toward a Genealogy of Black Female Sexuality: The Problematic of Silence." In *Feminist Genealogies, Colonial Legacies, Democratic Futures,* ed. M. Jacqui Alexander and Chandra Talpade Mohanty. New York: Routledge, 1997.

Hancock, Ange-Marie. *The Politics of Disgust: The Public Identity of the Welfare Queen.* New York: NYU Press, 2004.

Haney, Lynne. "Motherhood as Punishment: The Case of Parenting in Prison." *Signs* 39, no. 1 (2013).

Hansen, Beth E. "Invidiously Discriminatory Animus—A Class Based on Gender and Gestation under 42 U.S.C. 1985(3): Lewis v. Pearson Foundation, Inc." *Creighton Law Review* 24 (1991).

Harris, Lisa H. "Second Trimester Abortion Provision: Breaking the Silence and Changing the Discourse." *Reproductive Health Matters* 16, no. 31 (2008).

Harrison, Laura. *Brown Bodies, White Babies: The Politics of Cross-Racial Surrogacy.* New York: NYU Press, 2016.

Hartmann, Heidi I. "The Unhappy Marriage of Marxism and Feminism: Towards a More Progressive Union." *Capital and Class* 3, no. 2 (1979).

———. "The Family as the Locus of Gender, Class, and Political Struggle: The Example of Housework." *Signs* 6, no. 3 (1981).

Hartshorn, Peggy. *Foot Soldiers Armed with Love: Heartbeat International's First Forty Years.* Virginia Beach, VA: The Donning Company Publishers, 2011.

Harvey, David. *A Brief History of Neoliberalism.* New York: Oxford University Press, 2005.

Haugeberg, Karissa. *Women against Abortion: Inside the Largest Moral Reform Movement of the Twentieth Century.* Champaign: University of Illinois Press, 2017.

Hayley, Sarah. *No Mercy Here: Gender, Punishment, and the Making of Jim Crow Modernity.* Chapel Hill: University of North Carolina Press, 2016.

Hays, Sharon. *The Cultural Contradictions of Motherhood.* New Haven, CT: Yale University Press, 1996.

Herman, Ellen. *Kinship by Design: A History of Modern Adoption in the United States.* Chicago: Chicago University Press.

Hicks, Cheryl D. "'Bright and Good Looking Colored Girl': Black Women's Sexuality and 'Harmful Intimacy' in Early-Twentieth-Century New York." *Journal of the History of Sexuality* 18, no. 3 (Sept. 2009).

Hill, Ian T. "Improving State Medicaid Programs for Pregnant Women and Children." *HealthCare Financing Review,* Annual Supplement (1990).

Hinton, Elizabeth. *From the War on Poverty to the War on Crime: The Making of Mass Incarceration.* Cambridge, MA: Harvard University Press, 2016.

Hochschild, Arlie. *The Second Shift: Working Families and the Revolution at Home.* New York: Penguin Press, 1989.

Hoffman, S. L. "On Prisoners and Parenting: Preserving the Tie That Binds." *Yale Law Journal* 87, no. 7 (June 1978).

Holtzman, Benjamin. "'Shelter Is Only a First Step': Housing the Homeless in 1980s New York City." *Journal of Social History* 52, no. 3 (2019).

Hussey, Laura A. "Crisis Pregnancy Centers, Poverty, and the Expanding Frontiers of American Abortion Politics." *Politics and Policy* 41, no. 6 (2013).

Johnson, Elizabeth I., and Jane Waldfogel. "Parental Incarceration: Recent Trends and Implications for Child Welfare." *Social Service Review* 76, no. 3 (Sept. 2002).

Johnson, Tracey, and Elizabeth Fee. "Women's Participation in Clinical Research: From Protectionism to Access." In *Women and Health Research: Ethical and Legal Issues of Including Women in Clinical Trials*, vol. 2, ed. Anna C. Mastroianni, Ruth Faden, and Daniel Federman. Washington, DC: National Academies Press, 1994.

Kajstura, Aleks. *Women's Mass Incarceration: The Whole Pie, 2019*. Easthampton, MA: Prison Policy Initiative, Oct. 29, 2019.

Kaplan, Laura. *The Story of Jane: The Legendary Underground Feminist Abortion Service*. Chicago: University of Chicago Press, 1995.

Karpman, Hannah E., Emily H. Ruppel, and Maria Toress. "'It wasn't feasible for us': Queer Women of Color Navigating Family Formation." *Family Relations* 67, no. 1 (2018).

Kelly, Kimberly. "In the Name of the Mother: Renegotiating Conservative Women's Authority in the Crisis Pregnancy Center Movement." *Signs* 38, no. 1 (2012).

———. "Evangelical Underdogs: Intrinsic Success, Organizational Solidarity, and Marginalized Identities as Religious Movement Resources." *Journal of Contemporary Ethnography* 43, no. 4 (2014).

Kelly, Kimberly, and Amanda Gochanour. "Racial Reconciliation or Spiritual Smokescreens? Blackwashing the Crisis Pregnancy Center Movement." *Qualitative Sociology* 41 (2018).

Kenney, Sally J. *For Whose Protection? Reproductive Hazards and Exclusionary Policies in the United States and Britain*. Ann Arbor: University of Michigan Press, 1992.

Kerber, Linda K. *No Constitutional Right to Be Ladies: Women and the Obligations of Citizenship*. New York: Hill and Wang, 1998.

Kessler-Harris, Alice. *In Pursuit of Equity: Women, Men, and the Quest for Economic Citizenship in 20th-Century America*. New York: Oxford University Press, 2001.

Kimport, Katrina. "Pregnant Women's Reasons for and Experiences of Visiting Antiabortion Pregnancy Resource Centers." *Perspectives on Sexual and Reproductive Health* 52, no. 1 (2020).

Klein, Dorie. "The Etiology of Female Crime: A Review of the Literature." In *The Female Offender*, ed. Laura Crites. New York: Lexington Books, 1976.

Kohler-Hausmann, Julilly. *Getting Tough: Welfare and Imprisonment in 1970s America*. Princeton, NJ: Princeton University Press, 2017.

Koonin, Lisa M., Tedd V. Ellerbrock, and Hani K. Atrash. "Pregnancy Associated Deaths due to AIDS in the United States." *Journal of the American Medical Association* 261, no. 9 (1989).

Kornbluh, Felicia. *The Battle for Welfare Rights: Politics and Poverty in Modern America*. Philadelphia: University of Pennsylvania Press, 2007.

Kornbluh, Felicia, and Gwendolyn Mink. *Ensuring Poverty: Welfare Reform in Feminist Perspective*. Philadelphia: University of Pennsylvania Press, 2019.

Kluchin, Rebecca M. *Fit to Be Tied: Sterilization and Reproductive Rights in America, 1950–1980*. New Brunswick, NJ: Rutgers University Press, 2009.

Krause, Harry, "Bringing the Bastard into the Great Society—A Proposed Uniform Act on Legitimacy." *Texas Law Review* 44, no. 5 (1966).

———. "Legitimate and Illegitimate Offspring of *Levy v. Louisiana*—First Decisions on Equal Protection and Paternity." *University of Chicago Law Review* 36, no. 2 (1969).

———. *Illegitimacy: Law and Social Policy*. Indianapolis, IN: Bobbs-Merrill, 1971

———. "The Uniform Parentage Act." *Family Law Quarterly* 8, no. 1 (Spring 1974).

Kronebusch, Karl. "Children's Medicaid Enrollment: The Impacts of Mandates, Welfare Reform, and Policy Delinking." *Journal of Health Politics, Policy, and Law* 26, no. 6 (2001).

Kruttschnitt, Candace, and Rosemary Gartner. *Marking Time in the Golden State: Women's Imprisonment in California*. New York: Cambridge University Press, 2005.

Kunzel, Regina. *Criminal Intimacy: Prison and the Uneven History of Modern American Sexuality*. Chicago: University of Chicago Press, 2008.

Kuziemko, Ilyana, Jessica Pan, Jenny Shen, and Ebonya Washington. "The Mommy Effect: Do Women Anticipate the Employment Effects of Motherhood?" Cambridge, MA: National Bureau of Economic Research (NBER), Working Paper no. 24740. June 2019.

Landesman, Sheldon H., Howard L. Minkoff, and Anne Willoughby. "HIV Disease in Reproductive Age Women: A Problem of the Present." *Journal of the American Medical Association* 261, no. 9 (Mar. 3, 1989).

Lareau, Annette. *Unequal Childhoods: Class, Race, and Family Life*. Berkeley: University of California Press, 2011.

Laurence, Leslie, and Beth Weinhouse. *Outrageous Practices: The Alarming Truth about How Medicine Mistreats Women*. New York: Fawcett Columbine, 1994.

Law, Vikki. *Resistance behind Bars: The Struggles of Incarcerated Women*. Oakland: PM Press, 2009.

LefLouria, Talitha L. *Chained in Silence: Black Women and Convict Labor in the New South.* Chapel Hill: University of North Carolina Press, 2015.

Leheny, Mary F. "A Question of Class: Does 42 U.S.C. Section 1985(3) Protect Women Who Are Barred from Abortion Clinics." *Fordham Lew Review* 60 (1992).

Levenstein, Lisa. *A Movement without Marches: African American Women and the Politics of Poverty in Postwar Philadelphia.* Chapel Hill: University of North Carolina Press, 2010.

Lewis, Sophie. *Full Surrogacy Now: Feminism against Family.* London: Verso, 2019.

Lin, Vitoria, and Cynthia Dailard. "Crisis Pregnancy Centers Seek to Increase Political Clout, Secure Government Subsidy." *Guttmacher Report on Public Policy* 5, no. 2 (2002).

Lipton, Douglas S., Robert Martinson, and Judith Wilks. *The Effectiveness of Correctional Treatment: A Survey of Treatment Evaluation Studies.* New York: Praeger, 1975.

Lloyd, Jenna. *Health Rights Are Civil Rights: Peace and Justice Activism in Los Angeles, 1963–1978.* Minneapolis: University of Minnesota Press, 2014.

Lombroso, Cesare. *Criminal Woman, the Prostitute, and the Normal Woman.* Durham, NC: Duke University Press, 2004.

Ludlow, Jeannie. "The Things We Cannot Say: Witnessing the Trauma-tization of Abortion in the United States." *Women's Studies Quarterly* 36, no. 1/2 (2008).

Luker, Kristin. *Abortion and the Politics of Motherhood.* Berkeley: University of California Press, 1984.

———. *Dubious Conceptions: The Politics of Teenage Pregnancy.* Cambridge, MA: Harvard University Press, 1996.

———. *When Sex Goes to School: Warring Views on Sex—and Sex Education—since the Sixties.* New York: W. W. Norton, 2006.

Luna, Zakiya. *Reproductive Rights as Human Rights: Women of Color and the Fight for Reproductive Justice.* New York: NYU Press, 2020.

Maclean, Nancy. "Postwar Women's History: The 'Second Wave' or the End of the Family Wage?" In *A Companion to Post-45 America,* ed. Jean-Christophe Agnew and Roy Rosenzweig. Malden, MA: Blackwell, 2002.

Mamo, Laura. "Biomedicalizing Kinship: Sperm Banks and the Creation of Affinity-Ties." *Science as Culture,* 14, no. 3 (2005).

———. *Queering Reproduction: Achieving Pregnancy in the Age of Technoscience.* Durham, NC: Duke University Press, 2007.

———. "Fertility Inc.: Consumption and Subjectification in U.S. Lesbian Reproductive Practices," in *Biomedicalization: Technoscience, Health, and Illness in the U.S.,* ed. A. E. Clarke, L. Mamo, J. R. Fosket, J. R. Fishman, and J. K. Shim. Durham, NC: Duke University Press, 2010.

Mamo, Laura, and Eli Alston-Stepnitz. "Queer Intimacies and Structural Inequalities: New Directions in Stratified Reproduction." *Journal of Family Issues* 36, no. 4 (2015).

Mayeri, Serena. "Marital Supremacy and the Constitution of the Nonmarital Family." *California Law Review* 103 (2015).

———. "Foundling Fathers: (Non-)Marriage and Parental Rights in the Age of Equality." *Yale Law Journal* 125 (2016).

———. "Intersectionality and the Constitution of Family Status." *Constitutional Commentary* 32 (2017).

Mays, Vickie M., and Susan D. Cochran. "Issues in the Perception of AIDS Risk and Risk Reduction Activities by Black and Hispanic/Latina Women." *American Psychologist* 43, no. 11 (Nov. 1988).

McElroy, Meagan. "Protecting Pregnant Pennsylvanians: Public Funding of Crisis Pregnancy Centers." *University of Pittsburgh Law Review* 76 (2015).

McGovern, Theresa M., Martha Davis, and Mary Beth Caschetta. "FDA Policy on Women in Drug Trials." *New England Journal of Medicine* 329, no. 4 (1993).

McGuire, Maureen, and Nancy J. Alexander. "Artificial Insemination of Single Women." *Fertility and Sterility* 43, no. 2 (Feb. 1985).

McHugh, Gerald Austin. "Protection of the Rights of Pregnant Women in Prisons and Detention Facilities." *New England Journal on Prison Law* 6 (1980).

McIntire, Lisa. *Crisis Pregnancy Centers Lie: The Insidious Threat to Reproductive Freedom.* Washington, DC: NARAL Pro-Choice America, 2015.

Merkatz, Ruth B. "FDA: Making a Difference in Women's Health." *Journal of the American Medical Women's Association* 49, no. 4 (1994).

Merkatz, Ruth B., and Suzanne White Junod. "Historical Background of Changes in FDA Policy on the Study and Evaluation of Drugs in Women." *Academic Medicine: Journal of the Association of American Medical Colleges* 69, no. 9 (1994).

Merkatz, Ruth B., and Elyse I. Summers. "Including Women in Clinical Trials: Policy Changes at the Food and Drug Administration." In *Women's Health Research: A Medical and Policy Primer,* ed. Florence P. Haseltine and Beverly Greenberg Jacobson. Washington, DC: Health Press International, 1997.

Merkatz, Ruth B., Robert Temple, Solomon Sobel, Karyn Feiden, and David A. Kessler. "Women in Clinical Trials of New Drugs—A Change in Food and Drug Administration Policy." *New England Journal of Medicine* 329 (1993).

Mink, Gwendolyn. *Wages of Motherhood: Inequality in the Welfare State, 1917-1942.* Ithaca, NY: Cornell University Press, 1996.

———. *Welfare's End.* Ithaca, NY: Cornell University Press, 1998.

Minkoff, Howard, Jonathan D. Moreno, and Kathleen R. Powderly. "Fetal Protection and Women's Access to Clinical Trials." *Journal of Women's Health* 1, no. 2 (1992).

Mitchell, Janet L. "Recruitment and Retention of Women of Color in Clinical Studies." In *Women and Health Research: Ethical and Legal Issues of Including Women in Clinical Studies,* vol. 2. Washington, DC: National Academies Press, 1994.

Mittlestadt, Jennifer. *From Welfare to Workfare: The Unintended Consequences of Liberal Reform, 1945–1965.* Chapel Hill: University of North Carolina Press, 2005.

Montegary, Liz. *Familiar Perversions: The Racial, Sexual, and Economic Politics of LGBT Families.* New Brunswick, NJ: Rutgers University Press, 2018.

Moore, Lisa Jean. *Sperm Counts: Overcome by Man's Most Precious Fluid.* New York: NYU Press, 2007.

Moore, Mignon. *Invisible Families: Gay Identities, Relationships, and Motherhood among Black Women.* Berkeley: University of California Press, 2011.

Morgan, Jennifer. *Laboring Women: Reproduction and Gender in New World Slavery.* Philadelphia: University of Pennsylvania Press, 2004.

Morgen, Sandra. *Into Our Own Hands: The Women's Health Movement in the United States, 1969–1990.* New Brunswick, NJ: Rutgers University Press, 2002.

Mosley, W. Henry, and Lincoln C. Chen. "An Analytical Framework for the Study of Child Survival in Developing Countries." *Population and Development Review* 10 (1984).

Muhammed, Khalil. *The Condemnation of Blackness: Race, Crime, and the Making of Modern Urban America.* Cambridge, MA: Harvard University Press, 2011.

Mumola, Christopher J. "Bureau of Justice Statistics Special Report: Incarcerated Parents and Their Children." U.S. Department of Justice, Aug. 2000.

Murphy, Michelle. *Seizing the Means of Reproduction: Entanglements of Feminism, Health, and Technoscience.* Durham, NC: Duke University Press, 2012.

Murray, Christopher J. L. "Rethinking DALYs." In *The Global Burden of a Disease: A Comprehensive Assessment of Mortality and Disability from Diseases, Injuries, and Risk Factors in 1990 and Projected to 2020,* ed. Christopher J. L. Murray and Alan D. Lopez. Cambridge, MA: Harvard School of Public Health, 1996.

Murray, Melissa. "What's So New about the New Illegitimacy?" *American University Journal of Gender, Social Policy, and the Law* 20, no. 387 (2011).

———. "Loving's Legacy: Decriminalization and the Regulation of Sex and Sexuality." *Fordham Law Review* 86, no. 6 (2018).

Nadasen, Premilla. *Welfare Warriors: The Welfare Rights Movement in the United States.* New York: Routledge, 2005.

Nash, Jennifer. "From Lavender to Purple: Privacy, Black Women, and Feminist Legal Theory." *Cardozo Women's Law Journal* 11 (2005).

Nathan, Richard P., and Fred C. Doolittle. *Reagan and the States*. Princeton, NJ: Princeton University Press, 1987.

NeJaime, Douglas. "Marriage Equality and the New Parenthood." *Harvard Law Review* 129, no. 5 (Mar. 2016).

———. "The Nature of Parenthood." *Yale Law Journal* 126, no. 8 (2017).

Nelson, Alondra. *Body and Soul: The Black Panther Party and the Fight Against Medical Discrimination*. Minneapolis: University of Minnesota Press, 2011.

Nelson, Jennifer. *Women of Color and the Reproductive Rights Movement*. New York: NYU Press, 2003.

———. *More Than Medicine: A History of the Feminist Women's Health Movement*. New York: NYU Press, 2015.

Nelson, Roxanne. "Laboring in Chains: Shackling Pregnant Inmates, Even during Childbirth, Still Happens." *American Journal of Nursing* 106, no. 10 (2005).

Norwood, Christopher. *Advice for Life: A Woman's Guide to AIDS Risks and Prevention*. New York: Pantheon Books, 1987.

———. "Alarming Rise in Deaths: Are Women Showing New 'AIDS' Symptoms?" *Ms. Magazine* (July 1988).

Oberg, Charles N., and Cynthia Longseth Polich. "Medicaid: The Third Decade." *Health Affairs* 7, no. 4 (Fall 1988).

O'Connor, Alice. *Poverty Knowledge: Social Science, Social Policy, and the Poor in Twentieth Century U.S.* Princeton, NJ: Princeton University Press, 2001.

O'Donnell, Mary, Val Leoffler, Kater Pollock, and Ziesel Saunders. *Lesbian Health Matters!* Santa Cruz: Santa Cruz Women's Health Collective, 1980.

Ong, Aihwa. *Neoliberalism as Exception*. Durham, NC: Duke University Press, 2006.

Orleck, Annelise. *Storming Cesar's Palace: How Black Mothers Fought Their Own War on Poverty*. Boston: Beacon Press, 2005.

———. *Rethinking American Women's Activism*. New York: Routledge, 2015.

———. *"We Are All Fast-Food Workers Now": The Global Uprising against Poverty Wages*. Boston: Beacon Press, 2018.

Owens, Diedre Cooper. *Medical Bondage: Race, Gender, and the Origins of American Gynecology*. Athens: University of Georgia Press, 2017.

Owens, Emily A. "Reproducing Racial Fictions: Critical Meditations on (a) Lesbian Pregnancy." *Signs* 44, no. 4 (2019).

Padavic, Irene, Robin J. Ely, and Erin M. Reid. "Explaining the Persistence of Gender Inequality: The Work-Family Narrative as a Social Defense against the 24/7 Work Culture." *Administrative Science Quarterly* 65, no. 1 (2020).

Palmer, John L., and Isabel V. Sawhill, eds. *The Reagan Record: An Assessment of America's Changing Domestic Priorities*. Cambridge, MA: Ballinger, 1984.

Palmer, Richard. "The Prisoner Mother and Her Child." *Capital University Law Review* 1 (1972).

Parrenas, Rhacel. *The Force of Domesticity: Filipina Migrants and Globalization.* New York: NYU Press, 2008.

Patel, Raj, and Jason Moore. *The History of the World in Seven Cheap Things: A Guide to Capitalism, Nature and the Future of the Planet.* Berkeley: University of California Press, 2018.

Patton, Cindy. *Last Served? Gendering the HIV Pandemic.* London: Taylor and Francis, 1994.

Patton-Imani, Sandra. *Queering Family Trees: Race, Reproductive Justice, and Lesbian Motherhood.* New York: NYU Press, 2020.

Pearce, Diana. "The Feminization of Poverty: Women, Work and Welfare." *Urban and Social Change Review* 11, no. 28 (1978).

Pearce, Diana, and Harriette McAdoo. *Women and Children: Alone and in Poverty.* National Advisory Council on Economic Opportunity. 1981.

Perkoff, Gerald T. "Artificial Insemination in a Lesbian: A Case Analysis." *Archives of Internal Medicine* 145 (Mar. 1985).

Petchesky, Rosalind P. *Abortion and Woman's Choice: The State, Sexuality, and Reproductive Freedom.* Boston: Northeastern University Press, 1985.

Peterson, Janice. "The Feminization of Poverty." *Journal of Economic Issues* 21, no. 1 (Mar. 1987).

Pinnow, Ellen, Pellavi Sharma, Ameeta Parekh, Natalie Gevorkian, and Kathleen Uhl. "Increasing Participation of Women in Early Phase Clinical Trials Approved by the FDA." *Women's Health Issues* 19, no. 2 (2009).

Pleck, Elizabeth. *Not Just Roommates: Cohabitation after the Sexual Revolution.* Chicago: University of Chicago Press, 2012.

Pollak, Otto. *The Criminality of Women.* Philadelphia: University of Pennsylvania Press, 1950.

Poo, Ai-jen. *The Age of Dignity: Preparing for the Elder Boom in a Changing America.* New York: The New Press, 2016.

Poon, Rita, Keshav Khanijow, Sphoorti Umarjee, Emmanuel Fadrian, Monica Yu, Lei Zhang, and Ameeta Parekh. "Participation of Women and Sex Analyses in Late-Phase Clinical Trials of New Molecular Entity Drugs and Biologics Approved by the FDA in 2007–2009." *Journal of Women's Health* 22, no. 7 (2013).

Price, Barbara Raffel, and Natalie J. Sokoloff. *The Criminal Justice System and Women: Offenders, Prisoners, Victims, and Workers.* Boston: McGraw Hill, 2004.

Quadagno, Jill. *The Transformation of Old Age Security: Class Politics in the American Welfare State.* Chicago: University of Chicago Press, 1988.

———. *The Color of Welfare: How Racism Undermined the War on Poverty.* New York: Oxford University Press, 1994.

Randolph, Sherie M. *Florynce "Flo" Kennedy: The Life of a Black Feminist Radical*. Chapel Hill: University of North Carolina Press, 2015.

Reagan, Leslie. *When Abortion Was a Crime: Women, Medicine, and Law*. Berkeley: University of California Press, 1996.

Rensenbrink, Greta. "Parthenogenesis and Lesbian Separatism: Regenerating Women's Community through Virgin Birth in the United States in the 1970s and 1980s." *Journal of the History of Sexuality* 19, no. 2 (May 2010).

Rich, Adrienne. *Of Woman Born: Motherhood as Experience and Institution*. New York: W. W. Norton, 1986.

Richie, Beth E. *Arrested Justice: Black Women, Violence, and America's Prison Nation*. New York: NYU Press, 2012.

Riwder, Ines, and Patricia Ruppelt, eds. *AIDS: The Women*. Pittsburgh: Cleis Press, 1988.

Ritchie, Andrea J. *Invisible No More: Police Violence against Black Women and Women of Color*. Boston: Beacon Press, 2017.

Rivers, Daniel. *Radical Relations: Lesbian Mothers, Gay Fathers, and Their Children in the United States since World War II*. Chapel Hill: University of North Carolina Press, 2015.

Roberts, Dorothy E. *Killing the Black Body: Race, Reproduction, and the Meaning of Liberty*. New York: Vintage Books, 1999.

———. *Shattered Bonds: The Color of Child Welfare*. New York: Basic Civitas Books, 2002.

———. "Privatization and Punishment in the New Age of Reprogenetics." *Emory Law Journal* 54 (2005).

Ross, Loretta J. "Trust Black Women: Reproductive Justice and Eugenics." In *Radical Reproductive Justice: Foundations, Theory, Practice, Critique*, ed. Loretta J. Ross, Lynn Roberts, Erika Derkas, Whitney Peoples, and Pamela Bridgewater Toure. New York: Feminist Press, 2017.

Ross, Loretta J., Elena Gutierrez, Marlene Gerber Fried, and Jael Silliman. *Undivided Rights: Women of Color Organize for Reproductive Justice*. Boston: South End Press, 2004.

Ross, Loretta J., and Rickie Solinger. *Reproductive Justice: An Introduction*. Berkeley: University of California Press, 2017.

Rossi, Peter. "The Old Homeless and the New Homelessness in Historical Perspective." *American Psychologist* 45, no. 8 (1990).

Roth, Rachel. *Making Women Pay: The Hidden Costs of Fetal Rights*. Ithaca, NY: Cornell University Press, 2000.

Russo, Jennefer A., Kristin L. Schumacher, and Mitchell D. Creinin. "Antiabortion Violence in the United States." *Contraception* 86, no. 5 (2012).

Salamon, Lester. "Non-Profit Organizations: The Lost Opportunity." In *The Reagan Record: An Assessment of America's Changing Domestic Priorities*, ed. John L. Palmer and Isabel V. Sawhill. Cambridge, MA: Ballinger, 1984.

Sametz, Lynn. "Children of Incarcerated Women." *Social Work* 25, no. 4 (July 1980).

Sandomire, Hazel. "Women in Clinical Trials: Are Sponsors Liable for Fetal Injury?" *Journal of Law, Medicine, and Ethics* 21, no. 2 (1993).

Sawyer, Wendy. "The Gender Divide: Tracking Women's State Prison Growth." Prison Policy Initiative, Jan. 9, 2018. Accessed Sept. 15, 2019, https://www .prisonpolicy.org/reports/women_overtime.html.

Schoen, Johanna. *Choice and Coercion: Birth Control, Sterilization, and Abortion in Public Health and Welfare.* Chapel Hill: University of North Carolina Press, 2005.

———. *Abortion after Roe.* Chapel Hill: University of North Carolina Press, 2017.

Schupak, Terri L. "Women and Children First: An Examination of the Unique Needs of Women in Prison." *Golden Gate University Law Review* 16, no. 3 (1986).

Schwartz, Marie Jenkins. *Birthing a Slave: Motherhood and Medicine in the Antebellum South.* Cambridge, MA: Harvard University Press, 2006.

Scott, Douglas R., Jr. "The Making of Controversy: The History of the Conspiracy against Pregnancy Care Centers." *Life Decisions International* 3 (2000).

Scott, Folkers. "Lewis v. Pearson Foundation, Inc.: Does 42 U.S.C. §1985(3) Offer Protection to Women as a Class?" *South Dakota Law Review* 37 (1992).

Sechrest, Lee, Susan O. White, and Elizabeth D. Brown. *The Rehabilitation of Criminal Offenders: Problems and Prospects.* Washington, DC: National Academy of Sciences, 1979.

Self, Robert O. *American Babylon: Race and the Struggle for Postwar Oakland.* Princeton, NJ: Princeton University Press, 2003.

———. *All in the Family: The Realignment of American Democracy since the 1960s.* New York: Hill and Wang, 2012.

Shapiro, Donald, and Lisa Schultz. "Single-Sex Families: The Impact of Birth Innovations upon Traditional Family Notions." *Journal of Family Law* 24, no. 2 (1985).

Sherman, Linda Ann, Robert Temple, and Ruth B. Merkatz. "Women in Clinical Trials: An FDA Perspective." *Science* 269, no. 5225 (Aug. 1995).

Shields, Kristine, and Anne Drapkin Lyerly. "Exclusion of Pregnant Women from Industry-Sponsored Clinical Trials." *Obstetrics and Gynecology* 122, no. 5 (2013).

Simon, Kosali I., and Arden Handler. "Welfare Reform and Insurance Coverage during the Pregnancy Period: Implications for Preconception and Interconception Care." *Women's Health Issues* 18, no. 6 (2008).

Smith, Anne Marie. *Welfare Reform and Sexual Regulation.* New York: Cambridge University Press, 2007.

Smith, Shawn Michelle. *American Archives: Gender, Race, and Class in Visual Culture.* Princeton, NJ: Princeton University Press, 1999.

Singh, Gopal, and Stella Yu. "Infant Mortality in the United States: Trends, Differentials and Projections, 1950–2010." *American Journal of Public Health* 85, no. 7 (July 1995).

Sokoloff, Natalie J., Barbara Raffel Price, and Jeanne Flavin. "The Criminal Law and Women." In *The Criminal Justice System and Women: Offenders, Prisoners, Victims, and Workers,* ed. Barbara Raffel Price and Natalie J. Sokoloff. New York: McGraw Hill, 2004.

Solinger, Rickie. *Wake Up Little Susie: Single Pregnancy and Race before Roe v. Wade.* New York: Routledge, 1992.

———. *Beggars and Choosers: How the Politics of Choice Shapes Adoption, Abortion, and Welfare in the United States.* New York: Hill and Wang, 2001.

Solinger, Rickie, Paula C. Johnson, Martha L. Raimon, Tina Reynolds, and Ruby Tapia. *Interrupted Life: Experiences of Incarcerated Women in the United States.* Berkeley: University of California Press, 2010.

Somerville, Siobhan. "Scientific Racism and the Emergence of the Homosexual Body." *Journal of the History of Sexuality* 5, no. 2 (Oct. 1994).

Southern Governors' Association. *Coming of Age: Ten Years in the Campaign against Infant Mortality.* Southern Regional Project on Infant Mortality, 1984–1994, 1994.

Spar, Debora. *The Baby Business: How Money, Science, and Politics Drive the Commerce of Conception.* Cambridge, MA: Harvard Business School Press, 2006.

Staggenborg, Suzanne. *The Pro-Choice Movement: Organization and Activism in the Abortion Conflict.* New York: Oxford University Press, 1991.

Stanley, Eric A. and Nat Smith, eds. *Captive Genders: Trans Embodiment and the Prison Industrial Complex.* 2nd ed. Oakland: AK Press, 2015.

Steffensmier, Darrell J. "Sex Differences in Patterns of Adult Crime, 1965–1977: A Review and Assessment." *Social Forces* 58, no. 4 (1980).

Stein, Judith. *Pivotal Decade: How the United States Traded Factories for Finance in the Seventies.* New Haven, CT: Yale University Press, 2010.

Stern, Alexandra Minna. *Eugenic Nation: Faults and Frontiers of Better Breeding in Modern America.* Berkeley: University of California Press, 2005.

Stevens, Robert, and Rosemary Stevens. *Welfare Medicine in America: A Case Study of Medicaid.* New York: The Free Press, 1974.

Stoller Shaw, Nancy. "Preventing AIDS among Women: The Role of Community Organizing." *Socialist Review* 18, no. 4 (Fall 1988).

Stoy, Diane B. "Recruitment and Retention of Women in Clinical Studies: Theoretical Perspectives and Methodological Considerations." In *Women and Health Research: Ethical and Legal Issues of Including Women in Clinical Studies,* vol. 2. Washington, DC: National Academies Press, 1994.

Strong, Carson, and Jay S. Schinfeld. "The Single Woman and Artificial Insemination by Donor." *Journal of Reproductive Medicine* 29, no. 5 (May 1984).

Sugrue, Thomas J. *The Origins of the Urban Crisis: Race and Inequality in
Postwar Detroit*. Princeton, NJ: Princeton University Press, 1996.

Sutton, Stuart A. "The Lesbian Family: Rights in Conflict Under the California
Uniform Parentage Act." *Golden Gate University Law Review* 10 (Jan. 1980).

Swanson, Kara. "The End of Men, Again." *Boston University Law Review
Annex* 93 (2013).

———. *Banking on the Body: The Market in Blood, Milk and Sperm in Modern
America*. Cambridge, MA: Harvard University Press, 2014.

Swavola, Elizabeth, Kristine Riley, and Ram Subramanian. *Overlooked: Women
and Jails in an Era of Reform*. New York: Vera Institute of Justice, 2016.

Swinth, Kristen. *Feminism's Forgotten Fight: The Unfinished Struggle for Work
and Family*. Cambridge, MA: Harvard University Press, 2018.

———. "Post–Family Wage, Postindustrial Society: Reframing the Gender and
Family Order through Working Mothers in Reagan's America." *Journal of
American History* 105, no. 2 (Sept. 2018).

Sykes, Gresham M. *The Society of Captives: A Study of a Maximum Security
Prison*. Princeton, NJ: Princeton University Press, 1958.

Tani, Karen M. *States of Dependency: Welfare, Rights, and American Governance, 1935–1972*. New York: Cambridge University Press, 2016.

Taranto, Stacie. *Kitchen-Table Politics: Conservative Women and Family
Values in New York*. Philadelphia: University of Pennsylvania Press, 2017.

Taylor, Janelle S. *The Public Life of the Fetal Sonogram: Technology, Consumption, and the Politics of Reproduction*. New Brunswick, NJ: Rutgers University Press, 2008.

Temin, Carolyn. "Discretionary Sentencing of Women Offenders." *American
Criminal Law Review* 11 (1973).

Tenoso, Patricia, and Aleta Wallach. "Book Review." *UCLA Law Review* 19 (1972).

Theobald, Brianna. *Reproduction on the Reservation: Pregnancy, Childbirth,
and Colonialism in the Long Twentieth Century* Chapel Hill, NC: University
of North Carolina Press, 2019.

Thistle, Susan. *From Marriage to the Market: The Transformation of Women's
Lives and Work*. Berkeley: University of California Press, 2006.

Thompson, Charis. *Making Parents: The Ontological Choreography of Reproductive Technologies*. Boston: MIT Press, 2005.

Thuma, Emily. *All Our Trials: Prisons, Policing, and the Feminist Fight to End
Violence*. Chicago: University of Illinois Press, 2019.

Tober, Diane. *Romancing the Sperm: Shifting Biopolitics and the Making of
Modern Families*. New Brunswick, NJ: Rutgers University Press, 2018.

Treichler, Paula A. *How to Have Theory in an Epidemic: Cultural Chronicles of
AIDS*. Durham, NC: Duke University Press, 1999.

Turk, Katherine. *Equality on Trial: Gender and Rights in the Modern American Workplace*. Philadelphia: University of Pennsylvania Press, 2016.

Twine, France Winndance. *Outsourcing the Womb: Race, Class and Gestational Surrogacy in a Global Market*. New York: Routledge, 2011.

Vinovskis, Maris A. *An "Epidemic" of Adolescent Pregnancy? Some Historical and Policy Considerations*. New York: Oxford University Press, 1988.

Waggoner, Miranda R. *The Zero Trimester: Pre-pregnancy Care and the Politics of Reproductive Risk*. Berkeley: University of California Press, 2017.

Waldby, Catherine. *AIDS and the Body Politic: Biomedicine and Sexual Difference*. New York: Routledge, 1996.

Walker, Anders. *The Ghost of Jim Crow: How Southern Moderates Used Brown v. Board of Education to Stall Civil Rights*. New York: Oxford University Press, 2009.

Walker, Judith. "Mothers and Children." In *Women, AIDS, and Activism*, ed. ACT UP/NY Women and AIDS Book Group. Boston: South End Press, 1990.

Ward, David A., and Gene G. Kassebaum. *Women's Prison: Sex and Social Structure*. New Brunswick, NJ: Aldine Transaction, 1965.

Wegman, Myron. "Infant Mortality in the 20th Century, Dramatic but Uneven Progress." *Journal of Nutrition* 131, no. 2 (Feb. 1, 2001).

Weisman, Carol Sachs. *Women's Health Care: Activist Traditions and Institutional Change*. Baltimore: Johns Hopkins University Press, 1998.

West, Robin. "From Choice to Reproductive Justice: De-Constitutionalizing Abortion Rights." *Yale Law Journal* 118 (2009).

Weston, Kath. *Families We Choose: Lesbians, Gays, Kinship*. New York: Columbia University Press, 1997.

———. "Families in Queer States: The Rule of Law and the Politics of Recognition." *Radical History Review* 93 (Fall 2005).

Whetten, Kathryn, and Susan Reif. "Overview: HIV/AIDS in the Deep South Region of the United States." *AIDS Care* 18 (2006).

Whitmore, Suzanne K. "Epidemiology of HIV/AIDS among Non-Hispanic Black Women in the United States." *Journal of the National Medical Association* 97, no. 7 (July 2005).

Wildeman, Christopher, Anna Haskins, and Christopher Muller. "Implications of Mass Imprisonment for Inequality among American Children." In *The Punitive Turn: New Approaches to Race and Incarceration*, ed. Deborah McDowell, Claudrena N. Harold, and Juan Battle. Charlottesville: University of Virginia Press, 2013.

Winant, Gabriel. "A Place to Die: Nursing Home Abuse and the Political Economy of the 1970s." *Journal of American History* 105, no. 1 (2018).

———. *The Next Shift: The Fall of Industry and the Rise of Health Care in Rust Belt America*. Cambridge, MA: Harvard University Press, 2021.

Wright, Melissa W. *Disposable Women and Other Myths of Global Capitalism.* New York: Routledge, 2006.

Yang, Yongsheng, Alan S. Carlin, Patrick J. Faustino, Monica I. Pagan Motta, Mazen L. Hamad, Ruyi He, Y. Watanuki, E. E. Pinnow, and Mansoor A. Khan. "Participation of Women in Clinical Trials for New Drugs Approved by the Food and Drug Administration in 2000–2002." *Journal of Women's Health* 18, no. 3 (2013).

Zalba, Serapio R. *Women Prisoners and Their Families: A Monograph on a Study of the Relationships of a Correctional Institution and Social Agencies Working with Incarcerated Women and Their Children.* Los Angeles: Delmar, 1965.

Ziegler, Mary. *After Roe: The Lost History of the Abortion Debate.* Cambridge, MA: Harvard University Press, 2015.

———. *Beyond Abortion: Roe v. Wade and the Fight for Privacy.* Cambridge, MA: Harvard University Press, 2018.

Index

Founded in 1893,
UNIVERSITY OF CALIFORNIA PRESS
publishes bold, progressive books and journals
on topics in the arts, humanities, social sciences,
and natural sciences—with a focus on social
justice issues—that inspire thought and action
among readers worldwide.

The UC PRESS FOUNDATION
raises funds to uphold the press's vital role
as an independent, nonprofit publisher, and
receives philanthropic support from a wide
range of individuals and institutions—and from
committed readers like you. To learn more, visit
ucpress.edu/supportus.